Ophthalmic Photography

About the cover

The fundus image on the cover is a multi-image computer composite from multiple 60-degree fundus photographs—a FundusMap. The original 25 images were taken on slide film by Patrick J. Saine and were scanned onto a Kodak Photo-CD. The digital images were combined into a photo-illustration by Richard E. Hackel using Adobe Photoshop on a Macintosh computer. Lines were added that indicate the alignment procedure for the seven standard fields of view (circles). The term "FundusMap" describes this computer-based photo-illustrative method of combining fundus photographs to make a map.

The cover layout and typography are by Thane Kerner of Silverchair Science + Communications.

Ophthalmic Photography: A Textbook of Fundus Photography, Angiography, and Electronic Imaging

Patrick J. Saine, M.Ed, C.R.A., F.O.P.S.
*Senior Ophthalmic Photographer, Davis Duehr Dean
at Dean Medical Center, Madison, Wisconsin*

Marshall E. Tyler, C.R.A., F.O.P.S.
*Instructor of Surgical Sciences in Ophthalmology,
Bowman Gray School of Medicine of Wake Forest University,
Winston-Salem, North Carolina*

Butterworth-Heinemann
Boston Oxford Johannesburg Melbourne New Delhi Singapore

Butterworth-Heinemann

 A member of the Reed Elsevier group

Every effort has been made to ensure that drug dosage schedules within this text are accurate and conform to standard accepted at time of publication. However, as treatment recommendations vary in the light of continuing research and clinical experience, the reader is advised to verify drug dosage schedules herein with information found on product information sheets. This is especially true in cases of new or infrequently used drugs.

 Recognizing the importance of preserving what has been written, Butterworth-Heinemann prints its books on acid-free paper whenever possible.

Library of Congress Cataloging-in-Publication Data

Saine, Patrick J.
    Ophthalmic photography : a textbook of fundus photography,
    angiography, and electronic imaging / Patrick J. Saine, Marshall E.
    Tyler.
       p.   cm.
    Includes bibliographical references and index.
    ISBN 0-7506-9793-8 (alk. paper)
    1. Ophthalmic photography.   I. Tyler, Marshall E.   II. Title.
re79.P54S25 1996
617.7'07545—dc20   96-25989
                                                    CIP

British Library Cataloguing-in-Publication Data
A catalogue record for this book is available from the British library.

The publisher offers discounts on bulk orders of this book.

For information, please write:
Manager of Special Sales
Butterworth-Heinemann
313 Washington Street
Newton, MA 02158-1626
Tel: 617-928-2500
Fax: 617-928-2620

For information on all medical publications available, contact our World Wide Web home page at: http://www.bh.com/med

10 9 8 7 6 5 4 3 2 1

Printed in the United States of America

Contents

Contributing Authors

Timothy J. Martin, M.D.
Assistant Professor of Surgical Sciences in Ophthalmology, Bowman Gray School of Medicine of Wake Forest University, Winston-Salem, North Carolina

Lawrence M. Merin, R.B.P., F.I.M.I., F.O.P.S.
Instructor in Ophthalmology, Jones Eye Institute, University of Arkansas for Medical Sciences, Little Rock, Arkansas

Paula F. Morris, C.R.A., F.O.P.S.
Chief Photographer, John A. Moran Eye Center, University of Utah School of Medicine, Salt Lake City, Utah

Patrick J. Saine, M.Ed, C.R.A., F.O.P.S.
Senior Ophthalmic Photographer, Davis Duehr Dean at Dean Medical Center, Madison, Wisconsin

Stephen J. Sramek, M.D., Ph.D
Vitreoretinal Surgeon, Davis Duehr Dean at Dean Medical Center, Madison, Wisconsin

Marshall E. Tyler, C.R.A., F.O.P.S.
Instructor of Surgical Sciences in Ophthalmology, Bowman Gray School of Medicine of Wake Forest University, Winston-Salem, North Carolina

Preface

This book is predicated on the belief that ophthalmic photography is an exciting and challenging career. Photographing the retina has become both important and routine in the practice of ophthalmology ever since the first crude photographic attempts more than 100 years ago. The introduction of fluorescein angiography in 1961 ignited new interest in fundus imaging and has since revolutionized our understanding of the retina. Electronic imaging technology and indocyanine green angiography are examples of continued evolution in our field.

Like many photographic endeavors, the profession of ophthalmic photography is a collaborative blend of art and science. Ophthalmic photography's specific mix combines the animated art of patient interaction with the inherently formidable technical challenges of recording high-quality retinal images. To be successful, you must cheerfully convince the worried, wary, or weary patient to submit to yet another set of bright lights while you simultaneously juggle complicated technical concerns.

The best preparation for this career is college-level instruction integrating the life sciences with photography and communication skills. Increasingly, facility with computers and electronic imaging is also important.

Variety is the hallmark of every fulfilling career path. Ophthalmic photography offers many options. The subject of this textbook, imaging the retina, is but one part of the complete ophthalmic photographer's repertoire. External, corneal, and operating room photography procedures combine with the skills associated with general biomedical photography for a myriad of opportunities. Settings range from basic research laboratories to large hospitals to clinical doctor's offices. Each opportunity offers a distinctly different working environment.

This book is designed to help you use photographic expertise in the pursuit of quality ophthalmic health care. As an ophthalmic photographer, you will surely experience some thrilling moments—your first view of a vein pulsating on an optic nerve head, or glimpses of fluorescein dye as it ambles through ocular blood vessels. The challenges and frustrations of photographing anxious patients with compromised media will also be a part of your professional life. We sincerely hope that your career is filled with rewarding moments. You should be proud of your role in helping save a patient's vision. We encourage you to become a vital member of your eye care team.

Patrick J. Saine
Marshall E. Tyler

Acknowledgments

Much of this book is the work of a small, dedicated group of individuals who, having battled both words and images, have survived and included their names as authors and editors. We appreciate the vital contributions of our co-authors Timothy J. Martin, Lawrence M. Merin, Paula F. Morris, and Stephen J. Sramek. We graciously thank Elizabeth Willingham, Baylor Fooks, and Lisa Biggs of Silverchair for their fine editorial and composition expertise, as well as Susan Pioli and Mary-Kate Bourn of Butterworth-Heinemann for guiding this project to successful completion.

Many others shared in the creation of this work. We are each deeply indebted to the fine ophthalmologists with whom we work. The ophthalmologists at Davis Duehr Dean have been helpful and supportive. Especially important were Richard K. Dortzbach, M.D., who, by example and instruction, taught Pat to pursue and expect the best; and Michael B. Shapiro, M.D., who continues to encourage high standards and professional development. The support of the Wake Forest University Eye Center ophthalmologists has been equally important. We thank both Richard G. Weaver, M.D., for his clinical mentorship, which provided increased diagnostic depth to Marshall's career, and M. Madison Slusher, M.D., for providing a superb clinical setting for ophthalmic photography. Marshall also thanks Hollis N. Todd, professor at the Rochester Institute of Technology, for his foundation course on materials and processes in photography.

We are grateful to the ophthalmic photographers who have shared their expertise with us. The Ophthalmic Photographers' Society has helped us grow both professionally and personally. A special thank you to Don Wong, R.B.P., for his continuous sharing of knowledge as well as his role as an educator and friend. We acknowledge Johnny Justice, Jr., C.R.A., for his leadership in elevating ophthalmic photography from its infancy as an offshoot of biomedical photography to a profession that significantly participates on the ophthalmic clinical team.

Special thanks go to the photographers who have provided specific images or information for the book: Albert Aan De Kirk, Julie Balza, Tim Bennett, Mike Borgrud, Dennis Cain, Colin Clements, Brad Clifton, Mark Croswell, Denise Cunningham, William Fisher, B.J. Graham, Richard Hackel, Peter Hay, Ray Hendrickson, Charles Juarez, Csaba Martonyi, Paul Montague, Bill Nyberg, Michael Palczynski, and Tim Steffins. Thanks also to Dorie Roberts and Judith MacMillan for their generous support.

Our families, those forgiving eyewitnesses to our late-night struggles, deserve a special acknowledgment. A sincere thank you to Deb, Julie, and Beth, and to Alix and Christina for their understanding and support throughout this arduous process. They have helped us accomplish a very important goal.

For technical data—the camera was used faithfully.

—Minor White

Ophthalmic Photography

Chapter 1

Landmarks in the Development of Fundus Photography and Fluorescein Angiography

Patrick J. Saine

Introduction

In 1961 two medical students from Indiana, H.R. Novotny and D.L. Alvis, wrote a paper on retinal angiography techniques still in use today.[1] They described a fundus camera equipped with an exciter filter, barrier filter, and electronic flash to sequentially document the retinal blood flow following a sodium fluorescein injection. The development of this procedure began many years before this seminal report, however.

Fluorescein angiography was developed by combining the evolution of retinal imaging with the application of sodium fluorescein to ophthalmology. This chapter reviews published landmarks in the development of the fluorescein angiography by examining the historical use of dyes to view the retina, the evolution of retinal photography, and important work contemporaneous with Novotny and Alvis (Figure 1-1). It traces the history of fluorescein angiography through selected quotes from the publications of significant contributors. A list of resources is included—you are encouraged to further explore the historical record.

Beginnings

The foundation from which fluorescein angiography evolved includes anatomic drawings of the retina and the use of fluorescein dye to observe ophthalmic phenomena. Fundus photography was developed in pursuit of an accurate and specific graphic representation of the retina. Medical illustration has a long history of depicting the eye (Figure 1-2).[2] A landmark in the realistic graphic representation of the retina was an 1854 pub-

1850	**1854** The first color representation of the retina is published.
1860	
1870	**1871** Fluorescein is synthesized.
1880	**1881** The aqueous flow is examined with sodium fluorescein.
1890	**1886-98** In vivo retinal photography of human subjects is refined.
1900	**1899** High quality fundus photographs are shown.
1910	**1910** The choroid and retina are examined with sodium fluorescein.
1920	
1930	**1926** Fundus camera becomes commercially available. **1927** First fundus photography atlas published. **1930** Filters are used to observe dye in the retina.
1940	**1939** Dye flowing through retinal blood vessels is described. **1946** The electronic flash tube is invented.
1950	**1953** Electronic flash tube technology is applied to fundus photography.
1960	**1959** Sodium fluorescein is photographed in the cat retina with an exciter filter. **1960** Sodium fluorescein is used to determine a retinal diagnosis. **1961** Modern fluorescein angiography technique is described.

FIGURE 1-1
Timeline relating events leading to the development of fluorescein angiography.

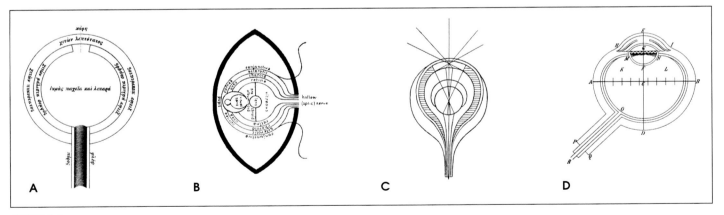

A   **B**   **C**   **D**

FIGURE 1-2
Medical illustration has a rich tradition of depicting the eye. Democritus (Greece, circa 400 B.C.) drew a simple, two-layer construction with a hollow tube connecting the eye to the brain (A). Hunain Ibn Ishak (Arabia, circa 1000 A.D.) incorporated the layers of the retina (B). Leonardo Da Vinci (Italian, circa 1500) added a three-dimensional aspect and the refraction of light to his representation of the eye (C). Greater anatomic accuracy began with the work of Scheiner in 1619 (D). (Reproduced from S Duke-Elder. *System of Ophthalmology.* Vol II. St. Louis: Mosby, 1961.)

lication by Van Trigt (Figure 1-3).[3] It is here that the story of modern fundus photography begins. From Duke-Elder:

> *The frontispiece to this volume is interesting. It is a photographic representation of the first coloured printed illustration of the fundus of the eye which appeared in the thesis of Adrian Christopher Van Trigt (1825–64), Dissertatio Ophthalmologica Inauguralis de Speculo Oculi in 1853…*[3]

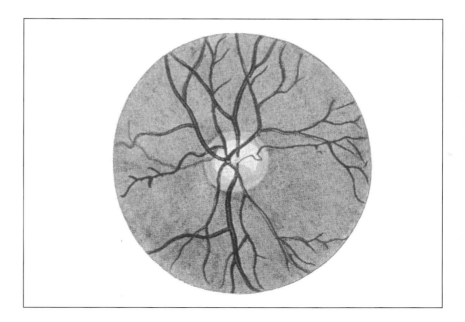

FIGURE 1-3
This realistic fundus illustration was originally drawn in color by Van Trigt in 1853. (Reproduced from S Duke-Elder. *System of Ophthalmology.* Vol X. London: Henry Kimpton, 1967.)

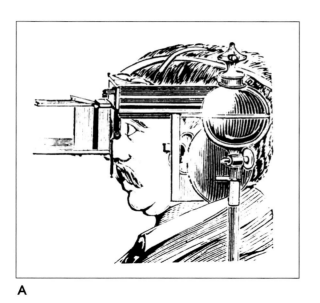

A

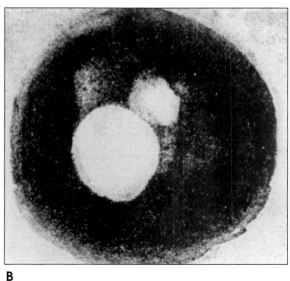

B

FIGURE 1-4
Jackman and Webster produced the first published human fundus photograph using an albo-carbon burner, an ophthalmoscopic mirror, and a 2½-minute exposure. Interpretation requires some imagination: The small upper white area is the optic disc, and the lower, larger light area is an artifact. Blood vessels cannot be defined. (Reproduced from WA Mann. History of photography of the eye. *Surv Ophthal* 1970;15:179.)

Jackman and Webster[4] and Bedell[5] note early attempts at retinal photography on anesthetized animals. The first published account of in vivo human retinal photography is by Jackman and Webster in 1886.[4] They describe the use of an ophthalmoscopic mirror (a curved mirror with a central hole) in conjunction with a 2-inch microscope objective (Figure 1-4). An albo-carbon light source provided illumination during the 2½-minute exposure. From their paper:

> *After considerable practice, and numerous experiments, we have at last succeeded in obtaining a very fair photograph of the blind spot and a few larger blood vessels of the living human retina.[4]*

As important as these early attempts were, the images were blurry. Improvements in instrumentation and technique were needed before high-quality fundus photography was to become routine.

Meanwhile, Adolf Baeyer, a 1905 Nobel laureate in chemistry, described methods for producing a number of new organic dyes—including sodium fluorescein—in 1871.[6] Ten years later, fluorescein dye was used by Ehrlich to examine the flow of the aqueous humor[7]; This was the first published use of sodium fluorescein in ophthalmology. Sodium fluorescein has since become an important ophthalmic tool. Ehrlich describes his methods:

I proceeded to inject 2 cc of fluorescein, and when the yellow absorbed—this happened in a few minutes—I saw an effect nearby. After ¼ to ½ minutes I could see a spot near the pupil border, soon the spot encircled the pupil and I saw an intense green fluorescent color which diffused throughout the anterior chamber within 2–3 minutes.[7]

Colored Dyes and the Eye

Erhlich's investigation of fluorescein in the eye was followed in 1910 by Burke's examination of the choroid and retina after the administration of fluorescein dye in coffee.[8] In 1930, Kikai viewed the retina with filtered light in an attempt to more clearly view injected dye.[9] It was not until 1939 that the path of dye in the retinal blood vessels was described.[10] While reading this next excerpt, imagine how the history of fluorescein angiography may have been changed if Sorsby had a specific interest in photographing the retina, or if his experiments had been carried out with a different patient population.

With these dyes whilst effective staining of the brain could be obtained in the intact animal, staining of the fundus was, as with the pure basic dyes, of the most transient character. The retinal vessels could be seen carrying a coloured blood stream for about two minutes, but the colouration of the fundus amounted to little more than a transient flushing....The experimental observation that the damaged retina retained the colour suggested the possibility that the diseased retina in man might behave similarly.[11]

The use of fluorescein dye in circulation studies of the intestine and skin were summarized by Lange and Boyd in 1942.[11] Their technique included the rapid injection of 2–4 ml of 5% sodium fluorescein in the antecubital vein. Using a purple light for excitation, they observed the effect of fluorescein dye on multiple tissues. Except for the lack of specifics describing ophthalmic imaging, their paper describes, in very general terms, modern fluorescein angiography:

If a definite section of tissue containing a small artery and vein is observed with the aid of a low power microscope after intravenous injection, one readily can watch the stain enter the artery, pass the capillaries, stain the surrounding tissue and return through the vein.[11]

Fundus Photography Refined

Rapid progress in fundus photography was made in the years just after Jackman and Webster's fuzzy fundus photographs were published. Dimmer describes the work of a number of scientists who attempted retinal

Table 1-1. The Work of Retinal Photography Pioneers*

Pioneers	Publication Date
Noyes	1862
Rosebrugh	1864, 1887
Liebreich	1874
T. Stein	1877
Dor	1884
Albertotti	1884
W. T. Jackman and J. D. Webster	1886
Panel	1887
L. Howe	1887, 1893
E. Starr	1887
H. Cohn	1888, 1889
Leroy	1888
S. Segal	1888
Bagneris	1889
T. Guilloz	1891, 1893
O. Gerloff	1891
W. Thorner	1896
Guinkoff	1896
E. Borghi	1897, 1898
W. Nikolaew & J. Dogiel	1900
S. Jackson	1901

*As summarized in Dimmer's 1907 treatise on ophthalmic photography.

photography near the end of the nineteenth century (Table 1-1).[12] Howe and Barr both made progress toward better quality, as evidenced in the next three quotes[13, 14]:

> The photograph to which I venture to call attention is here presented. It will be seen that the disc is perfectly distinct, even the shading of the different parts is well defined. Moreover, the vessels are so clearly shown over at least a third of the fundus that the arteries can be distinguished from the veins....For while it must be admitted that the results here presented are not entirely satisfactory, on the other hand this is, as far as I can learn, the first time that any photographs of the interior of the eye have been produced in which the details were even recognizable, and as such, they at least give promise of results of great practical value in the future.[13]

The next quote is taken from the uncredited discussion published directly following Howe's paper:

> Letter A Carbutt's dry plate is used with ten minutes exposure to an ordinary gas light, giving an unretouched and unremagnified negative...

Barr wrote:

> Up to the present time, so far as I am able to learn, attempts to photograph the interior of the human eye have not yielded very encouraging results. In the Philadelphia Photographer, of June 5, 1886, Drs. Jackman and Webster, of Coggestall, Essex, England, give results of their experiments. They succeeded in showing the end of the optic nerve and an indistinct outline of a part of one or two large vessels....I began experimenting to obtain a photograph of the interior of the human eye, and the results are better than others I have seen, showing the optic nerve and vessels quite well....The lens in the camera has a focus of only three inches, and this I think is important, for it makes a very bright image, and consequently a very short exposure—six to ten seconds—is sufficient....[14]

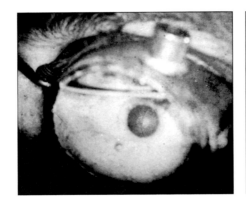

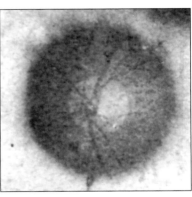

FIGURE 1-5
In 1891, Gerloff published a low-magnification retinal photograph that was much clearer than earlier efforts. (Reproduced from O Gerloff. *Ueber die Photographie des Augenhintergrundes.* Klin Monatf Augenheil 1891;29:397.)

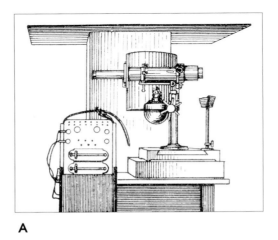

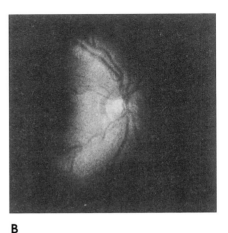

A   **B**

FIGURE 1-6
Thorner's camera (A) provided fundus photographs (B) with adequate detail but lacking even illumination. (Reproduced from F Dimmer. *Ueber die Photographie des Augenhintergrundes.* Wiesbaden, Germany: Bergmann, 1907.)

In 1891, Gerhoff used flash powder to illuminate a low-magnification fundus photograph (Figure 1-5).[15] Thorner wrote a 1903 book outlining his fundus photography techniques (Figure 1-6).[16]

Accurate, high-quality fundus photography began at the turn of the twentieth century with the work of Frederick Dimmer. Bedell wrote that Dimmer "electrified the 9th International Congress (1899) with his marvelous pictures...."[5] Dimmer's 1907 treatise on fundus photography described his cumbersome apparatus, which used carbon arc illumination (Figure 1-7).[12] He was the first to incorporate fundus photography into a basic ophthalmic textbook and the first to publish a photographic atlas.[17, 18]

Only one of Dimmer's cameras was ever produced. Modern fundus camera design grew from the work of Helmholtz, who introduced the direct ophthalmoscope in 1851.[19] Its design was improved by Thorner in 1899 and Gullstrand in 1910.[20, 21] Nordenson introduced a camera based on Gullstrand's principles in 1925.[22] The Carl Zeiss Company marketed Nordenson's design as the first commercially available fundus camera in 1926 (Figure 1-8).[23] This camera had a 10-degree field of view and required a one-half second exposure with color film.[24]

Color fundus photography was attempted as early as 1929, the same year Bedell published the first stereo atlas of fundus photographs.[25, 26] In

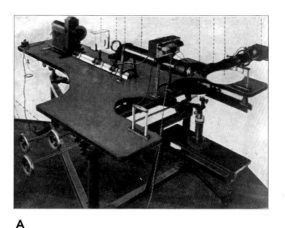
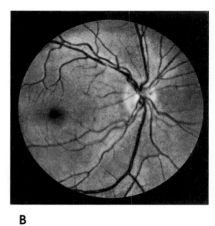

A   **B**

FIGURE 1-7
Dimmer's fundus camera (A) was used to create this fine retinal photograph of a normal eye (B). (Reproduced from F Dimmer, A Pillat. *Atlas photographischer Bilder des Menschlichen Augenhintergrundes.* Leipzig, Germany: F Deuticke, 1927.)

FIGURE 1-8
An advertisement for the Zeiss fundus camera from 1932. Fundus cameras have changed dramatically in the last 50 years. Advertising copy has not. (Reproduced from *Am J Ophthalmol* 1932;32:1214.)

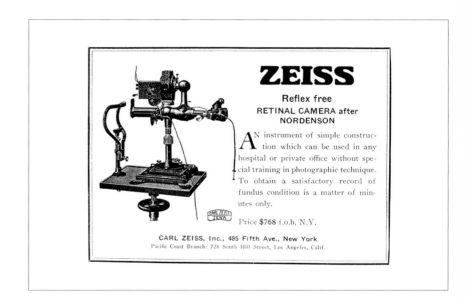

June 1935, Bedell delivered the chairman's address at the Eighty-Sixth Annual Session of the American Medical Association[5] and described the current state of fundus imaging:

> *Direct color photography has attracted attention and some excellent pictures have been presented, but because of the expense and the difficulty of reproduction, it is not as yet popular. Eventually, drawings will be supplanted and even the most skillful artist will be forced to admit the superiority of photographs. For several years I have been taking colored photographs.[5]*

Limitations in clinical use of fundus photography in the 1930s and 1940s can be directly attributed to the difficulty in obtaining quality images. Slow film speeds and long shutter speeds were the rule with the then current carbon arc illumination system. Although Hartinger described a modification of the fundus camera by the addition of an electrical lamp, carbon arc fundus cameras continued to be used through the 1940s.[27, 28] A bright, instantaneous light source was needed for high-quality, routine fundus photography. External eye photographs taken with

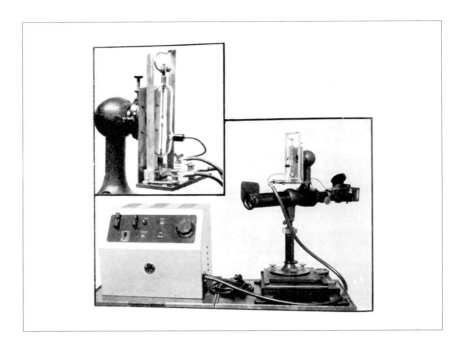

FIGURE 1-9
Hansell and Beeson adapted an electronic flash tube to a Zeiss fundus camera. (Reproduced from P Hansell, EJG Beeson. Retinal photography in color. *Br J Ophthal* 1953;37:65.)

a "lightning illumination process" were produced by Cohn and DuBois-Reymond in 1888.[29] In 1946, Edgerton developed the electronic flash tube, and in 1949 Rizzutti introduced its use to ophthalmology.[30, 31] Electronic flash was adapted to the fundus camera in 1953 in both Britain and the United States (Figure 1-9)[28, 32]:

> *The application of a new compact xenon arc lamp (FA5) to retinal photography in colour is described. The circuit required for pulse operation of the lamp is given and some modifications of the Zeiss-Nordenson retinal camera are mentioned....By these means standard and comparable records of the fundus oculi may be obtained on Kodachrome colour film at exposures of ⅕ sec.[28]*

> *By using again the ring of light just within the pupil to illuminate the retina, and photographing directly through the center of the pupil, one can obtain pictures which are reflex-free. Because the flash exposure of the tube is of the order of 0.0001 second, the problems of blinking and of the movements of the eye being photographed are eliminated. The use of the flash-tube technique also is less fatiguing and annoying to the patient.[32]*

By the early 1950s, fluorescein dye had been observed flowing through the retina, filters had been used to enhance the visualization of the retina filled with dye, and flash-adapted fundus cameras were a reality. A flurry of activity in the late 1950s preceded Alvis and Novotny's important paper.

Fluorescein Angiography

In early 1959, Chao and Flocks described a method for measuring the "retinal circulation time" in cats.[33] Using a stopwatch, ophthalmoscopy, and tryptan blue, they found that the circulation time of the cat retina was approximately 2 seconds. Their discussion concluded with this observation:

We do not yet know whether more innocuous indicator solutions such as fluorescein can be used so that the method could be adapted to the human retina. If it could be, it is conceivable that the study of retinal circulation time might be of value in such pathologic conditions as retinitis pigmentosa, diabetic retinopathy, and macular degeneration.[33]

Later that year, Flocks, Miller, and Chao published a refinement of their technique including the addition of a motion picture camera, an exciter filter, and fluorescein dye[34]:

If a cobalt-blue filter is inserted in the ophthalmoscope, the retina appears dark purple in color and the vessels black. When intravenously injected fluorescein reaches the central retinal artery, it lights up the artery to a fluorescent yellow if viewed through the cobalt-blue filter....The idea was conceived that the end points could be ascertained more precisely by means of motion picture photography using a motion picture film viewer and editor to examine leisurely the individual frames of the film. With this technique the unavoidable error due to the reaction time of the person pressing the stop watch would be eliminated and, in addition, a permanent objective record of the circulation time and of the retinal circulation would be obtained....[34]

Their attempts at fundus cinephotography of sodium fluorescein in humans failed:

Two attempts to determine the retinal circulation times in human beings using motion pictures were unsuccessful because of insufficient light. Motion pictures of the retina of cats is much easier to make than the motion pictures of the human retina. We are currently trying to improve the optical system of our apparatus so that this method can be applied to the study of human retinal circulation time....[34]

The future of fluorescein angiography was not in the determination of circulation time but rather in the evaluation and differential diagnosis of chorioretinal disease. In 1960, MacLean and Maumenee published this landmark description of fluorescein angioscopy—the first published case of sodium fluorescein being used to obtain a diagnosis[35]:

The patient, Stanford University Hospital No E-1234719 J.G., a white man, truck driver, 30 years of age, was first seen in consultation on February 16, 1955. He stated that three years prior to that time he had noted spots and flashes of light in front of his left eye. He had seen an optometrist who prescribed glasses for him. Four weeks prior to his examination visual acuity in his left eye had suddenly decreased....A cobalt blue filter was placed in front of the beam of the Haag-Streit slit lamp and the patient was given 2 cc of 5.0 percent fluorescein intravenously. A dozen small spots in the central portion of the tumor fluoresced within 30 seconds....A diagnosis of hemangioma of the choroid was made....[35]

The final piece of the puzzle was published in the journal *Circulation* by Novotny and Alvis.[1] The description of the technique used to create the first successful fluorescein angiogram (Figure 1-10) was published in 1961:

The purpose of this paper is to describe a method for the study of retinal blood flow in man by the use of intravascular fluorescein and retinal photography, and to report some preliminary observations made with this method....Serial fluorescence-photography of the human retinal vasculature

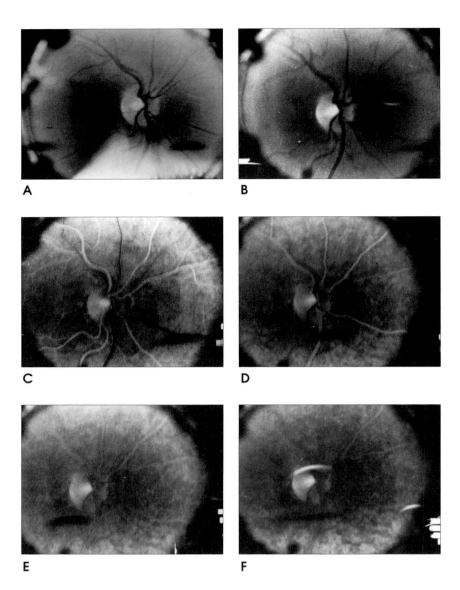

FIGURE 1-10
Harold Novotny produced the first fluorescein angiogram by recording fluorescein dye in the retinal blood vessels of David Alvis in 1959. Note the use of match sticks to signify print sequence. (Courtesy of T. Steffins.)

provides a dynamic record and increased visibility of the vascular pattern and blood flow by means of a simple technic....Separate arteriolar and venous filling phases, an arterio-venous shunt, sluggish choroidal circulation, stratified flow of fluorescein, and rapid central retinal circulation times were observed in normal retinas. Similar findings were seen in hypertensive and diabetic patients, and, in addition, neovascularization was clearly defined, and some cotton-wool patches, but not hemorrhages, were found to fluoresce.[1]

Resources

We encourage you to examine the original texts of the above citations, as well as the following books and reviews.

Early Books and Photographic Atlases

Allen L, Braley AE. *Stereoscopic Manual of the Ocular Fundus in Local and Systemic Disease.* St. Louis: Mosby, 1964.

Bedell AJ. *Photographs of the Fundus Oculi.* Philadelphia: FA Davis, 1929.

Bothman L, Bennett RW. *Fundus Atlas—Stereoscopic Photographs of the Fundus Oculi.* Chicago: Year Book, 1939.

Cattaneo D. *Oftalmoangioscopia.* L. Bologna, Italy: Cappelli, 1947.

Dimmer F. *Ueber die photographie des Augenhintesgrundes.* Wiesbaden, Germany: Bergmann, 1907.

Dimmer F, Pillat A. *Atlas photographischer Bilder des Menschlichen Augenhintergrundes.* Leipzig, Germany: F Deuticke, 1927.

Shikano S, Shimuzu K. *Atlas of Fluorescence Fundus Angiography.* Philadelphia: Saunders, 1968.

Thorner W. *Die theory des augenspiegels und die photographie des Augenhintergrundes.* Berlin, Germany: Hirschwald, 1903.

Tillé H. *Atlas clinique d'ophtalmoscopie photographique, syndromes cliniques du fond de l'oeil.* Paris: A. Couadau, 1939.

Historical Reviews

Alvis MD, Julian KG. The story surrounding fluorescein angiography. *J Ophthal Photog* 1982;5:6.

Bedell AJ. Stereoscopic fundus photography. *JAMA* 1935;105:1502.

Dimmer F. *Ueber die Photographie des Augenhintesgrundes.* Wiesbaden, Germany: Bergmann, 1907.

Englebert M. Uber die photographie des augenhintesgrundes. *Tecnische Roundschau* 1965;39:57.

Hurtes R. Evolution of Ophthalmic Photography. In J Justice (ed), *Ophthalmic Photography.* Boston: Little, Brown, 1982.

Liesenfeld H. Uberblick uber die entwicklung der augenhintergrundsphotographie. *Ophthalmologica* 1959;137:390.

Mann WA. History of photography of the eye. *Surv Ophthal* 1970;15:179.

Meyer-Schwickerath GRE. Ophthalmology and photography. *Am J Ophthal* 1968;66:1011.

Saine PJ. Landmarks in the historical development of fluorescein angiography. *J Ophthal Photog* 1993;15:17.

Saine PJ. Ophthalmic photography books: an historical bibliography. *J Ophthal Photog* 1994;16:78.

Shatz H, Burton TC, Yannuzzi LA, Rabb MF. *Interpretation of Fundus Fluorescein Angiography.* St. Louis: Mosby, 1978.

Van Cader TC. History of ophthalmic photography. *J Ophthal Photog* 1978;1:7.

Wong D. *Textbook of Ophthalmic Photography.* New York: Inter-Optics Publications, 1982.

References

1. Novotny HR, Alvis DL. A method of photographing fluorescence in circulating blood in the human retina. *Circulation* 1961;24:82.
2. Duke-Elder S. *System of Ophthalmology.* Vol II. St. Louis: Mosby, 1961.
3. Duke-Elder S. *System of Ophthalmology.* Vol X. London: Henry Kimpton, 1967.
4. Jackman WT, Webster JD. On photographing the retina of the living human eye. *Philadelphia Photographer* 1886;23:275.
5. Bedell AJ. Stereoscopic fundus photography. *JAMA* 1935;105:1502.
6. Baeyer A. Ueber eine neue klasse von farbstoffen. *Ber Dtch Chem Gzellshaft* 1871;4:555.
7. Ehrlich P. Ueber provocirte fluorescenzerscheinungen am auge. *Dtsch Med Wochenschr* 1882;8:21.
8. Burke A. Die klinische, physiologische und pathologische bedeutung der fluoreszenz in auge nach darreichnung von uranin. *Klin Monasbl Augenheilkd* 1910;48:445.
9. Kikai K. Uber die vitalfarbung des hinteren bulbussabschnittes. *Arch Augenheilkd* 1930;103:541.
10. Sorsby A. Vital staining of the retina; preliminary clinical note. *Br J Ophthal* 1939;23:20.
11. Lange K, Boyd LJ. The use of fluorescein to determine the adequacy of the circulation. *Med Clin North Am* 1942;26:943.
12. Dimmer F. *Ueber die Photographie des Augenhintergrundes.* Wiesbaden, Germany: Bergmann, 1907.
13. Howe L. Photography of the interior of the eye. *Trans Am Ophthal Soc* 1887;23:568.
14. Barr E. On photographing the interior of the human eyeball. *Am J Ophthal* 1887;4:181.

15. Gerloff O. Ueber die photographie des augenhintergrundes. *Klin Monat f Augenheil* 1891;29:397.
16. Thorner W. *Die theory des Augenspiegels und die Photographie des Augenhintergrundes.* Berlin, Germany: Hirschwald,1903.
17. Dimmer F. *Der Augenspiegel und die Ophthalmoskopische Diagnostik.* Leipzig, Germany: F Deuticke, 1921.
18. Dimmer F, Pillat A. *Atlas photographischer Bilder des Menschlichen Augenhintergrundes.* Leipzig, Germany: F Deuticke, 1927.
19. Helmholtz H. *Bescreibung eines Augenspiegels zur untersuchung der Netzhaut in lebenden Auge.* Berlin, Germany: Forstner, 1851.
20. Thorner W. A new stationary ophthalmoscope without reflexes. *Am J Ophthal* 1899;16:376.
21. Gullstrand A. Neue methoden der reflexlosen ophthalmoskopie. *Ber Dtsch Ophth Ges* 1910;36:75.
22. Nordenson JW. Augenkamera zum stationaren ophthalmoskop von Gullstrand. *Ber Dtsch Ophth Ges* 1925;45:278.
23. Van Cader TC. History of ophthalmic photography. *J Ophthal Photog* 1978;1:7.
24. Ridley H. Retinal photography. *Trans Ophthamol Soc UK* 1957;77:417.
25. Nida. Essai sur la photographie en couleurs du fond de l'oeil, XIII Concilium Ophthalmologicum. *Hollandia* 1929;1:39.
26. Bedell AJ. *Photographs of the Fundus Oculi.* Philadelphia: FA Davis, 1929.
27. Hartinger H. Ein neue reflexfreie ophthalmoskoplinse fur die zeiss-nordenonsche netzhautkammer. *Z Ophthalmol Optik* 1936;24:137.
28. Hansell P, Beeson EJG. Retinal photography in color. *Br J Ophthal* 1953;37:65.
29. Cohn P, DuBois-Reymond C. Photograms of the eye. *JAMA* 1888;10:540.
30. Edgerton HE. Photographic use of electrical discharge flashtubes. *J Optical Soc Am* 1946;36:390.
31. Rizzutti AB. High speed photography of the anterior ocular segment. *Arch Ophthal* 1950;43:365.
32. Ogle KN, Rucker CW. Fundus photographs in color using a high speed flash tube in the Zeiss retinal camera. *Arch Ophthal* 1953;49:435.
33. Chao P, Flocks M. The retinal circulation time. *Am J Ophthal* 1958;46:8.
34. Flocks M, Miller J, Chao P. Retinal circulation time with the aid of fundus cinematography. *Am J Ophthal* 1959;48:3.
35. MacLean AL, Maumenee AE. Hemangioma of the choroid. *Am J Ophthal* 1960;50:3.

Chapter 2

Fundus Photography: Instrumentation and Technique

Patrick J. Saine

A. Introduction
B. Instrumentation
    1. Sub-Systems
    2. Types of Fundus Cameras
    3. Selecting a Fundus Camera
    4. Fundus Camera Controls
    5. Fundus Camera Maintenance
C. Fundus Photography Technique: Step By Step
    1. Prepare
    2. Align
    3. Expose
    4. Follow-up
D. Focusing The Fundus Camera: A Clinical Approach
    1. The Fundus Camera's Focusing System
    2. Sharp Fundus Photographs
    3. Focusing Technique
E. Errors in Fundus Photography: Artifacts
    1. Causes of Artifacts
    2. Describing Artifacts
F. Managing the Challenging Patient
    1. Illumination problems
    2. Unsharp Subjects
    3. The Light-Sensitive Patient
    4. Eyelids
    5. Children
G. Advanced Techniques
    1. The Periphery
    2. Photographs After Laser Treatment
    3. Fundus Photography with Filters
    4. Fundus Photographs for Torsion
    5. Hand-Held Fundus Cameras
    6. Not Necessarily the Fundus
    7. Auxiliary Lenses at the Photo Slit Lamp

Introduction

Fundus photography documents the retina, the neurosensory tissue in the eye that translates optical images into electrical impulses the brain understands. The retina can be photographed directly, as the pupil is

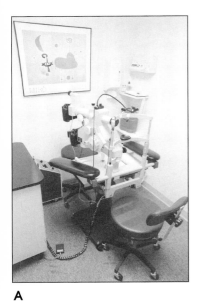
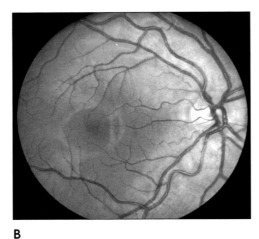
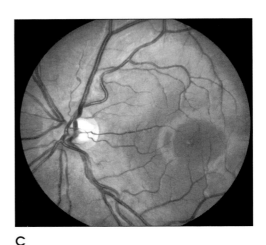

A   B   C

FIGURE 2-1
A typical fundus camera (A) is shown with normal
fundus photographs of a right (B) and left eye (C).

used as both an entrance and exit for the fundus camera's illuminating and imaging light rays. Ophthalmologists use the resulting retinal photographs to follow, diagnose, and treat eye diseases.

This chapter begins by discussing the instrumentation used to perform fundus photography. A step-by-step description of clinical technique is followed by a detailed explanation of the focusing process. Practical tips for avoiding artifacts and managing challenging patients are presented. Advanced fundus photography techniques conclude the chapter.

Instrumentation

The optical instrument used to document the visual condition of the retina is called a fundus camera. It is a specialized low-power microscope with an attached camera (Figure 2-1).

Subsystems

All automobiles have a steering wheel, engine, and wheels. The steering wheel guides you, the engine provides the energy, and the wheels get you where you want to go. Likewise, all fundus cameras share three interrelated subsystems: mechanical, optical, and electrical. The joystick steers the camera while the optical system creates the image from light energy provided by the electrical system.

MECHANICAL
Support for the fundus camera is provided by the mechanical subsystem. The heavy optical head is mounted on a height-adjustable table, the most versatile of which is wheelchair accessible. Standardized patient interface and camera positioning are provided by the mechanical subsystem. The chin rest and forehead rest reduce patient head movement. During the procedure, the precise positioning of the fundus camera is controlled by the joystick and optical head height control.

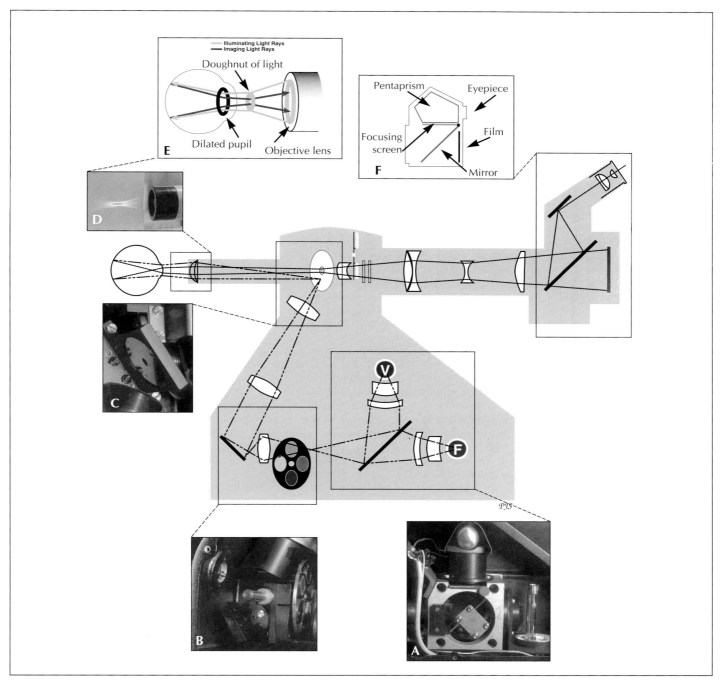

FIGURE 2-2
The optical pathway of the fundus camera. Light generated from either the viewing lamp or the electronic flash (A) is projected through a set of filters and onto a round mirror (B). This mirror reflects the light up into a series of lenses that focus the light. A mask on the uppermost lens shapes the light into a doughnut. The doughnut-shaped light is reflected onto a round mirror with a central aperture (C), exits the camera through the objective lens, and proceeds into the eye through the cornea. When the illuminating light is seen from the side, you can appreciate the complexity and precision of the optical scheme (D). Assuming that both the illumination system and the image are correctly aligned and focused, the resulting retinal image exits the cornea through the central, unilluminated portion of the doughnut (E). The light continues through the central aperture of the previously described mirror, through the astigmatic correction device and the diopter compensation lenses, and then back to the single lens reflex camera system (F).

OPTICAL

The retinal image is accurately and efficiently transferred to both the photographer and the film using the optical subsystem. The classic fundus camera design features an aspheric objective lens precisely aligned with a 35-mm single lens reflex camera body (Figure 2-2). Simply stated, the

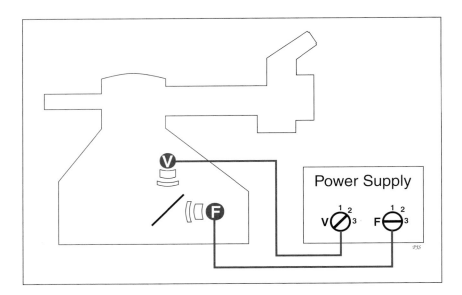

FIGURE 2-3
The flash tube and the viewing lamp are controlled by separate electrical subsystems. Increase the flash setting if your pictures are too dark; increase the view lamp setting if your view of the fundus is dark.

optical system of the fundus camera projects a ring of illumination through the dilated pupil; the light then reflects off the retina, exits the pupil through the center of the illumination ring, and continues through the fundus camera optics to form an image at the film plane. The viewfinder and the film back or digital recording device are integral parts of this subsystem.

ELECTRICAL

The fundus camera's electrical subsystem provides two sources of illumination. Distinctly different circuitry coexists for viewing the fundus and exposing the film (Figure 2-3). Viewing the retina requires a continuous light source that can be adjusted according to the patient's level of comfort and the photographer's ability to distinguish fine retinal detail. The viewing light is usually a tungsten bulb that is specific to the particular camera model and its manufacturer. Changing the viewing lamp intensity has no effect on the exposure of the final fundus photograph.

A xenon-filled flash tube provides a brief burst of intense light to expose the fundus photograph. The gas in the flash tube is ionized by the high voltage that is stored in the capacitors of the camera's power unit. Changing the intensity of the flash setting has no effect on the viewing illumination.

Types of Fundus Cameras

A wide variety of fundus cameras is available from a number of different manufacturers. The particular brand of camera may be identified by its image shape and identification tab (Figure 2-4).

Fundus cameras are described by the angle of view—the optical angle of acceptance of the lens (Figure 2-5). An angle of 30 degrees, considered the normal angle of view, creates a film image 2.5 times larger than life. Wide-angle fundus cameras capture images between 45 and 140 degrees and provide proportionately less retinal magnification. A narrow-angle fundus camera has an angle of view of 20 degrees or less. Normal-angle cameras have smaller illuminating annuli, making them more suitable for patients with narrow pupils. The inner diameter of the illuminating ring in wide-angle cameras is larger, making it more difficult to photograph patients with small pupils.

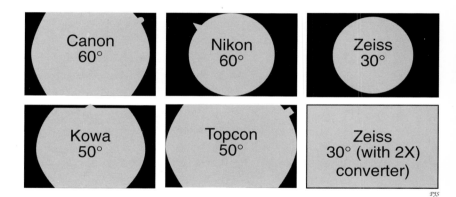

FIGURE 2-4
The shape and location of identification tabs help identify the brand of fundus camera. The actual size and shape of the image mask and the location of the identification tab may vary with the year of manufacture.

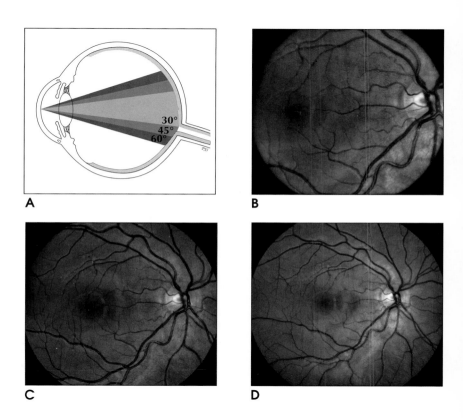

FIGURE 2-5
Angles of view. The greater the angle of view, the larger the retinal area contained in the photograph (A). The smaller the angle of view, the greater the magnification. The same eye is photographed at 20 degrees (B), 35 degrees (C), and 50 degrees (D).

Interchangeable lenses are important tools for the general photographer. The ability to vary the angle of view allows the ophthalmic photographer the same flexibility. Fundus cameras may ("multiple-angle cameras") or may not ("single-angle cameras") have the ability to internally alter their angle of view. Accessory teleconverter-type optics can be inserted in front of the film back to increase the versatility of some single-angle cameras (Figure 2-6).

There are two strategies for obtaining multiple angles of view. Either more than one single-angle fundus camera (e.g., a normal-angle and a wide-angle) or just one multiple-angle camera may be used. The optics of single-angle fundus cameras are optimized for a particular magnification and will provide higher-quality images than multiple-angle cameras. Multiple angle cameras offer versatility. However, usually only one angle of view (usually the widest) is sharp; alternate angles are less

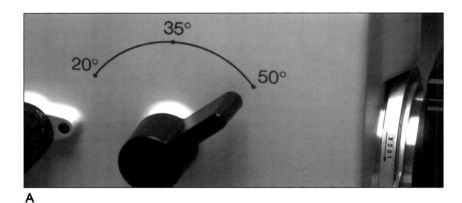

A

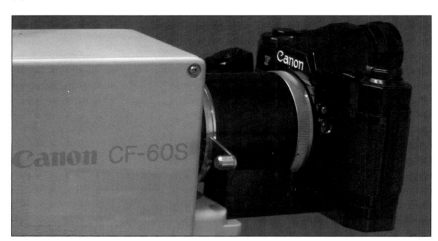

B

FIGURE 2-6
In multiple-angle cameras, select the angle of view by flipping a switch that inserts a different lens internally (A). In single-angle fundus cameras, place auxiliary teleconverter type optics between the camera body and lens to modify the angle of view (B).

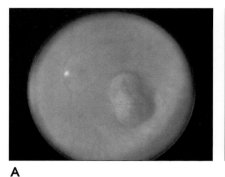

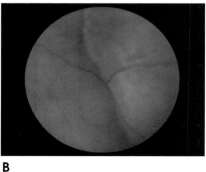

A   **B**

FIGURE 2-7
This 150-degree fundus photograph (A) of a tumor illustrates relative size and location. Multiple 30-degree photographs (B) would be needed to convey the same information.

critically sharp. The choice here is the familiar dilemma, pitting high quality against convenience and cost.

There are a number of specialized fundus camera designs. Extreme wide-angle cameras have an angle of acceptance of over 150 degrees and are used when large retinal areas need to be documented (Figure 2-7). Their small magnification minimizes fine retinal detail.

Simultaneous stereo fundus cameras use one exposure to place two images side by side on a single 35-mm frame (Figure 2-8). Their standardized stereo base allows longitudinal studies of retinal topography as well as detailed electronic analysis of retinal topography.

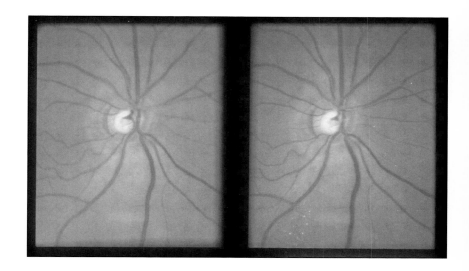

FIGURE 2-8
Simultaneous stereo cameras record two slightly different views of the retina side by side on a standard 35-mm film.

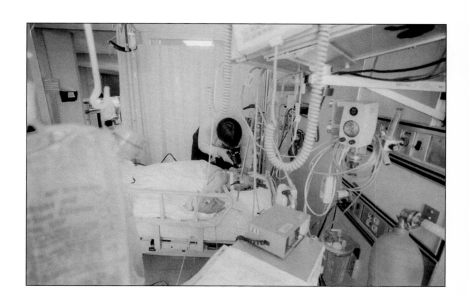

FIGURE 2-9
Hand-held fundus cameras are useful when patient positioning makes it difficult to use a standard fundus camera.

Hand-held fundus cameras provide maximum portability (Figure 2-9). They are useful for photographing bedridden, infant, and animal patients (see the section below on hand-held fundus cameras).

Both mydriatic and nonmydriatic fundus cameras are available. Mydriatic fundus cameras require patient dilation. Their versatility allows both sequential stereo fundus photography and fluorescein angiography. Nonmydriatic fundus cameras exploit the patient's natural dilation in a dark room. The photographer views the fundus using an infrared light source and an infrared video camera. Only a single image is captured, usually on instant film. Because the patient's pupil will take some time to naturally dilate again, multiple-image procedures are impossible. Nonmydriatic cameras are useful as screening devices.

Like much of the rest of the imaging world, ophthalmic photography is currently in a state of flux. Traditional silver-based imaging (film) is being challenged by the silicon-based technology of electronic imaging using computers. See Chapter 7 for a discussion of this new technology.

Choosing a Fundus Camera

1. How much versatility or specialization is required for your ophthalmic practice? Will the practice be growing or changing soon? Is this the practice's first or only fundus camera? If this is a second or third camera, should it be identical (for compatibility) or different (to expand the photographic capabilities or take advantage of technological advances)?

2. Will the optics of this camera provide adequate or superior sharpness and contrast? What angles of view are available and of what quality?

3. What are the clinical needs of the physician who will be evaluating the photographs? Will extremely fine macular detail be required in all images?

4. What type of patients will be photographed? Will their pupils be widely or poorly dilated? What is the minimum pupil size required for a good fundus photograph on a particular camera model?

5. Will patients be reasonably comfortable during the procedure? Can physically challenged patients be accommodated? Is portability an issue?

6. Are the camera's controls well balanced, adequately marked, and ergonomically placed? How easy or difficult is the viewing or focusing system to use?

7. Is this a reliable model? How sturdy does the camera feel? If this camera breaks down, how will it be repaired? How much time is involved? What is the cost, expected life, and availability of viewing lamps and flash tubes?

8. What is the initial cost of the unit? Is a used camera of the same model available?

9. What experience have other photographers had with this camera model? Is the photographer's preference to view with or without the barrier filter during fluorescein angiography?

10. Will the photographer using the camera be pleased with it?

Cleaning Your Lens

The best fundus photographs are taken using a fundus camera with a clean front element (Figure 2-11). Recommendations for cleaning your objective lens are available from your fundus camera manufacturer. Most lenses will not be harmed by over-the-counter "photographic" or "coated lens" cleaners and good-quality photographic lens cleaning tissue. Avoid products that leave a residue.

Begin cleaning your lens by inserting the negative diopter lens and focusing on the dust on the front element. Use a bulb syringe to blow off any loose dust. Place a few drops of lens-cleaning solution on a piece of lens tissue or natural cotton (never on the lens itself, and never on a commercial cotton swab manufactured with glue). Using gentle pressure, wipe in circular motions beginning in the center of the lens and spiraling to the outside.

(continued)

Selecting a Fundus Camera

Choosing a fundus camera is similar to buying an automobile. A family minivan is selected because of its versatility: It can transport people and haul larger loads. It's not flashy, nor particularly fast, and it won't get the best gas mileage. A minivan is most like a medium-priced multiple-angle fundus camera. It offers respectable sharpness in a variety of optical angles and is suitable for the general ophthalmic practice.

A minivan will never outrace a sports car. Built for performance first and price second, the sports car is analogous to the normal-angle fundus camera favored by the retinal specialist. It is designed to produce sharp photographs of the macula and does so extremely well. Its small illumination doughnut facilitates photographing through narrow pupils, and the astigmatic compensation device is useful for peripheral views.

Minimal-feature, entry-level cameras and used models are inexpensive purchase options. Special-use fundus cameras can be compared to pick-up trucks or all-terrain vehicles. These include extreme wide-angle, simultaneous stereo, and hand-held fundus cameras.

Pay careful attention to your specific needs when surveying the market. Compare and test drive competing camera models during fundus photography workshops such as those sponsored by the Ophthalmic Photographers' Society. The questions in the sidebar on choosing a fundus camera may help you prioritize fundus camera features and your practice's needs.

Fundus Camera Controls

Each time you perform fundus photography, you will be adjusting a complex optical instrument in a darkened room filled with strangers. Your mission: to completely familiarize yourself with each of your camera's controls. The alternative? Turning the light repeatedly on and off while searching for the appropriate setting, all the while cursing under your breath. Not a pretty picture.

Read your manual cover to cover. Memorize it. Contact the manufacturer to obtain a copy of a missing manual.

Figure 2-10 provides an overview of the controls found on most fundus cameras. Rely on your manual for the location and function of specific or specialized controls.

Fundus Camera Maintenance

The proper maintenance of a fundus camera involves skills as simple as changing a light bulb and procedures as complex as aligning optics.

A properly maintained fundus camera will provide years of reliable service. You should be able to handle simple maintenance such as cleaning the front surface of the objective lens or cleaning the film transport chamber (see the sidebar on cleaning your lens). Surfaces that come into direct contact with the patient should be disinfected after each procedure and at the end of every day. Consult a member of your infection control team or your physician for current recommendations of appropriate antimicrobial agents.

Always have two spare viewing lights, flash tubes, and fuses readily available. Know when and how to change them. Your fundus camera's instruction manual should contain detailed installation procedures. Alternately, contact the manufacturer's technical representative.

The 35-mm camera body is the fundus camera's most frequently repaired component. Its shutter fires and its film transport gears rotate each time a photograph is exposed. Keep a spare camera body available.

Cleaning Your Lens *(continued)*

Follow each damp lens tissue with a dry one, wiping in the same way. It may take a few passes to clean your lens well: Be patient and resist the urge to "scrub" the glass. Complete the process by breathing gently on the lens before the final wipe with a dry tissue.

Use common sense when cleaning your camera's lens. Clean regularly (but not after each patient) and gently (not vigorously).

After cleaning, the best way to keep your front element clean is to actively use the lens cap. Place the lens cap over the lens between each patient and whenever you leave the room—even when changing film!

It is wise to have your optics checked regularly by the manufacturer's service technician. Refer the cleaning of internal optics to a trained professional.

You may experience some residue that does not yield to these instructions. More extreme measures are described below. Caution: Because each different manufacturer uses different optical glass and lens coatings, check with your technical representative before using any of the following cleaning solutions. In addition, because these chemicals may pose a health hazard, use them with caution. Observe proper Occupational Safety and Health Administration (OSHA) regulations concerning both use and material safety data sheets (MSDS) documentation.

If your lens has a particularly nasty spot, these solutions, listed in order of least to most potent, may prove useful:

- Denatured alcohol
- Equal parts denatured alcohol and acetone
- Acetone
- Lacquer thinner followed by acetone

Of course, your front element is not the only place your fundus camera needs to be cleaned. External surfaces that come into contact with your patients should be disinfected both between each patient and at the end of the day.

FIGURE 2-10
Controls on three different fundus cameras are labeled to correspond with the numbered descriptions below (A, B, C). Your controls may vary according to the specific make and year of your fundus camera. You should be completely familiar with the function of all of your fundus camera's dials, knobs, and switches; consult the manual or the manufacturer if you are not. (Courtesy of Canon USA, Nikon, Inc., and Topcon USA.)

1. **Angle selection lever.** Inserts lenses into the optical pathway, which either increases or decreases the angle of view (or magnification). You should be familiar with the retinal area circumscribed by each setting, as well as the relative sharpness of each.
2. **Anterior segment lens.** Inserts a positive lens into the optical pathway, allowing for a more accurate imaging of the external eye or name tag. The diopter compensation lens performs this function on some cameras.
3. **Astigmatism compensation control.** Inserts an adjustable cylindrical lens into the optical pathway. It is especially useful when patients have a large amount of astigmatism or when photographing the periphery of the retina.

Fundus cameras that are used daily should have yearly inspections by factory-trained technicians. Consider returning your camera to the factory for complete optical realignment and refurbishment every 5–10 years. Mobile cameras may need service more often.

Fundus Photography Technique: Step By Step

The time involved in obtaining a good fundus photograph is significantly longer than the tiny fraction of a second it takes to expose the film. Like the athlete who is judged on split-second decisions, you should recognize that proper preparation, standardized technique, and careful follow-through are vital to successful fundus photography.

Fundus photography is actually a multistep procedure (Table 2-1). We will explore each of the following four major steps in detail:

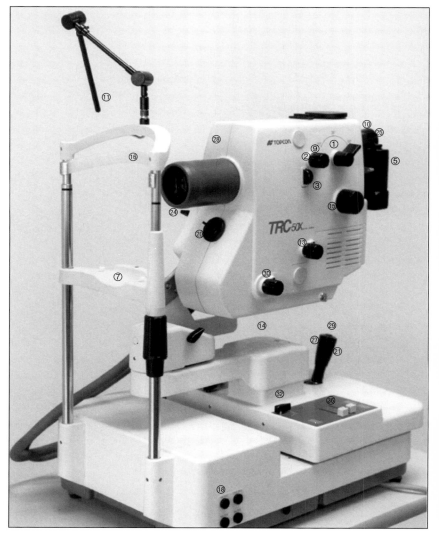

A

FIGURE 2.10 (*continued*)

4. **Barrier filter slide.** Positions a yellow barrier filter (for fluorescein angiography) in front of the film, but after the image has left the patient's eye. Some camera models position the barrier filter directly in the throat of the 35-mm camera back; some place it further forward in the optical system.

5. **Camera back.** Conventionally, this is a light-tight container that holds the film and contains the shutter. Modern fundus cameras offer a choice of film (silver-based imaging), video, or a digital chip (electronic imaging). Use separate camera backs for color film (for fundus photography) and black and white film (for fluorescein angiography). An instant film back may also be available.

6. **Camera back selection switch.** Selects between multiple camera backs. This is one of those simple switches that, if left in the incorrect position, can sabotage your session by sending images to the wrong camera body.

7. **Chin rest.** Stabilizes the patient. This should be cleaned after each patient.

8. **Data card port.** Positions a patient data card for recording information on the film next to the fundus images. Most photographers prefer to expose a separate name tag between patients.

9. **Diopter compensation lens.** Places positive and negative lenses into the optical pathway, extending the focusing range to permit the photography of patients with unusually long or short eyes. The plus setting can also be used for external or anterior segment photographs.

10. **Eyepiece diopter adjustment.** Sets the eyepiece, allowing the photographer to view the reticle in sharp focus. The eyepiece must be correctly set and the reticle must be in sharp focus to obtain sharp fundus photographs. Proper adjustment of the eyepiece is a critical element in successful fundus photography.

11. **External fixation light.** Used to direct patient fixation, this small light is universally positionable. Fixation lights can be green, red, or white; can have a focusable target; and sometimes blink.

12. **Filter slide.** Allows the addition of optional filters into the optical pathway (see number 13, filter wheel, for insertion of standard filters). These filters affect the light that enters the eye.

13. **Filter wheel.** Inserts the clear (color fundus photographs), green ("red-free" photographs), blue (exciter filter for fluorescein angiography), or red (choroidal photography) filter into the optical pathway in front of the light source (i.e., before the light enters the patient's eye).

14. **Flash intensity control.** Adjusts the amount of illumination emitted from the electronic flash. This control has no effect on the viewing illumination.

15. **Focusing knob.** Adjusts the distance between the front element and the focusing screen/film plane to maximize sharpness.

16. **Forehead rest.** Stabilizes the patient. It should be cleaned immediately after patient contact.

17. **Forehead rest adjustment.** Moves the patient toward and away from the front element. Used to position the fundus camera's illumination system with the patient's eye.

18. **Fuse.** Know the location of all of your camera's fuses and keep spares readily available. If the fuses on your power supply are unmarked, label them for future reference.

19. **Instruction booklet.** Full of important information, this should be read studiously from cover to cover.

20. **Internal fixation device.** Small pointer that can be introduced into the optical pathway. It is useful for obtaining fixation in the eye you are photographing, for recording the retinal location of patient fixation, or as a pointer in a teaching slide. When not serving a specific purpose, it should be removed from the optical pathway before the picture is taken.

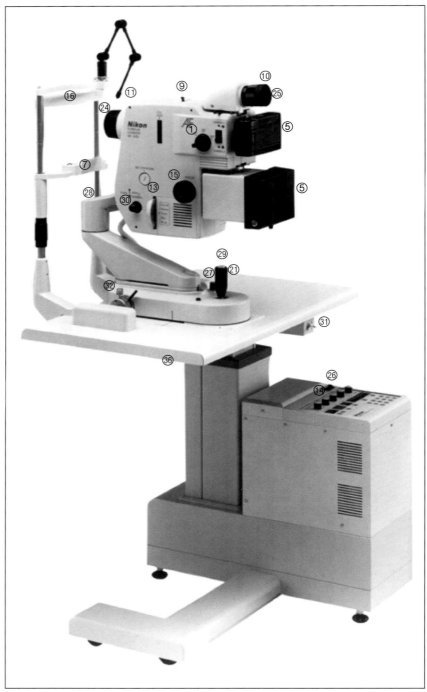

B

- Prepare
- Align
- Expose
- Follow-up

Prepare

1. *Prepare the room.* The room should be clean and tidy. All billing, departmental, and other paperwork should be completed before escorting the patient to the camera. Adjust the stool height and the

FIGURE 2.10 *(continued)*

21. **Joystick.** Controls the side-to-side and forward-to-backward motion of the optical head during photography. Using this control becomes second nature with experience.
22. **Joystick tension control.** Adjusts the ease of moving the joystick.
23. **Lens cap.** Protects the front element. It should be placed over the lens whenever photographs are not being taken and immediately after each patient session.
24. **Objective lens.** The expensive, aspheric lens that is primarily responsible for imaging the retina. Both the front and the rear surface should be kept scrupulously clean and dust-free.
25. **Ocular (eyepiece).** Allows you to view and judge the image before it is exposed. During fundus photography, keep both of your eyes open, relaxed, and focused on infinity. (See also number 10, eyepiece diopter adjustment.)
26. **On/off power switch.** Obvious, but essential—master switch that controls all electrical functions.
27. **Optical head height adjustment.** Raises or lowers the optical head in relation to the patient's eye.
28. **Pivot point.** The fundus camera rotates about this point, facilitating the visualization of nasal or temporal retina.
29. **Shutter release.** When pressed, exposes the photograph by initiating a series of events that includes raising the eyepiece mirror and opening the shutter, which triggers the flash.
30. **Small pupil device.** Slightly decreases the diameter of the illumination ring on a wide-angle camera, improving photographs imaged through a smaller pupil. This device is usually ambitiously named; a single, normal-angle camera is the best choice in small pupil situations.
31. **Table adjustment.** Raises or lowers the table height manually or with an electric motor.
32. **Table lock.** Holds the table steady during photography or while transporting the fundus camera.
33. **Tilt mechanism.** Rotates the camera up and down, facilitating inferior or superior retinal views.
34. **Timer reset.** Resets the angiogram timer to zero.
35. **Timer start.** Begins the angiogram timer.
36. **Viewing illumination control.** Adjusts the intensity of the viewing light. It has no effect on the brightness or darkness of the final fundus photograph.

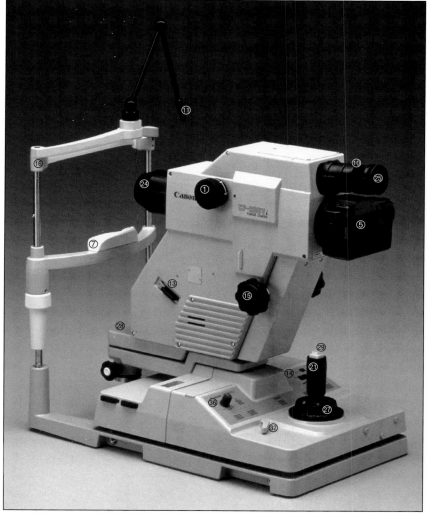

C

FIGURE 2-11
This fundus photograph was not taken during a blizzard. Keep your front element scrupulously clean. Blurry white circles appearing in the image are images of dust, dirt, or tears on the front of your objective lens. Dirty lenses are more noticeable in photographs of patients with smaller pupils and with off center camera alignment.

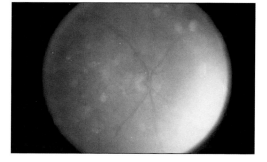

fundus camera's mechanical controls to their approximate midpoints. Select the appropriate camera back and load it with color slide film (see the sidebar on choosing film). Check that the illumination and flash settings, the filter wheel, and the diopter compensation control are in their standard positions.

2. *Adjust the eyepiece.* Follow the step-by-step procedure described in the sidebar on setting your reticle. Each time you look through the fundus camera, you should see the reticle in sharp focus. A full

Which Film Should I Use?

Choosing a film involves making two decisions. First, the general type must be determined, and then a specific brand must be chosen.

One way to describe film is by listing opposing characteristics (Figure 2-12). You know that film is available in black and white and color. It is also available as positive (or slide film: black records as black) and negative film (black records as white). Of course, both black and white film and color film are available in positive and negative emulsions. Slow film (ISO 25: less sensitive to light but finer grain and better image quality) and fast film (ISO 400: more sensitive to light but coarser grain and lesser image quality) are options in each of the above categories. Finally, film can vary in its spectral sensitivity or light balance—daylight, tungsten, and infrared emulsions being available. Most ophthalmic photographers choose a 35-mm slow (ISO 25) or medium (ISO 100) speed transparency film balanced for daylight for routine fundus photography.

If you are unsure about the film characteristics described above, a basic photography course will help.

Which specific brand or speed of film should you use? That question is best answered through empirical testing. While each film records physical reality, no pair of films ever records it in quite the same way. Each brand and speed of film has its own specific color cast, resolution, acutance (the transition between black and white when a straight edge is imaged), and "look" (Figure 2-13). The same brand of film (e.g., Kodachrome) is sold in different film speeds (e.g., 25, 64, and 200), each of which has different image charateristics.

Before settling on a film, perform a film test. Photograph the same volunteer or patient using a number of different films (keeping other factors constant, of course). Both you and the physician should evaluate the choices without knowing the names of the films used, using a daylight balanced light box. After selecting the best choice, determine its practicality: Is the film and processing readily available at a reasonable price? Are the archival properties of the chosen film adequate (Figure 2-14)?[1]

Film manufacturers are continually improving their film stocks. We suggest keeping current with emulsion changes and testing new films regularly.

FIGURE 2-12
Choosing a film. Listing opposing characteristics will help you identify the film of choice for a particular application. With your final application in mind, follow the arrows: Fundus photography requires a color film that is positive (slides), has a slow or medium speed (for fine grain), and is daylight-balanced (flash illumination). Once these broad characteristics are defined, the choice of brand is a practical matter. Select the film with the best image quality, truest color balance, greatest convenience, and best value.

Table 2-1. Fundus Photography: Step by Step*

Prepare	Prepare the room Adjust the eyepiece Plan the photographs
Patient contact time ⟶	Seat the patient Inform the patient Position the patient Position the photographer
Align	Establish fixation Focus the illumination system Adjust the joystick Select the area of interest Select the angle of view Check the focus
Expose	Double-check everything Expose the film Close the session
Follow-up	Process the film/edit the images Edit the film/archive the data Deliver the finished product Review your work

*Review these steps before or during the procedure to help establish your routine. Post a copy of these steps near your fundus camera for reference.

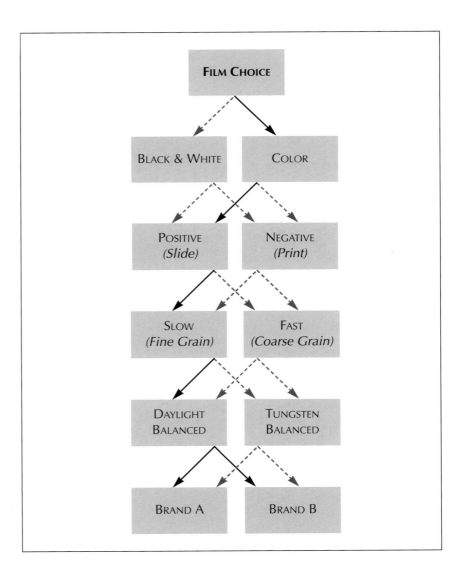

Setting Your Reticle

To obtain a sharp view of the reticle, your eyepiece must be correctly set. Here is a step- by-step procedure for eyepiece adjustment:

1. Have your eyes corrected for their best visual acuity. You may choose to photograph with or without glasses or contact lenses if your correction is spherical. Remember, however, that the correct eyepiece setting will be different depending on whether you wear your corrective lenses. If you have astigmatism, you should wear your corrective lenses while adjusting the eyepiece. Alternatively, correct the eyepiece itself by securing the appropriate trial lens directly over the eyepiece.[2] Do not wear reading glasses.

2. Eliminate any subject matter from the camera's field of view. Set your camera to the farthest focusing extreme and hold or tape a piece of white cardboard in front of the objective lens. When you look through the viewfinder, you should see a blurry reticle on a white field. The illumination level should be adjusted to a medium or low setting (approximately the same intensity as when viewing the retina). If the picture is too bright, it may cause your pupil to constrict, bringing depth of field into play and making an accurate setting difficult.

3. Set the eyepiece adjustment to the maximum plus diopter setting. This will blur any image of the focusing reticle. When looking through the viewfinder, you should see an evenly illuminated white field.

4. Relax your eyes. Blink and look at something far away— perhaps down a long hall or at a reflection. It is extremely important that your eyes be focused on infinity to obtain the correct setting. Keeping both eyes open may help keep you from accommodating.

5. Peer through the viewfinder and begin turning the eyepiece ring toward the zero setting. Smoothly rotate the ring. Rotate at a slow enough rate that you perceive the reticle becoming sharper, but not so slowly that your eyes accommodate for the change. Remember to keep both eyes open and focused at infinity.

6. Stop rotating when the reticle is just in sharp focus. If you continue to rotate the reticle after you achieve sharp focus, or if you begin to search for sharpness by rotating the reticle back and forth, then accommodation may be influencing your decision. If your eyes are at their best correction, your setting will probably be within a diopter or so of the zero mark. If your diopter setting is a high minus, chances are

(continued)

FIGURE 2-13
Comparing different films. Film and processing have a major impact on the color of your final fundus photographs. These three photographs of the same patient were exposed with the same camera on the same day but using different brands of film. Because commercially available film emulsions may change frequently, regularly test new film products.

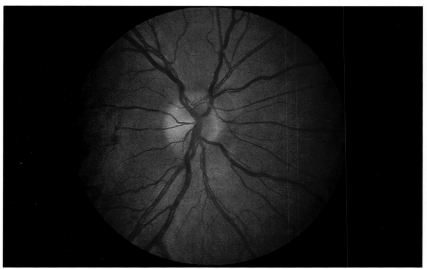

A

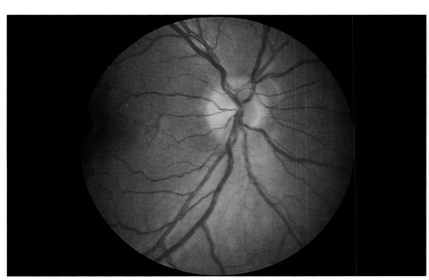

B

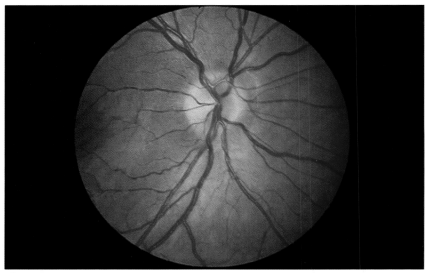

C

Setting Your Reticle (continued)

that you have accommodated. If you are wearing no correction, the setting should be within a diopter of your best correction.

7. Repeat, repeat, repeat. Continue setting the eyepiece until three successive, near-normal settings agree. Note the most consistent position of the eyepiece ring. Remember to correctly set the eyepiece before each patient session. New photographers should repeat this exercise daily until they are confident that their eyepiece setting is accurate.

   Each fundus camera should be set individually by each photographer. The correct setting for each camera (especially if brands vary) may be slightly different for the same photographer, and the correct setting for a single camera will vary between photographers in the same office. If an instrument has more than one user, a signal can be developed to alert alternate users of possible eyepiece setting changes (perhaps an empty film box placed over the eyepiece).

8. Check the eyepiece setting and reticle before each patient. It cannot be overemphasized that once your personal setting has been ascertained, it is imperative to check it before each patient. Be aware of the focusing screen's reticle throughout each photographic procedure. Only conscientious use of the eyepiece/reticle focusing system will assure consistently sharp fundus photographs.

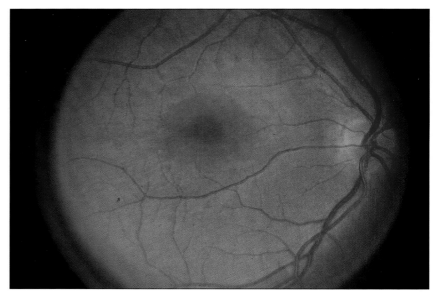

A

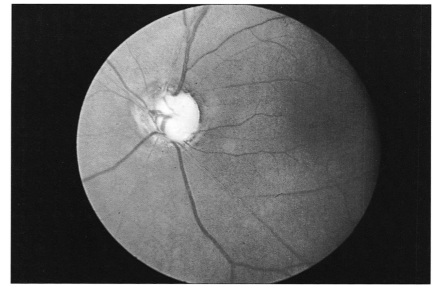

B

FIGURE 2-14
Archival properties of film. Are your images exposed on color film that will not fade or discolor with time? Both of these fundus photographs were exposed in the 1960s. By the mid-1990s, A has faded considerably while B has not. Investigate the archival properties of your film of choice.

explanation of how the reticle system works is found in the section on focusing the fundus camera. Photograph a name tag before the patient enters the room. A name tag is simply a photograph of the patient's name and chart number; you may use the patient's chart or routing slip or, alternately, handwrite or type the information. The name tag assures you that the camera is functioning properly and serves as a guidepost during editing. You won't be looking into the eyepiece again until Step 9.

3. *Plan the photographs.* Take a moment to prepare yourself for the procedure. You should be familiar with the basic anatomy of the eye (Figure 2-15). Review the photo request form (Figure 2-16), consulting with the referring physician as needed. Remember that you will be creating a permanent record of the patient's fundus at a particular moment in time. Your photographs should be complete enough to convey the condition of the retina to the physician.

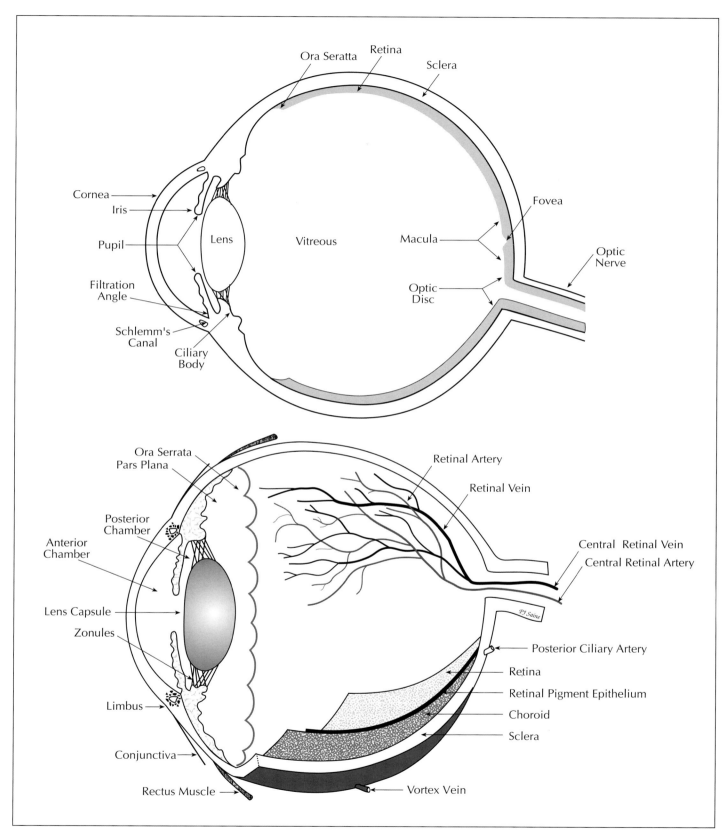

FIGURE 2-15
Basic eye anatomy. A thorough knowledge of the anatomy of the eye is a prerequisite for successful fundus photography.

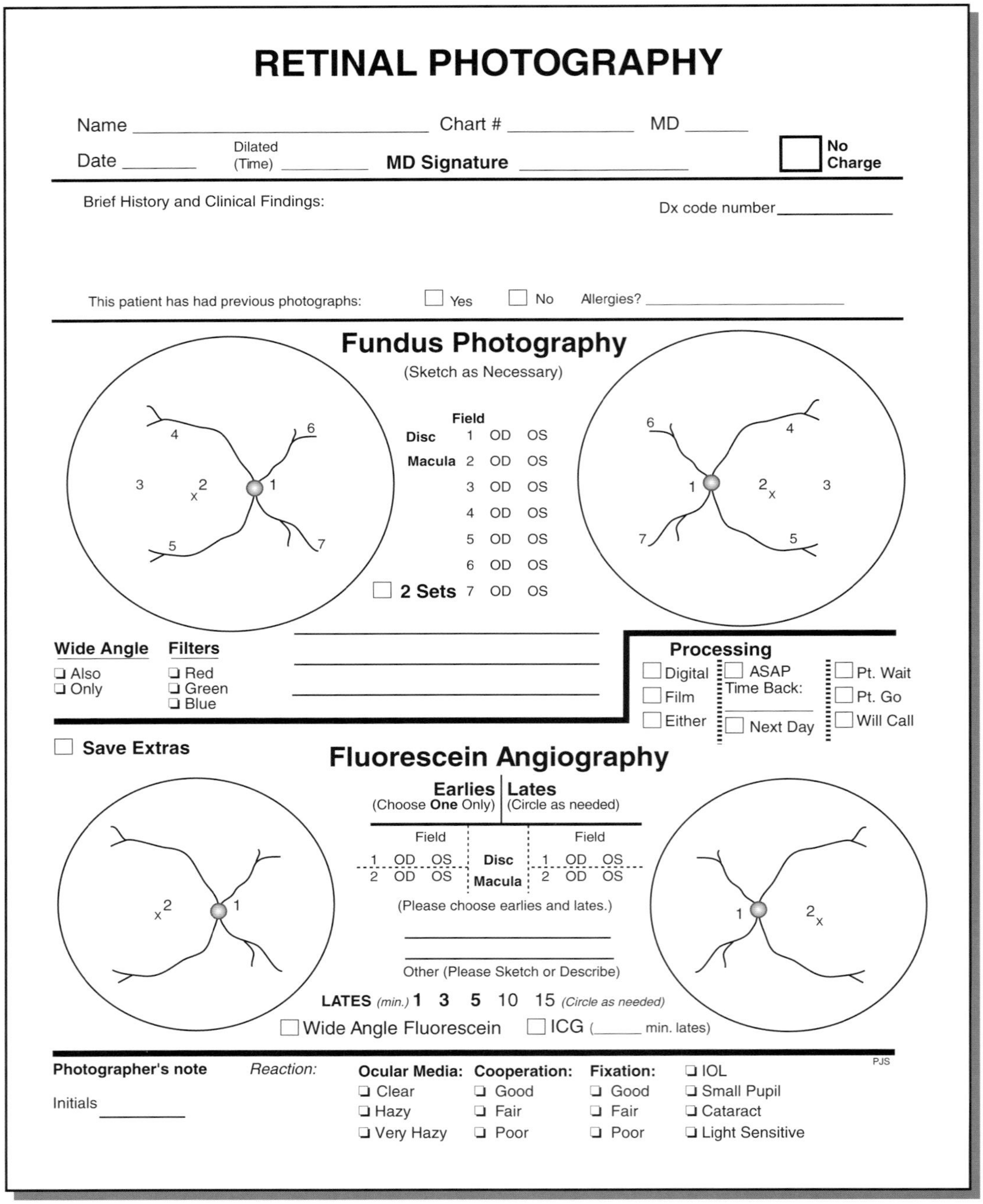

RETINAL PHOTOGRAPHY

Name _____ Chart # _____ MD _____

Date _____ Dilated (Time) _____ **MD Signature** _____ ☐ **No Charge**

Brief History and Clinical Findings: _____ Dx code number _____

This patient has had previous photographs: ☐ Yes ☐ No Allergies? _____

Fundus Photography
(Sketch as Necessary)

Field

Disc	1	OD	OS
Macula	2	OD	OS
	3	OD	OS
	4	OD	OS
	5	OD	OS
	6	OD	OS
☐ **2 Sets**	7	OD	OS

Wide Angle
☐ Also
☐ Only

Filters
☐ Red
☐ Green
☐ Blue

_____
_____
_____

Processing
☐ Digital   ☐ ASAP   ☐ Pt. Wait
☐ Film   Time Back: ☐ Pt. Go
☐ Either   ☐ Next Day   ☐ Will Call

☐ **Save Extras**

Fluorescein Angiography

Earlies (Choose **One** Only) | **Lates** (Circle as needed)

Field				Field		
1	OD	OS	**Disc**	1	OD	OS
2	OD	OS	**Macula**	2	OD	OS

(Please choose earlies and lates.)

_____
_____

Other (Please Sketch or Describe)

LATES (min.) 1 3 5 10 15 (Circle as needed)

☐ Wide Angle Fluorescein   ☐ ICG (_____ min. lates)

Photographer's note   *Reaction:*

Initials _____

Ocular Media:
☐ Clear
☐ Hazy
☐ Very Hazy

Cooperation:
☐ Good
☐ Fair
☐ Poor

Fixation:
☐ Good
☐ Fair
☐ Poor

☐ IOL
☐ Small Pupil
☐ Cataract
☐ Light Sensitive

PJS

FIGURE 2-16
Photo request form. Using a photography request form facilitates communication between the physician and the photographer. One form should be completed for each patient photography session.

Examine prior photographs and notes made by the previous photographer or the physician. Note the patient's visual acuity and working diagnosis. Will the patient have trouble fixating because of a macular problem? Which fields should be photographed? On which retinal level should the camera be focused? Should the periphery be scanned for retinal changes? Will another photographic procedure better document this particular disease entity? Should today's images match the magnification and fields of previous photographs? You should have a photographic plan in mind

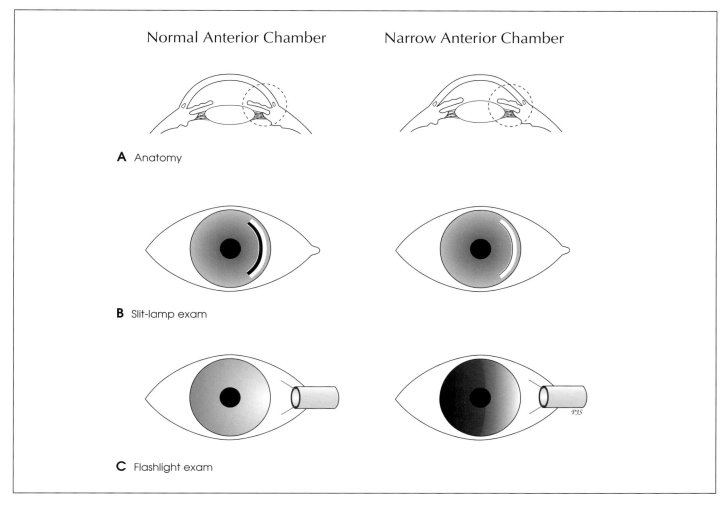

Normal Anterior Chamber

Narrow Anterior Chamber

A Anatomy

B Slit-lamp exam

C Flashlight exam

FIGURE 2-17
Estimating anterior chamber depth. The anterior chamber depth of each patient should be estimated before introducing dilation medication. Normal anterior chambers will not close during routine dilation. Narrow anterior chamber angles, however, often close upon routine dilation, causing increased intraocular pressure and an episode of medication-induced closed-angle glaucoma. Anatomically, the normal iris is well separated from the trabecular network (A). The iris and trabecular meshwork are more closely positioned in patients with narrow angles. Angle depths are estimated using a 0 (closed angle) through 4 (large, fully open angle) scale. Slit lamp examination is the best method for estimating anterior chamber depth. If a slit beam is projected at a 45-degree angle, then the aqueous space is indicated by unilluminated space (the black line between the two white lines) between the corneal reflection and the beam's projection on the iris (B). The normal anterior chamber will reveal a wide space, the narrow anterior chamber, a narrow distance. A flashlight projected at the limbus in the same plane as the iris can also be used to estimate the depth of the anterior chamber (note: the flashlight technique has fallen out of favor with many ophthalmologists). Normal chambers cast little or no shadows. A bowed iris in a shallow anterior chamber projects a wide shadow across the pupil to the limbus (C). Careful slit lamp or flashlight examination is necessary on all patients before dilation. Always check with the ophthalmologist before dilating a patient with a narrow anterior chamber angle.

before you escort the patient into the room. This plan should include your camera and angle of view selections, the areas of the patient's retina you intend to document, and any specialized techniques that may be useful.

4. *Escort the patient.* Your patient's pupils must first be dilated in accordance with the attending physician's orders (Figure 2-17) (see the sidebar on dilating your patient's pupils). Mentally evaluate your patients while escorting them to the fundus camera. Do they seem to be in good or poor general health? Are there any obvious physical disabilities? Retinal photography patients are often mature: Familiarize yourself with typical age-related hearing and visual changes. Become aware of your patient's disposition. Some patients will be uncomfortable merely because they are in a doctor's office.

Table 2-2. Medications Used for Routine Dilation

Generic Name	Trade Names	Action	Maximal Effect	Duration
Tropicamide	Mydriacyl Opticyl Tropicacyl	Mydriasis and cycloplegia	20–30 mins	4–6 hrs
Cyclopentolate hydrochloride	AK-Pentolate Cyclogel	Mydriasis and cycloplegia	15–30 mins	24 hrs
Phenylephrine hydrochloride	Efricel AK-Dilate Mydfrin Neo-Synephrine	Mydriasis	20–40 mins	3 hrs

Dilating Your Patient's Pupils

DILATION MEDICATION

An obvious prerequisite to creating any photograph is the ability to record the light that reflects off of the subject matter. This is taken for granted under ordinary circumstances. We are confronted with a biological system that is designed to counteract our best efforts when we attempt to photograph the retina, however. Because the eye has no internal light source, to photograph the retina we must shine a light into the patient's eye. This causes the iris to constrict—in effect, closing the window through which we are attempting to view. Extinguishing the light allows the pupil to become larger, and we are unable to record or even see in the resulting darkness. Clearly, we must counteract the iris' natural reaction to light if we are to obtain retinal photographs.

The solution to this fundamental problem is to artificially dilate the patient's pupils using topical medication. When we "dilate a patient," we instill drops that will counteract the pupils' normal reaction to light. This increases the size of the patient's pupil, allowing the illuminating light rays to be projected in and the imaging light to independently exit the eye.

The size of the pupil is controlled by the iris sphincter muscle and the dilating muscle. We can manipulate the normal reactions of these muscles by using two different types of medications: mydriatics and cycloplegics (Table 2-2). Mydriatics are sympathomimetics that dilate the pupil (or affect mydriasis) by causing the dilator muscle to contract. They also cause vasoconstriction and should be used with caution in individuals with a history of hypertension or heart problems. A commonly used mydriatic is phenylephrine. Available in both 2.5% and 10% solutions, maximal pupil dilation begins in 20 minutes and lasts for approximately 3 hours.

Cycloplegics are parasympatholytics that cause mydriasis by paralyzing the iris sphincter muscles. They also arrest accommodation (or cause cycloplegia) by paralyzing the ciliary muscle. A commonly used cycloplegic is tropicamide. Available in both 0.5% and 1% solutions, maximal pupil dilation occurs at about 30 minutes and lasts for 4–6 hours. Some offices prefer cyclopentolate. Available in 0.5%, 1%, and 2% solutions, it causes pupil dilation in 15–20 minutes and lasts for 24 hours. Other cycloplegics include atropine, homatropine, and scopolamine; each is available under various trade names.

(continued)

Others may be in low spirits because they just received some unpleasant news from the doctor. Your demeanor should be bright but professional. Offer to take a coat or other personal items, setting them on the available shelf or hook. Invite your patients to be seated and introduce yourself with a smile. (*"My name is ____, and I'd like to take some pictures of your eyes for Dr. ____."*) Speak in a clear, calm voice to put your patients at ease. Remember that this may be their first experience with fundus photography—they will be looking to you to guide them through the procedure. Talk to your patients throughout the procedure; reassure them and let them know what to expect.

5. *Inform your patient.* Informed patients are cooperative patients. Explain the procedure, acquainting them with the impending bright flashes and with your expectations. Let them know that it is fine for them to blink and breathe normally. Reassure them that the multicolored spots they will see afterward are nothing to worry about. Remind them that it is just like looking into a flash when they are having their picture taken and that no x-rays are involved. A mounted photograph should be available for simple explanations. Invite questions and answer them appropriately. Remember, however, that your role as a photographer precludes you from dispensing specific medical information. Diplomatically refer appropriate questions back to the referring physician.

6. *Position your patient.* Comfortable patients are cooperative patients. Adjust the patient's chair height, then the height of the camera, and finally the height of your chair (Figure 2-18). Instruct the patient to place his or her chin in the chinrest and forehead against the bar. Raise or lower the table height or adjust the chin rest as needed. When correctly positioned at the fundus camera, your patient should have a straight back and be leaning slightly forward. The height of his or her eyes should approximately correspond to the height of the objective lens. A mark on the side of your head rest may indicate this height. (Some photographers place a mark at the lowest and highest lens objective height setting to help gauge appropriate patient alignment at a glance.) Be sure to ask the patient whether he or she is comfortable. (*"Can I raise or lower the camera to make you more comfortable?"*) This question helps put your patient at ease by extending the same courtesy we would expect if we were in the patient's position.

7. *Position yourself.* After the patient has been made comfortable, you should do likewise. Your eye should be at the same height as the viewfinder; raise or lower your seat as appropriate. A typist uses

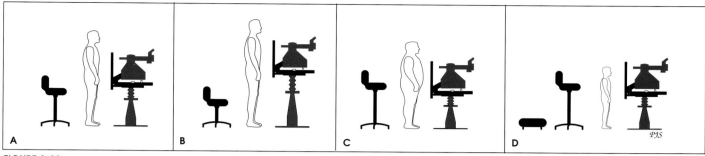

FIGURE 2-18
Seating the patient. Patient comfort is affected by the height of the patient's chair and the height of the fundus camera. Both the chair and the camera are adjusted to their midpoint for the average-sized patient (A). Lower the stool and raise the camera for tall or long-bodied patients (B). Raise the stool and lower the camera for heavy or short patients (C). A child's height will dictate the best seating strategy. The child may be comfortable while standing flat on the floor or on a short step stool (D). Younger children may sit or kneel either on their parent's lap or directly on a raised patient chair. Remove the head rest and lay papoosed babies on their side, or use a hand-held fundus camera for infant fundus photography.

Dilating Your Patient's Pupils   *(continued)*

A word of caution and an editorial: It is important to recognize the photographer's role in the health care setting. Ophthalmic photographers are surrounded by licensed individuals who specialize in understanding drugs and their effect on the body. These individuals should guide us in the use of all of the medications we administer to our patients. No drug should be administered to any patient without a physician's order. If a reaction occurs, refer the patient to a licensed health care worker. This does not mean that as ophthalmic photographers we are "just photographers." Ophthalmic photographers are highly trained professionals who specialize in acquiring images of the eye. We should use the strengths of other health care workers just as we expect them to recognize our areas of expertise.

INSTILLING EYE MEDICATION

Some important cautions: Read the medication insert completely for a description of contraindications and side effects. The administration of dilating drops is contraindicated in patients who are at risk for narrow-angle glaucoma. Estimate the anterior chamber depth before instilling dilation medication (Figure 2-17). Check with your physician before dilating patients with iris-fixated intraocular lenses. Children and infants should be dilated using ophthalmic medications that contain lower concentrations of active ingredients; consult the physician for specific instructions.

Educate your patients about the normal side effects of dilation. Remind them that the drops may sting (we jokingly remind patients that "these drops just sting on (insert day of the week)...." and tell older pediatric patients to "close your eyes and count backwards from 20: the stinging will be over by then"). Warn the patients of increased light sensitivity due to their enlarged pupils. Offer them inexpensive, disposable sunglasses. Patients should be counseled that reading may be difficult because their near vision will be blurry. Reassure them that their distance vision should be minimally affected. We suggest patients bring a driver if they will be dilated.

Begin by washing your hands with soap and water and instructing the patient to tilt his or her head back. Gently pull the lower eyelid down slightly to create a small space between the lid and the globe. Place a single drop in this pouch, being careful not to contaminate the

(continued)

the "home row" to standardize interaction with the typewriter. In the same way, you are encouraged to find your own "home keys." Grip the joystick with your dominant hand. If the optical head height adjustment is a separate control, place your other hand on it. The second hand also easily extends upward to the focusing knob or the external fixation device. The index finger of the joystick hand or the right foot triggers the shutter release. The hand closest to the power supply is used for any adjustments there.

Align

8. *Establish fixation.* Slide the fundus camera in front of the eye to be photographed (see the sidebar on which eye should be photographed first). Ask the patient to look straight ahead. Present the external fixation device to the eye that is not being photographed. Ask the patient if he or she can see the little light straight ahead. You may need to move the external fixation device quickly back and forth to gain the patient's attention (see the sidebar on establishing patient fixation). Ask the patient to keep looking at the little light while you shine another light into the other eye. Let the patient know that the small light will be in the middle of the bigger light once you have everything centered (Figure 2-19).

9. *Position the illumination system.* Turn the room lights down. Grossly align the fundus camera from side to side until the viewing light is centered on the cornea. Keep the joystick upright and use the optical head height adjustment as needed. Position the illumination system by moving the forehead rest adjustment (and patient) toward or away from the objective lens until the doughnut of light is centered on the pupil and focused on the cornea (or eyelid). Upon looking through the viewfinder with your dominant eye, you should see a blurry fundus image with an overlapping reticle (Figure 2-20). The image you see will probably be out of focus and may have a crescent-shaped artifact. Focus quickly (keeping the image of the reticle sharp and turning the focusing knob until the retina looks sharp), knowing that you will make fine focusing adjustments later. The crescent-shaped artifact indicates that the distance between the objective lens and the cornea is nearly correct. An unsharp or fuzzy artifact implies that the illumination system is improperly aligned.

10. *Adjust the joystick.* The location of the crescent indicates your centration in the pupil (Figure 2-21). If the crescent is found on the right

Dilating Your Patient's Pupils   *(continued)*

bottle by allowing it to touch the patient. (The drop may be applied inside the lower eyelid, on the sclera, or on the cornea. The patient's blink will distribute the medication.) Instill a second drop if you are not sure that the first was successful. One properly placed drop is sufficient: Avoid flooding the patient's eyes. After the drop has been instilled, ask the patient to close his or her eyes for a moment (without squeezing the eyelids). Blinking in moderation is acceptable. Patients may gently dab their closed eyes with a clean tissue but should avoid applying pressure. Replace the cap or dropper immediately after use. Wait 1 or 2 minutes between different eye medications.

Pay careful attention to the expiration date of your dilating medications. Never instill outdated or discolored medication. Consider dating the bottles when opened and then disposing of opened bottles after 30 days of use.

DIFFICULT CLINICAL SITUATIONS

Large pupils permit easier fundus photography. Unfortunately, dilating medication is not equally effective in all individuals. Be prepared to photograph through smaller pupils in patients who:

- Have darkly pigmented irises
- Are older
- Are taking glaucoma medication
- Have iritis with posterior synechia
- Have diabetes

You may encounter patients whose pupils constrict when you begin fundus photography. This could be the result of a number of different clinical situations. For example, the patient may have been dilated only with tropicamide. This dilation regimen is appropriate for routine direct ophthalmoscopy but inadequate for fundus photography. Patients being examined for closed-angle glaucoma are often dilated with only tropicamide. Another example is the patient who has been dilated much earlier that day. Routine dilation medication can last as little as 4–6 hours; if a patient has been dilated more than 3 hours earlier, his or her pupils may constrict during fundus photography. The patient may have a darkly pigmented iris and require a second set of drops for adequate dilation. Our routine for all of these situations is identical: We consult with the referring ophthalmologist to determine whether additional dilating drops may be safely administered. If so, fundus photography is resumed approximately 15 minutes after their administration. If additional dilating drops are not recommended, then fundus photography is resumed, the most important fields being imaged first. A note concerning the poor dilation is made on the order sheet, as it may affect the quality of the photographs.

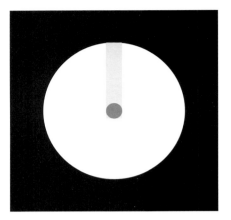

FIGURE 2-19
This diagram illustrates the normal patient's view when the retina is photographed. The patient will fuse the bright fundus camera light with the less bright fixation light. When fused, the small light will be perceived to be inside of the large light. The small light will be centered for macula photographs.

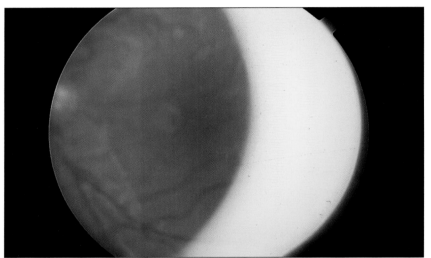

A

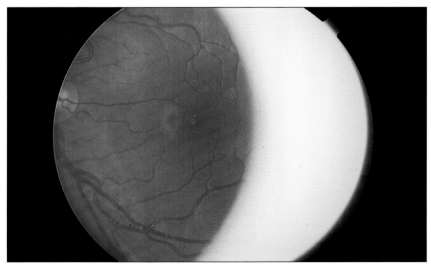

B

FIGURE 2-20
Just after aligning the optical system, your look through the viewfinder will probably look blurry and contain artifacts (A). After a quick focus (B), move up and down or side-to-side to eliminate all crescent artifacts (C), then move forward and backward to find the maximum color saturation (D). Finally, focus carefully on the retina.

Which Eye Should Be Photographed First?

When both eyes are to be photographed, one convention dictates that the macula of the right eye (OD) be photographed first. This establishes a routine introduction to the patient both at the camera and at the editing table. This approach is often favored for novice fundus photographers because of its simplicity.

Another approach is to photograph the affected eye first. This is the eye the physician is most interested in; it may have been chosen for the transit phase of a fluorescein angiogram. In this system, if the session ends early (e.g., if the camera breaks or if a very young patient declines further photography), the most important images have been captured. Additionally, the second eye photographed often exhibits increased light sensitivity.

It matters little which specific system you choose as long as you establish a logical and systematic approach to your patients.

Establishing Fixation

There are a number of reasons why your patient may not be able to fixate on the external fixation light, the most obvious of which is that your patient probably has vision problems! If you are having trouble establishing fixation using the external fixation device, try one of the following practical suggestions:

1. *Clarify your instructions.* Patients may look to the side and see the fixation light with the eye you are photographing (as opposed to the fixating eye). They will ask you which of the two lights you want them to look at—the one to the side or the one straight ahead. Instruct them to look at the little light in the middle of the big light, or at the small light straight ahead, not at the light to the side.

2. *Alter the visual stimulus.* A moving or blinking stimulus commands attention better than a stationary stimulus. Try moving the fixation light from side to side using short, quick movements. If your camera doesn't have a blinking fixation light, then simulate blinking by rapidly moving your finger back and forth in front of the fixation light.

3. *Change the fixation light location.* Younger patients may attempt to fixate with both of their eyes. These patients will cross their eyes, making it difficult for you to obtain the proper field of view. If your instructions to look straight ahead fail, try adjusting the distance between the fixation light and the patient's eye. Some patients will straighten their eyes if you move the fixation light further away, effectively hiding it from the eye being photographed. Alternately, rotate the fixation light in slightly and move it closer toward the inner canthus. The fixating eye will remain crossed, but the eye being photographed will be looking straight ahead.

4. *Use the internal fixation device.* Insert your internal fixation device into the optical pathway where it will cast a shadow onto the patient's fundus. This stick-like shadow will look in focus to the patient when it looks in focus.

(continued)

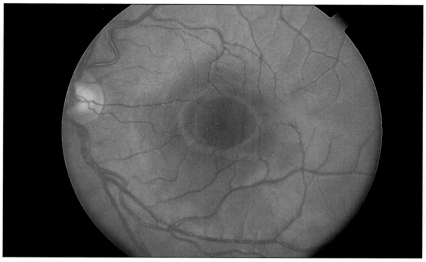

C

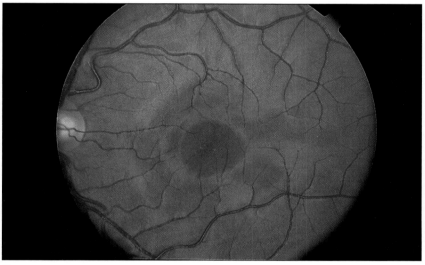

D

FIGURE 2-20 *(continued)*

side of the fundus image, the camera is off-center to the right side of the pupil. In this case, use the joystick to shift the camera slightly to the left, centering the doughnut in the pupil. These crescent artifacts can occur above, below, and to each side. Using the joystick, move in the opposite direction of the crescent to recenter the camera in the pupil (and eliminate the artifact). (See Chapter 3 on stereo fundus photography to learn the importance of finding and using these artifacts.) Once your view is free from crescent-shaped artifacts, seek proper color saturation. Moving the joystick toward and away from the patient, check for the most even, most fully saturated view. Remember that the reticle should still be sharp.

Two simple guidelines affect positioning artifacts during fundus photography: (a) moving the joystick from side to side and moving the optical head up and down controls the centration of the illuminating ring in the pupil and therefore controls the presence or absence of crescent shaped artifacts, and (b) moving the joystick in and out controls the color saturation of the image.

Establishing Fixation   *(continued)*

to you. In most cases you will want to remove the internal fixation device before the fundus photograph is exposed. This fixation strategy is especially useful if the eye being photographed has better vision than the fixating eye, or when the patient is monocular.

5. *Instruct the patient verbally.* If you have difficulty obtaining fixation with either fixation target, try asking the patient to look straight ahead in the middle of the light (for macula views). Alternately, have the patient look straight ahead at you (or your nose, voice, or the back wall). Simple directions (left, right, up, and down) or clock hours may help when peripheral photographs are requested. The patient's hand or thumb can be used to direct the patient's gaze.

6. *Move the camera.* If no reliable fixation can be obtained, simply instruct the patient to hold his or her eyes still. Use your fundus camera's adjustments to swing, tilt, or otherwise move until you locate the area of interest.

7. *Nystagmus.* Attempt to define a null point (the position of gaze at which the patient's eye movement decreases or stops) in patients with nystagmus. Alternately, adjust the camera to image the fundus at an extreme of travel (the furthest point at which the eye moves and must reverse direction), and time your photographs to coincide with the patient's eye movements.

8. *Do your best.* Some of your most challenging patients will be those that your ophthalmologist could not examine. The hope is that you will be able to provide at least one good photograph to help your physician examine the patient's retina. Young patients may not have reliable fixation. Using a wide angle of view maximizes the possibility that your final photograph will include the area of interest (assuming appropriate dilation). Use your ingenuity in other difficult cases. Adopt the attitude of the Canadian Mounties: *Always get your fundus photograph.*

FIGURE 2-21
Centering the camera. When the camera is centered on the pupil (A), you will see no position-related artifacts. Moving the camera slightly to the right (B) causes a reflection from the edge of the dilated pupil. Moving slightly further to the right (C) eliminates this reflection but results in a slightly darker, unevenly illuminated image (the result of a smaller portion of the doughnut being used to illuminate the retina). Further movement to the right (D) places the illuminating doughnut outside the pupil, effectively eliminating the retinal image. This same phenomenon happens along each axis. If we were to imagine a plane containing all centered and decentered fundus photographs of a specific retinal field, their composite would form a bulls' eye (E). This bull's eye is narrower in poorly dilated patients. Reproducing this series (with both a well-dilated and a poorly dilated patient) is a useful exercise for the intermediate photographer. Each fundus camera's angle of view and illuminating circle make the specific bull's eye different for each camera model (F). Normal-angle cameras have wider concentric rings of acceptable imaging, allowing a wider stereo base. Wide-angle cameras generally have narrower "bull's eye" rings. This results in less side-to-side movement and a smaller stereo base.

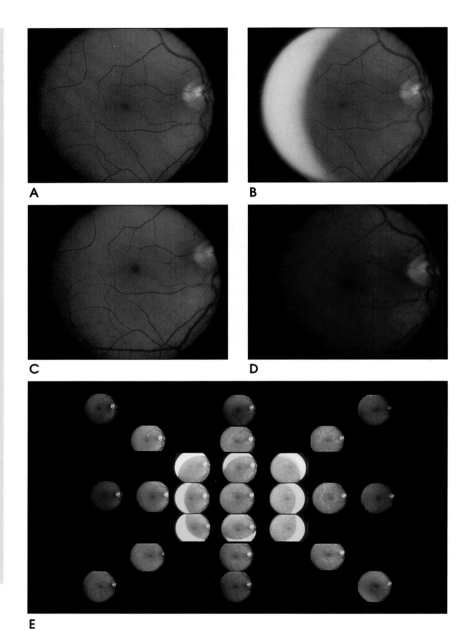

A   B

C   D

E

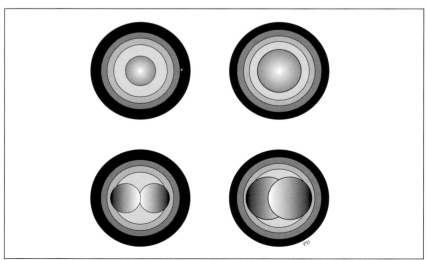

F

Determining the Correct Exposure

The correct exposure for a fundus photograph is the exposure that most clearly communicates the visual condition of the retina to the referring physician. Many factors influence the exposure. The photographer chooses the film stock and selects the flash intensity. Pupil size and fundus coloration are patient-related exposure factors. The judgment of the interpreting physician is important—does the physician prefer fully saturated or lighter fundus images?

Determining the correct exposure for fundus photography is an empirical process. First determine your standard exposure (Figure 2.26). Choose a slow or medium-speed color slide film and a standardized processing method. Using a well-dilated volunteer, expose two fundus photographs at each of your fundus camera's flash settings. Some fundus camera power supplies are calibrated in full stop increments, while some change by one-third or one-half stop between settings. A neutral-density filter (available from a photographic retailer) may assist you in achieving a precise exposure. Review this series of photographs with the physician to determine the best standard exposure.

Note the date and the exposure in the front of your camera manual. File the photographs for future reference.

Use the standard exposure on all patients who have the same pupil and fundus coloration characteristics as your model. You may need to increase this exposure by one or two steps if a particular patient:

- Has a small pupil
- Has a fundus with significantly darker pigmentation
- Has a large retinal hemorrhage
- Needs higher magnification (e.g., 2×) photographs

Decrease your exposure for:

- Young children
- Patients with significantly lighter pigmentation than your standard subject
- Patients with highly reflective fundi (e.g., Coats' disease, choroiderimia, albinism).

Repeat this test each time you make a significant change in your procedure (e.g., a change in film types or processors). Individually test each of your fundus cameras; each fundus camera–power supply combination can exhibit unique exposure characteristics. If you notice an exposure drift toward darkened images over time, consider scheduling a thorough cleaning of your fundus camera's internal optics.

11. *Select the area of interest.* Your photographic plan (step 3) should specify the areas you intend to photograph (Figure 2-22). If no posterior pole photographs have been requested, we routinely photograph the macula of the right eye first to ensure a familiar landmark during the editing process. Adjust the external fixation device until the area of interest is centered in the field of view. Some patients may require just disc photographs, while others need complete documentation of the posterior pole and periphery. Glaucoma and age-related macular degeneration are examples of conditions that may only require posterior pole photographs. Diabetic retinopathy, artery and vein occlusions, and retinitis pigmentosa are examples of conditions that may need peripheral documentation. When recording a peripheral nevus, be sure to include a photograph of the posterior pole and a photograph that contains both the nevus and a major blood vessel for orientation. All borders of a nevus should be visible in the final set of photographs. It is usually better to err on the side of too many photographs than too few.

12. *Select the angle of view.* Your choice of magnification depends on both the patient and the characteristics of the pathology. A normal angle of view is used to document retinal details (Figure 2-23). Recording the extent of a retinal condition requires a wide angle of view (Figure 2-24). Consider using multiple angles of view (Figure 2-25): Fundus photographs depicting the extent of a vein occlusion may benefit from a wide angle of view, while photographs of macular edema in the same eye may be more appropriate using a narrower angle of view.

Alternate factors may affect angle selection. A small pupil may preclude the use of a wide-angle camera, as the larger doughnut may not evenly illuminate the retina. You may choose to photograph an uncooperative child with a wide field of view to improve the chance that the final photograph will include a specific area of interest.

13. *Check the focus.* Look critically at the reticle and the fundus image. Adequate tear film is important to maximize clarity: Ask the patient to blink if he or she is not doing so naturally. Begin turning the focusing knob and the retinal image will sharpen. While remaining aware of the focusing reticle, keep turning the knob and the major blood vessels will become sharp. Concentrate on the next smaller blood vessel branches, and then the next smaller branches. In very clear eyes, you may be able to distinguish extremely fine blood vessels. Eyes with cataracts or other media opacities may reveal only the major blood vessels. Focus as best as you can, remembering that not every patient has clear media.

A brighter viewing light may make retinal details easier to distinguish; however, you should balance this need with patient comfort and cooperation. If you need a brighter light to focus with, try turning the viewing light up to focus and then turning it down again for final alignment.

A full discussion of focusing technique (including the rationale, a description of the mechanism, and a guide for focusing on different layers of the retina) is found later in this chapter.

Expose

14. *Double-check everything.* Develop the habit of quickly reviewing major variables just before the exposure. Make sure that both the reticle and the retina are in focus. Double-check the flash setting (Figure 2-26) (see the sidebar on determining the correct exposure).

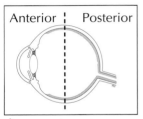

A Anterior/Posterior

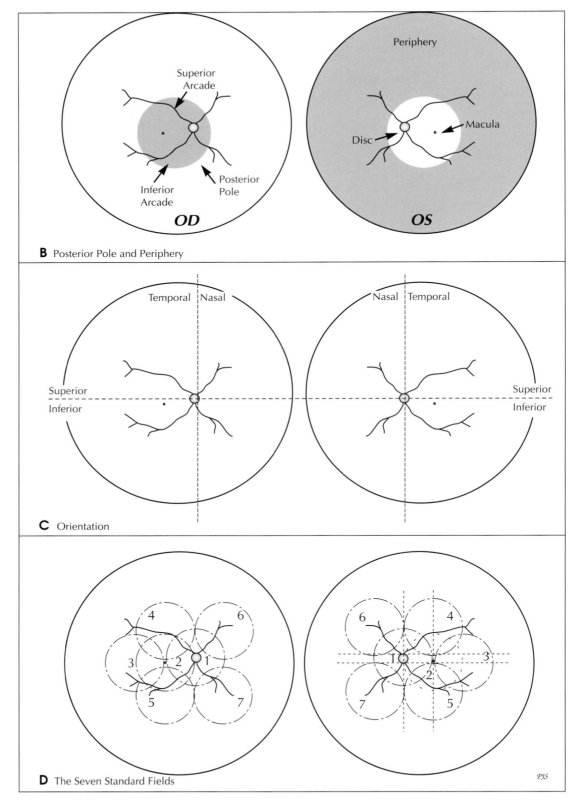

FIGURE 2-22
Finding your way. Items located in the front half of the eye are labeled anterior; those in the rear half of the globe are labeled posterior (A). A retinal lesion may be located in the posterior pole (the disc, macula, and the area enclosed within the inferior and superior arcades) or within the periphery (the area outside of the arcades) (B). The macula lies just below the midline of the disc. The macula is always temporal to the disc. Directions such as temporal (toward the temple), nasal (toward the nose), inferior, and superior allow greater specificity (C). Clock hours can also be used to specify location. Disc diameter (the width of the disc) is a convenient measuring stick. In a normal patient, the macula lies approximately 2.5 disc diameters temporal to the disc, and just below the a line which bisects the disc. The seven standard fields describe specific retinal locations as imaged by a 30-degree fundus camera (D).

How Many Photographs Should I Take?

The answer to this question depends on the patient, your skill level, and your practice. The desired outcome of the procedure is a good fundus photograph. Patients routinely blink, shift fixation, move their head, and in general make it difficult to guarantee that any single exposure will succeed. Most experienced photographers expose at least two photographs (or two stereo pairs) of each requested retinal field. It is less expensive to use an extra frame of film for insurance than to repeat the session. Film is actually a small part of the total procedure cost, especially when you consider the capital expense for the fundus camera and the wages and benefits of a skilled ophthalmic photographer.

A young child or an extremely light-sensitive patient may make it difficult to expose multiple photographs. In these cases, you should attempt to capture the best single image you can, concentrating all of your patient management and camera-positioning skills on the few photographs you will be able to expose.

Novice fundus photographers may need to expose more images to obtain a single good fundus photograph. This is encouraged: Experience is your best teacher. Film use will decrease as skill level increases.

Interesting or rare pathology deserves a few additional photographs. If your practice includes physicians or photographers who routinely lecture or publish, increase your number of exposures. Originals are always better than duplicate slides for teaching, reproduction, or sending to a referring physician.

You will need additional original exposures to build a portfolio of interesting patient photographs displaying fine technique. A portfolio is required for certification and for most job interviews.

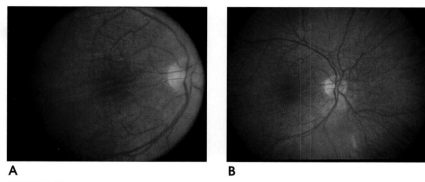

A   **B**

FIGURE 2-23
Normal- or narrow-angle fundus photographs excel in showing the fine details of a retinal problem. This 30-degree photograph (A) reveals more macular detail than this 60-degree photograph (B).

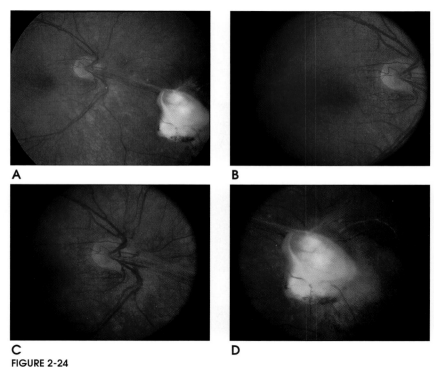

C   **D**

FIGURE 2-24
Wide-angle cameras are useful for showing the extent of a retinal problem. Here a single 60-degree fundus photograph (A) tells the same story as three 30-degree fundus photographs (B, C, D).

Fine-tune your focusing and field of view. Monitor the image for maximum color saturation and the absence of artifacts.

15. *Expose the film.* Press down on the shutter release button to take a picture (it's as easy as that!). Take multiple photographs of all necessary fields in each eye (see the sidebar on how many pictures to take), then proceed with the patient's other eye.

16. *Close the session.* Let your patients know that they did well (even if they did not) and that you obtained the needed photographs (which you should have). Remind them that the colors they are seeing are normal. Reassure them that the spots will go away soon. Suggest that fundus photography is just like looking into a flash

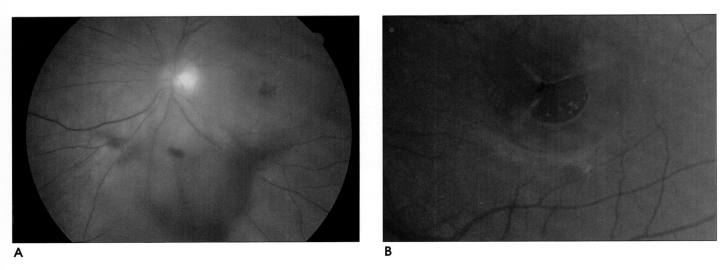

A   B

FIGURE 2-25
Consider using multiple angles of view in the same patient. Combining a wide-angle view (A) with a narrow-angle view (B) is effective in showing the retinal damage from this industrial laser accident.

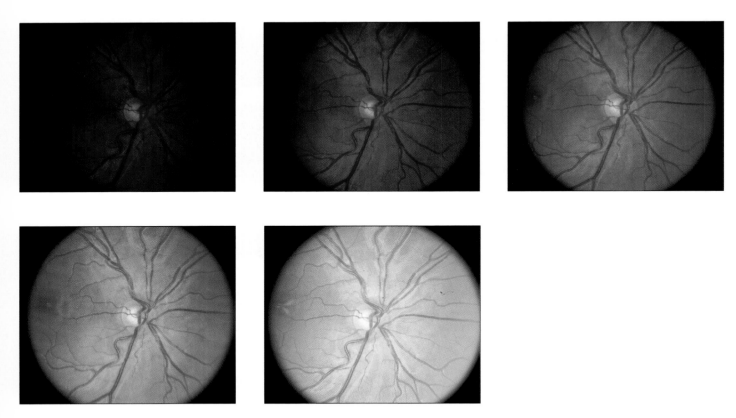

FIGURE 2-26
Exposure test. Create a series of photographs using each of the flash settings on your power pack. Carefully evaluate the pictures with the physician to determine a standard exposure.

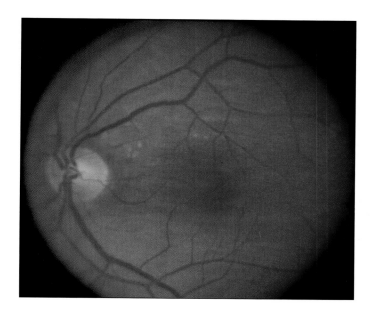

FIGURE 2-27
This unusable fundus photograph was damaged by the film processor.

when they get their picture taken. Release the patient with a smile, making sure that he or she feels fine and knows where the next clinic stop is. Complete all paperwork, including signing the chart. An uncharted procedure is an incomplete procedure. To avoid confusion, finish completely with one patient before beginning another.

Follow-Up

17. *Process your film.* Have your color film promptly developed by a professional processing laboratory. Quality processing and timely delivery are two important factors to consider when selecting a film processing vendor. Remember that the quality of *your* work will be judged by the quality of *their* processing (Figure 2-27).
18. *Edit and label your photographs.* Edit the film promptly after it is returned from the processor; keep the best images and discard the rest. If only a single mediocre photograph of a needed retinal field is available, then by all means include it. Otherwise, do not dilute your good photographs with poor images. Remember that good photographers don't just *take* good pictures; good photographers *show* good pictures. Label each slide with the patient's number, the date taken, and the referring physician. Some offices label each slide with the patient's diagnosis. Always take some time during the editing process to examine your work with an eye toward quality control. How could this photograph have been more effective? What could have been done to eliminate that artifact?
19. *Deliver the finished product.* Deliver the patient's photographs and chart for physician review in a timely manner.
20. *Review your work.* You should endeavor to understand not only pertinent photographic principles but also the various disease processes and their effect on the eye. Learn to look at photographs from your physician's point of view. Schedule regular conferences or ask impromptu questions, but regularly review your work with your employer. Your professional competence will benefit from this dialogue, as well as your value to your practice or institution.

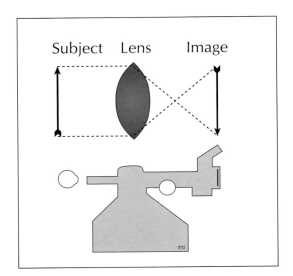

FIGURE 2-28
A sharp fundus photograph is created when a specific retina layer is the object, the fundus camera optics serve as a lens, and the film plane coincides with the plane of sharp focus.

Focusing the Fundus Camera: A Clinical Approach

Ophthalmic photography is a system of information transfer. Fundus photography transfers a visual description of the retina onto film. This two-dimensional representation is used by the physician to make judgments about the health and treatment of the patient's retina. Your goal is an accurate representation of the three-dimensional retinal and choroidal tissues. A sharp, well-focused retinal image is essential to successful fundus photography.

This section describes the fundus camera's aerial image–focusing system and its correct use. The well-focused fundus photograph is described, and proper focusing technique is related to retinal anatomy and pathology.

The Fundus Camera's Focusing System

In their most basic form, optical systems require light, a subject, a lens, a receiving plane, and an observer. Light reflects off the subject, is refracted (bent) by the lens, and is projected onto a receiving plane, where it is viewed. In fundus photography, the patient's retina becomes the subject, the optics of the patient's eye and the fundus camera replace the simple lens, the focusing screen or the film becomes the receiving plane, and you, the photographer, become the observer (Figure 2-28). Focusing the fundus camera consists of adjusting the relationship between the subject and lens so that the subject lies within the lens' depth of field and the receiving plane lies within the depth of focus of the image.

Most fundus cameras use a single lens reflex (SLR) viewing system. You should become familiar with the SLR design and the fundus camera's aerial image–viewing system (Figure 2-29).

SINGLE LENS REFLEX VIEWING SYSTEM

The objective lens of the fundus camera transmits light for both viewing the subject and exposing the film (Figure 2-30). The hinged mirror is positioned differently for viewing and taking the picture. First the image is evaluated through the viewfinder with the mirror in the down position. Then the mirror flips up and out of the way, the shutter opens, the flash is tripped, and the film is exposed to light.

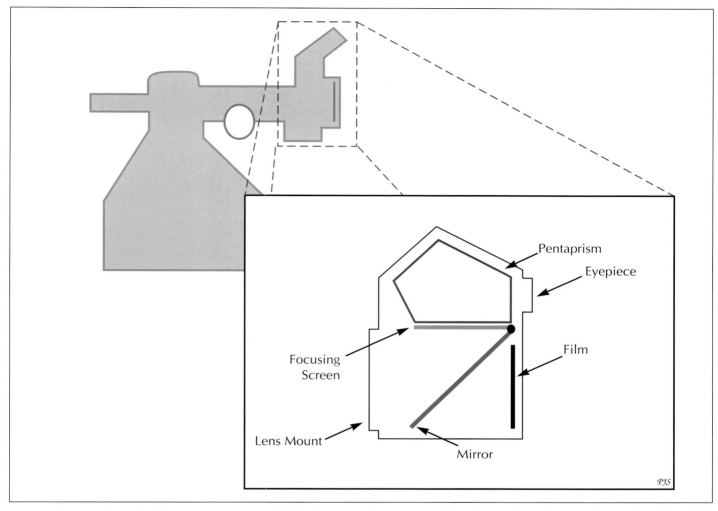

FIGURE 2-29
Most modern fundus cameras use a single lens reflex (SLR) system for viewing the fundus image. Standard components of an SLR system are identified in this simplified version of the fundus camera's SLR viewing system.

The focusing screen helps the photographer judge image sharpness before exposing the film. It is always located the same distance from the objective lens as the film plane. When an object appears sharp on the focusing screen, its image will also be sharp at the film plane. In standard 35-mm cameras, the focusing screen glass is either ground glass or a fresnel surface.

Light intensity decreases as it is scattered by the patterned glass focusing screen, an effect which is of little importance to most photographers. However, in fundus photography, a number of factors make it difficult to use these focusing screens:

1. *Relatively small amounts of light must be used when viewing the eye.* The possibility of retinal damage increases as the quantity and duration of illumination increases.[3] Many patients are sensitive to bright lights, making examination with bright light difficult.
2. *High magnifications* (e.g., 2.5× in a 30-degree fundus image) are used to photograph the retina. Light energy from a small portion of the subject is distributed over a physically greater image area when the image is magnified. This results in a relatively lower level of light available for imaging any particular portion of the subject.

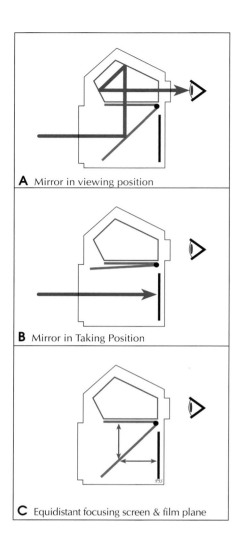

A Mirror in viewing position

B Mirror in Taking Position

C Equidistant focusing screen & film plane

FIGURE 2-30
Using a single lens reflex (SLR) camera. A. To preview a scene before you take a photograph, the light from the lens enters the camera body and reflects off the hinged, 45-degree mirror through the pentaprism and up to the focusing screen. You view the image on the focusing screen while looking through the viewfinder. B. When you choose to expose an image, depress the shutter release. This initiates a series of steps (specifics may vary according to the particular camera and flash) that include the mirror flipping up and out of the way, momentarily darkening the viewfinder. This allows the same light that you saw to expose the film. C. An SLR system is basically a "what-you-see-is-what-you-get" system. The distance between the focusing screen and the lens system is equal to the distance between the film plane and the lens system. When the image appears sharp on an SLR camera's focusing screen, it will also appear sharp on the film.

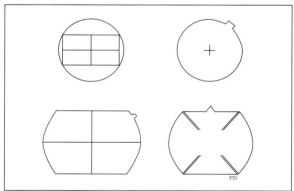

FIGURE 2-31
Various designs of focusing reticles. The reticle for your specific camera may vary according to manufacturer, camera model, and date.

3. *The grainy structure of a ground-glass focusing screen breaks up the fine detail of the fundus image.* The relatively large size of the grains in a ground-glass focusing screen make it difficult to focus on the fine retinal blood vessels.

Fundus cameras replace the patterned glass of a standard 35-mm SLR camera system with a clear glass focusing screen containing etched lines (Figure 2-31). The clear glass maximizes the light entering the photographer's eye. The etched black lines (called the *focusing reticle*) assist the photographer in focusing on the correct plane.

Because the image in the viewfinder is not "captured" by the focusing screen, but rather floats in the air space both in front of and behind the clear glass, it is termed an *aerial image*. Learning to focus this aerial image using the reticle is essential to obtaining sharp images with a fundus camera.

VIEWING THE AERIAL IMAGE

When you look through the fundus camera's viewfinder with your best corrected vision, you will see one of four possible views. The image inside the viewfinder may be totally out of focus, without distinct reticle lines or sharp areas of retina. The image alone may be in focus, only the black reticle lines may be in focus, or both the image and the black reticle lines may be in focus. Only in the last case will a sharp retinal image be recorded on film (Figure 2-32).

If both the focusing reticle and the fundus image are completely out of focus, then one of two conditions may exist. First, your eyes may not be corrected for their best visual acuity. A routine eye examination is recommended when you begin your career and at regular intervals thereafter. Second, the fundus camera's reticle and focus adjustment may be improperly set (see the section on obtaining a sharp fundus photograph below). Of course, a combination of the above circumstances may occur.

ACCOMMODATION

Accommodation is the normal mechanism your eye uses for focusing on near objects. In simple terms, the ciliary muscle tugs or releases tension on the lens zonules, modifying the refractive power of the lens. At the same time, the near reflex causes miosis and convergence. The ability to accommodate lessens with age.

A significant cause of unsharp fundus photographs is accommodation by the photographer during the focusing procedure. When you look through the camera eyepiece and accommodate, you may see a sharp image of the retina but not see a sharp image of the focusing reticle. If you accommodate to perceive a sharp image of the retina, then the optical system of your eye is used to obtain sharpness, rather than the optical system of the fundus camera. You may attempt to sharpen the image using the focusing knob, but a blurry photograph will result.

The tendency to accommodate when focusing is especially prevalent in fatigued or novice fundus photographers, and in experienced photographers who are under 40 years of age. Strategies for safeguarding against accommodation problems during fundus photography procedures include the following:

1. Highly trained photographers can "feel" themselves accommodate. You may want to test this yourself. Find a quiet room with no distractions. Fully relax your mind and body while focusing your eyes on an object at least 20 feet away. Bring your index finger about 18 inches from your nose. When you focus on your index finger, notice that the background becomes unsharp. Keeping your finger in focus, move it toward your nose slowly. The background will become increasingly less sharp and the edges of your visual field will constrict. You will feel your eyes converge and you may feel a sensation in the anterior section of your eyes. Focus on the distant object again and repeat. With practice, you will become more aware of your personal sensation during accommodation. Awareness of this sensation during fundus photography will alert you to the

PHOTOGRAPHER'S VIEW IN EYEPIECE	DIAGRAMMATIC EXPLANATION	FINAL FILM IMAGE

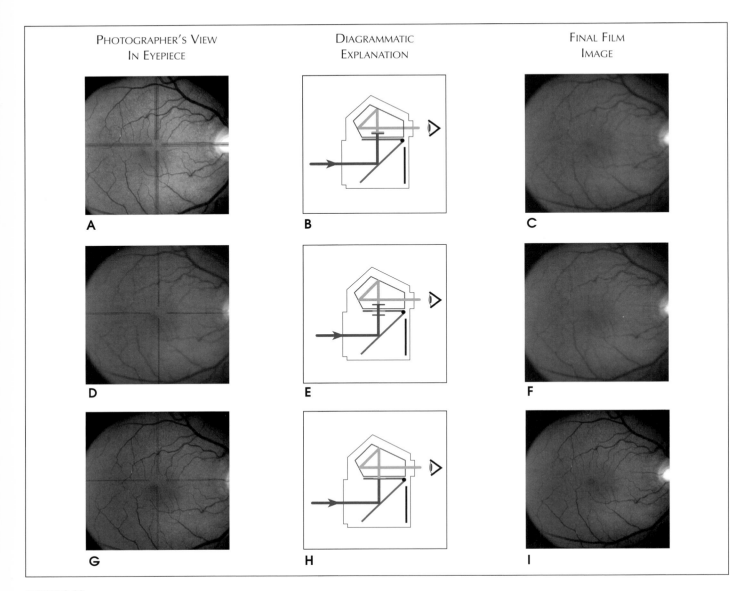

FIGURE 2-32
Using the reticle to focus. This figure illustrates the relationship between sharpness in the reticle, your fundus view, and the sharpness in the final fundus photograph. When you focus the image without regard to the sharpness of the focusing reticle, you will perceive the fundus image as sharp while the reticle image appears blurry (A). The image you see is focused by your eyes above the focusing screen, closer than infinity (B). Even though you see a sharp image in the viewfinder, the exposed photograph will be blurry (C). When you view through a correctly adjusted eyepiece before the fundus has been focused on, the fundus appears blurry while the reticle is distinctly sharp (D). You have correctly focused on the reticle, but the camera's image has not yet been adjusted to coincide with the receiving plane (E). If a picture is taken, the resulting image will be as unsharp as you see it in the viewfinder (F). After correctly adjusting the eyepiece and the fundus camera's focusing mechanism, both the fundus image and the reticle appear sharp and clear (G). Your eyes are focused on the reticle, and the image from the fundus camera corresponds with the film plane (H). Only this final combination will yield a sharply focused fundus photograph (I).

possibility of accommodation and the unsharp photographs that may result.

2. If you think you are accommodating during a procedure, look away from the eyepiece. Merely blinking or closing your eyes may help reset their focus. Upon looking again into the viewfinder, concentrate on the thin black lines of the focusing reticle. Intentionally blurring the fundus image (move the plane of focus into the vitreous by rotating the focusing knob) may help you concentrate on the reticle image.

3. Try to keep both eyes open throughout the procedure, preferably with the non-eyepiece eye focused across the room. A well-placed

visual (of a landscape or distant scene) on the opposite wall of the fundus photography room will promote distance focusing. If the room is especially small, a mirror (or the glass from the above print) may be used to reflect the image from a visual hanging directly behind the photographer. Glancing at this reflection will better approximate distance focusing in a small room. Viewing exciting scenery through a window in a fundus photography room may seem tempting. However, the darkness necessary during procedures precludes this option.

4. A full day of fundus photography may distort the normal accommodative process, causing your eye to be "stuck" in near-focus. Accommodative excess is the result of "prolonged and intense periods of near work," which may result in eyestrain and headaches.[4, 5] Persistent focusing on infinity may help retard this near-focus spasm. Consciously focus across the distance of the waiting room (or down a long hall) when you call patients. Practice focusing on infinity out a window during breaks or at lunch. Make a point of looking at distant scenery or buildings while commuting to and from work.

Of course, your eyes should always be corrected to their best visual acuity. You may find that one eye is sharper than the other. Keep your eyeglasses or contacts scrupulously clean.

Certain physiologic conditions may also distort the focusing process. Extreme changes in blood sugar may alter the thickness of the diabetic photographer's lens, making distance vision unsharp. Certain drugs may produce pseudopresbyopia.[6] Maintaining a healthy diet and good physical condition will also help your focusing abilities.

Sharp Fundus Photographs

DEFINITION

Sharpness in a photograph is a visual phenomenon that is difficult to quantify. Both contrast and resolution play a role in our subjective evaluations of sharpness. An image is described as sharp when the borders defining the subject are distinct and clear. An unsharp image contains borders between adjacent areas that overlap or are difficult to distinguish. A sharp fundus photograph results when the fundus camera's plane of sharp focus coincides with the specific pathology in question.

When photographing the retina, remember that, like most photographic subjects in our three-dimensional world, the posterior segment of the eye has depth. The vitreous, retina, and choroid may be described histologically as overlapping layers of gel, tissue, and blood vessels that are located at specific levels* within the eye (Figure 2-33).

Five distinct levels (the vitreous, inner retina, central retina, outer retina, and choroid) may be distinguished using white-light, 30-degree stereo fundus photography in many patients with diseased or swollen retinas.

Short wavelength color filters (e.g., exciter and barrier filters for fluorescein angiography, blue filters for retinal nerve fiber layer photography, and green filters for "red-free" photography) enhance the photographic separation of retinal levels.[7] Thickened diseased retina,

---

*The term *layer* is used when referring to histologic sections, while the term *level* is reserved for discussion of the fundus camera image.

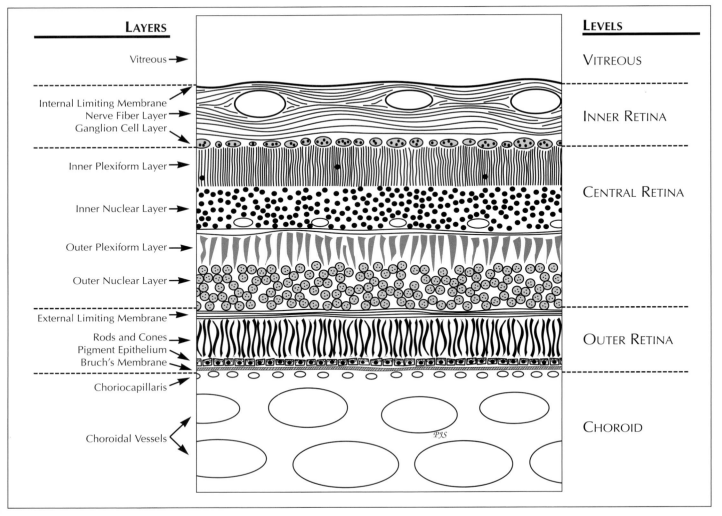

LAYERS		LEVELS
Vitreous →		VITREOUS
Internal Limiting Membrane Nerve Fiber Layer → Ganglion Cell Layer →		INNER RETINA
Inner Plexiform Layer →		CENTRAL RETINA
Inner Nuclear Layer →		
Outer Plexiform Layer →		
Outer Nuclear Layer →		
External Limiting Membrane →		OUTER RETINA
Rods and Cones → Pigment Epithelium → Bruch's Membrane →		
Choriocapillaris →		CHOROID
Choroidal Vessels		

FIGURE 2-33
Layers and levels. A 10-layer histologic representation of the retina and choroid is related to the five levels that may be distinguished when viewing either through a narrow-angle fundus camera viewfinder or the final stereo fundus photograph. Each of these five levels may or may not be able to be distinguished depending on the thickness and pathology of a particular patient's retina.

normal-angle fundus camera optics, and stereo imaging also facilitate the recognition of retinal levels and expedite their differential focusing (Figure 2-34).

Monocular (single-image) photography, wide-angle fundus cameras, and inaccurate focusing inhibit our ability to distinguish five separate retinal levels. The levels' thinness combined with the depth of field of the fundus camera may make it difficult to distinguish each of the five levels in patients with normal or thin retinas.

A sharp fundus photograph is precisely focused on a specific subject within a specific level of the retina. The objective appearance of clear, distinct borders in a fundus photograph does not in itself certify the sharpness of that photograph. A fundus photograph may be sharp, but not at the appropriate retinal level (Figure 2-35). Focusing too far forward (into the vitreous) or too far backward (into the outer retina or choroid) will result in a fundus photograph that does not accurately document the pathology of concern.

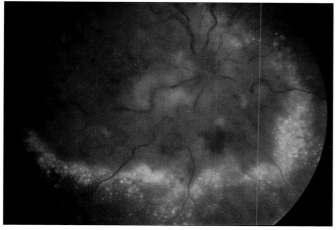
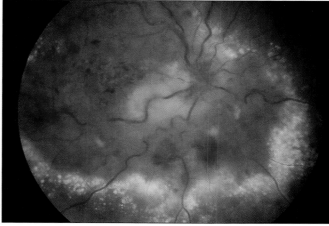

FIGURE 2-34
Multiple retinal levels may be appreciated when this photograph is viewed in stereo.

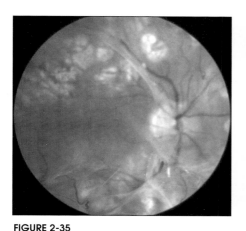
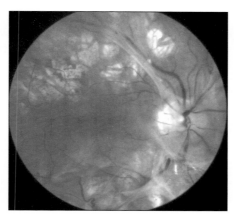
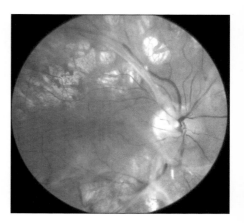

FIGURE 2-35
This eye was photographed at three different planes of focus. All three images contain areas that may be considered sharp. If the macula is the intended subject of the photograph, however, only the center image can be judged a sharp fundus photograph.

How can we achieve optimal focus at the appropriate layer within the eye? An understanding of retinal anatomy is essential to achieving sharp fundus photographs.

RETINAL ANATOMY: LAYERS AND LEVELS
Accurately adjusting the fundus camera's focus requires an awareness of the layered aspect of the eye's anatomy. The vitreous gel fills the posterior segment of the eye. The retina is a three-dimensional tissue described histologically as 11 separate layers. The choroid contains two layers of blood vessels.

The vitreous is positioned anterior to the retina. In the normal eye, the vitreous cannot be imaged with a standard fundus camera. However, when documentation of a diabetic neovascular frond, a retinal detachment, or asteroid hyalosis is necessary, the fundus camera should be focused "up" into the vitreous, rather than "down" on the retina (Figure 2-36).

The internal limiting membrane, the nerve fiber layer, and the ganglion cell layer combine to form the inner retina. It is visualized as the nerve fiber layer and the reflections from the large retinal blood vessels. Cotton-wool spots, nerve fiber defects, myelinated nerve fibers, and flame-shaped hemorrhages occur at this level.

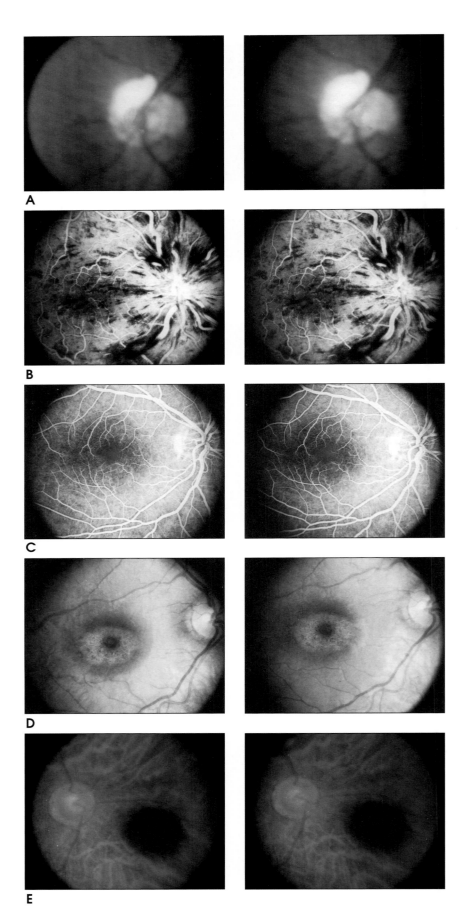

FIGURE 2-36
Clinical examples of focusing on different levels of
the retina are shown in these stereo pairs. A.
Focusing the fundus camera in the vitreous allows
the ophthalmic photographer to document various
opacities. B. The flame-shaped hemorrhages found
in the inner retina are in sharp focus in this photograph. C. The avascular zone surrounding the fovea
may be best appreciated when the central portion
of the retina is the object of focus. D. The outer retina
has been focused on for this stereo pair of a young
girl's bull's eye maculopathy. E. Maximum information at the level of the choroid is achieved through
the use of a red (650-nm) filter and careful focusing
on the choroidal nevus.

Table 2-3. Patient Diagnosis and Retinal Levels*

Patient's Diagnosis	Examples of Possible Abnormalities	Retinal Level
Asteroid hyalosis	Lipid deposits	Vitreous
Diabetic retinopathy	Neovascular fronds	
Retinoschisis	Elevated retinal sensory layers	
Retinal detachment	Elevated retina	
Diabetic retinopathy	Cotton-wool spots	Inner retina
Glaucoma	Nerve fiber layer defects, optic disc borders	
Hypertensive retinopathy	Cotton-wool spots	
Macular role	Edges of macular hole	
Preretinal membrane	Cellophane maculopathy	
Retinal hemorrhage	Preretinal hemorrhage, subhyaloid hemorrhage	
Retinal vein occlusion	Flame-shaped hemorrhages	
Cystoid macular edema	Swelling	Central retina
Diabetic retinopathy	Microaneurysms, hard exudates, dot and blot hemorrhages, macular edema	
Retinal artery occlusion	Blocked artery	
Retinal vein occlusion	Neovascularization	
Retinitis pigmentosa	Bone spicule-like pigment	
Age-related macular degeneration	Subretinal neovascular membranes, drusen	Outer retina
Central serous retinopathy	Pigment epithelium defect	
Hereditary abnormalities	Angioid streaks	
Presumed ocular histoplasmosis syndrome	Subretinal neovascular membranes, punched out hypopigmented areas	
AMPPE	Choroidal disturbance	Choroid
Nevus	Surface texture	
Optic nerve head drusen	Drusen under disc	
Choroidal tumor	Surface texture	

*Sample patient diagnoses are listed and related to the retinal layers visible through the fundus camera. Examples of possible retinal abnormalities (which may or may not be evident in each specific patient) are correlated. To target the focus to a specific layer, note the patient's diagnosis and focus on the specific abnormalities. If the retina is abnormally thick, you may be able to focus on the same retinal field at different levels. Double-check the focus with each field change.

The inner and outer plexiform layer and the inner and outer nuclear layer form the central portion of the retina. The central retina contains the smaller blood vessel branches, hard exudates, and diabetic microaneurysms. The capillary net surrounding the foveal avascular zone is imaged during fluorescein angiography when the fundus camera is properly focused on this middle level of the retina.

The outer retinal level includes the rods and cones, the pigment epithelium, and Bruch's membrane. Subretinal neovascular membranes, drusen, presumed ocular histoplasmosis scars, and angioid streaks occur at this level.

The choriocapillaris and major choroidal blood vessels lie below the retina. The surface of nevi and choroidal tumors can be imaged by focusing "down" into the choroid.

TARGETING FOCUS

It is difficult to distinguish 10 different retinal layers when looking through the eyepiece of the fundus camera. However, you can target the focus of the final fundus photograph to a specific level by recognizing its visual contents. Table 2-3 relates common retinal disorders, the affected retinal level, and examples of possible corresponding retinal abnormalities. Targeting focus to a specific level is a matter of recognizing retinal pathology and optimizing the focus to the appropriate retinal depth.

Focusing on the highlights reflected from the large blood vessels will result in a sharp photograph of the inner retina. The central retina will appear clear in the fundus photograph if the photographer first seeks

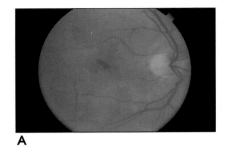
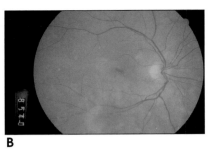

A   **B**

FIGURE 2-37
When narrow- (A) and wide-angle (B) photographs
(asteroid hyalosis) are compared, the wide-angle
image appears to have greater depth of field
because of its smaller magnification.

sharpness in the larger blood vessels, then their branches, and their branches, and so forth. If the granular appearance of the pigment epithelium is focused on, then the outer retina becomes the subject of the photograph. When photographing a subretinal neovascular membrane (located in the outer level of the retina), an unsharp photograph of the offending blood vessels will result if you focus on the larger, main retinal blood vessels (found in the inner level of the retina). A sharp image can be obtained by focusing on the drusen that lay directly on the pigment epithelium.

Multiple levels of focus may be chosen in a retina with diabetic macular edema. If you focus on the inner surface of the retina, the photograph will document the elevation of the retina but may render much of the posterior pole blurred. A deeper focus may depict the surface of the swollen macula unsharply but will clearly reveal any hard exudates and/or blot hemorrhages. Focusing in the central retina will accurately document the leaking retinal blood vessels in a fluorescein angiogram.

The fundus camera's depth of field is a focusing consideration. When focusing a fundus camera, only the single level that has been targeted will be in critically sharp focus. When we view the final photograph however, more than one level may appear acceptably sharp. This range of acceptably sharp focus extends both in front of and behind the actual plane of sharp focus.

Wide-angle fundus cameras produce a greater depth of field than do normal-angle cameras, if the same eye is photographed and the exposed film area is identical (Figure 2-37). It is not the angle of the optics but rather the decrease in magnification that contributes to the increased impression of sharpness.[8]

A working knowledge of depth of field will help you when documenting the retina. Focusing on the central retina (in a normal, clear eye) will yield a final photograph in which the outer and possibly the inner retina are acceptably sharp. However, if you focus on the granular appearance of the pigment epithelium, then the inner retina will most likely not be in sharp focus.

Depth of focus is found at the film plane and usually mirrors the depth of field located at the subject plane. The depth of focus in most traditional imaging systems is relatively flat. This corresponds with the flatness of the film that is used as a receiving plane (Figure 2-38). The depth of field in most fundus camera lens systems is curved to mimic the shape of the normal retina. In well-corrected fundus camera optical systems, the curved plane of the subject's detail is translated into a flat plane for maximum interface with the film plane. In less well-corrected fundus camera lens systems, the plane of the depth of focus is just as curved as the depth of field. Fundus cameras that exhibit this curved depth of focus yield film images that are unsharp at the edges when the camera is focused centrally (and are unsharp centrally when focused on the edges). The intended subject will appear sharp on the film only with careful composition and focus.

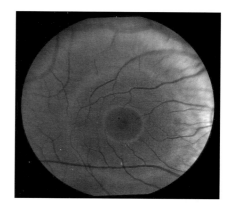

FIGURE 2-38
Images from a well-corrected fundus camera closely match the curvature of the retina, increasing the visual accuracy of the fundus photograph. Learn the limitations of your particular camera by carefully focusing on the fovea of a clear eye and then evaluating the actual sharpness at the edges of the processed photograph.

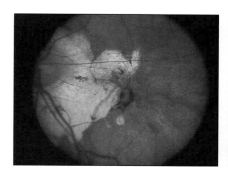 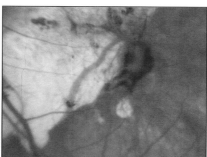

FIGURE 2-39
Although the sharpness and contrast of magnified images are compromised, they may still provide useful information.

SHARPNESS LIMITATIONS OF THE CAMERA

The sharpness of a final fundus photograph is, of course, limited by the sharpness of the specific camera's optical system. Unfortunately, objective tests comparing the relative sharpness of various fundus cameras are unavailable. Fortunately, experience with multiple cameras in a clinical setting has yielded some general guidelines.

Resolution of fine detail decreases as the magnification decreases because less film area is used for creating an image of a particular detail. When two fundus cameras have imaging circles of equal size, the wide-angle fundus camera (over 45 degrees) will be less able to resolve fine detail than the normal-angle camera (30 degrees). When two fundus cameras have optics of equal quality, the fundus camera with higher magnification will achieve better definition of fine retinal details.

Resolution and contrast decrease with the introduction of angle-changing lens systems. Multiple-angle cameras typically have one best setting—often the widest angle. An optical departure from this angle of view degrades image quality. However, greater magnification may yield details not perceived under low magnification (Figure 2-39). Use your professional judgment to determine the most appropriate angle of view for a specific fundus photograph.

Wide-angle cameras suffer greater losses in resolution from local areas of potential blurriness (e.g., a cataract or a corneal scar) than do normal-angle cameras. This phenomenon is due to the larger bundle of returning image-forming rays that constitute the wide-angle image. The thinner bundles of normal-angle camera optics are more likely to permit you to select small pockets of clear media.

A fundus camera's cost is not directly proportional to the sharpness of its optics. Lens performance, cost, and ease of use must each be considered separately. While a low price and ergonomic design should be considered when purchasing a fundus camera, actual lens performance is critical.

Only the publication of unbiased data detailing the actual performance of many different fundus cameras will allow fair comparisons to be made. Until such tests are designed and implemented, the opinions of other ophthalmic photographers and personal experience must guide us.[9]

Focusing Technique

If you conscientiously use the reticle and practice a deliberate focusing procedure, you will produce consistently sharp fundus photographs. The eyepiece must be correctly set to obtain a sharp view of the reticle. Instructions for adjusting the eyepiece are found in the sidebar on setting your reticle. A suggested focusing procedure is as follows:

1. Review the patient's photo request form and prior photographs. Note the working diagnosis.
2. Seat the patient at the instrument and explain the procedure.
3. Adjust the head rest, chin rest, joystick, and camera head height while looking around the side of the camera. Align the patient and camera so that the retina and the film plane are parallel. Project the doughnut of light into the center of the dilated pupil. Position the illumination system by obtaining a sharp image of the viewing light's filament on the cornea or closed outer eyelid.
4. Turn out the room lights. Your view through the viewfinder will brighten, and your eye's depth of field will decrease as a result of your slightly dilated pupils. It will be easier for you to discriminate between retinal layers with this shallower depth of field. In addition, the darkened room enhances the figure-ground relationship between the external fixation light and its background. This allows the patient to follow the external fixation device more easily.
5. Establish patient fixation (focusing on a moving target is difficult).
6. Look through the ocular and visualize the focusing reticle. Constant awareness of this reticle throughout the focusing procedure is necessary for obtaining sharp fundus photographs. Dust specks may be visible in the viewfinder. If these dust specks are on the same plane as the etched lines, use them like the reticle. If you are unsure of their precise location, consult a knowledgeable service technician to either clean the dust specks or to determine the specific plane on which they rest.
7. Adjust the image for maximum color saturation and minimum artifacts. Move the fixation light to visualize the requested retinal field.
8. Begin turning the focusing knob. You will see the retinal image begin to sharpen. Check the sharpness of the focusing reticle and decide on which retinal level to focus. Myopic, hyperopic, and aphakic patients may require you to adjust the compensation lens system (diopter control). Myopic patients (long axial length) may need a minus diopter compensation. Hyperopic patients (short axial length) and patients without their natural lenses may require a plus diopter correction. The small black antireflection dot in the front element is often imaged in patients with high myopia. Both this artifact and the use of the diopter compensation lens system can be eliminated by requesting highly myopic patients to wear their contact lenses while being photographed.[10]

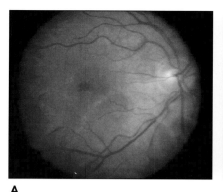
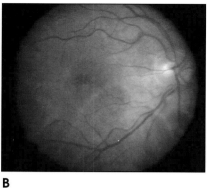

A   **B**

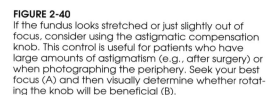

FIGURE 2-40
If the fundus looks stretched or just slightly out of focus, consider using the astigmatic compensation knob. This control is useful for patients who have large amounts of astigmatism (e.g., after surgery) or when photographing the periphery. Seek your best focus (A) and then visually determine whether rotating the knob will be beneficial (B).

9. As the plane of sharpness travels inward with the rotation of the focusing knob, the vitreous, inner retina, central retina, outer retina, and finally choroidal levels will become sharp in turn. The focusing reticle must always remain sharp.

10. Stop focusing inward as the targeted level is passed and becomes unsharp again.

11. "Rock" the focus (with tiny forward and backward movements of the focusing knob) until the sharpest focus has been obtained. Check the sharpness of the focusing reticle.

12. Patient fixation or camera position is adjusted until the desired field of view is obtained. Recheck crosshair sharpness and retinal focus. The area of primary importance should be photographed first, as the best images are often obtained at the beginning of the photo session when both you and the patient are fresh. Many patients require photographs of both the macula and disc. Focusing on the macula first will approximate more closely the general depth of the retina.

13. Evaluate the need for the astigmatism control (if available). If the image of the fundus seems not quite sharp, or if the blood vessels appear elongated in a single direction, then a small rotation of the astigmatism control may be helpful (Figure 2-40). Sharp posterior pole photographs of patients with keratoconus, patients with large amounts of corneal astigmatism, and peripheral photography may require astigmatic correction. Imaging rays may traverse an oblique cross section of the lens and cornea in peripheral fundus photography, creating an image that appears smeared or stretched in a single direction.

14. Constantly monitor the focus throughout the procedure. Recheck the focus each time you change fields; a diseased retina may or may not be swollen in different areas (Figure 2-41). Monitor the focus during side-to-side changes in camera position during stereo photography. Peripheral fundus photography necessitates a change in the camera-cornea distance and will require focus adjustment. The axial length of most patients' eyes will vary slightly from right to left. If alternating photographs of the right and left eye are required and a large focusing discrepancy exists between the two eyes, then a small piece of tape on the right and left focusing knobs may be used to mark each side's correct adjustment.[11] While these landmarks will help you adjust the camera more quickly as the alternate eyes are photographed, always check your viewfinder for a final focus.

Focusing is an acquired skill requiring both practice and a keen understanding of the retinal landscape. Constant awareness of the focusing

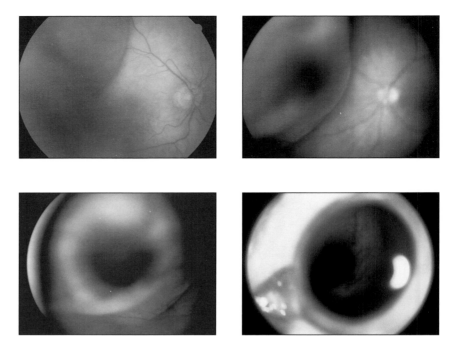

FIGURE 2-41
Be prepared to alter your focus or alignment to capture items of interest extending into the vitreous. Documenting the extent of this tumor required both changing the focus and pulling the camera away from the patient's eye.

reticle and precisely targeting the focus to a specific retinal level are keys to success.

Errors in Fundus Photography: Artifacts

Successful fundus photographs are obtained through the mutual interaction and proper alignment of the patient, the camera, and the photographer. The patient contributes a cooperative attitude and clear media. The camera must faithfully translate the fundus image using integrated optical, mechanical, and electrical subsystems. The photographer must elicit a cooperative response from the patient, correctly align and set the camera controls, and make decisions concerning film choice and processing procedures. Each of these factors must be taken into consideration when evaluating a fundus photograph.

Causes of Artifacts

The ideal fundus photograph is an accurate visual representation of the retina. Of course, as with any complex process, many things may go wrong. If the error alters the ideal image (i.e., if the error can be seen in the final fundus photograph), it is called an *artifact*. Artifacts are portions of the image that arise from the process—not from the patient's retina. Typical artifacts include yellow or orange crescents, white or blue haze at the edge of the photograph, blinks, dust on the front element, and poor focus (Figure 2-42).

The fundus camera generates a flash that is projected into the patient's eye, reflects off the fundus, and then travels through the camera's optical system to the film. Each step in this process has the potential to compromise image quality. If we follow the pathway of image-forming energy from its point of origin (*the electrical wall socket*) to its final destination (*the finished fundus photograph*), we can identify specific problem areas where technical difficulties could occur.

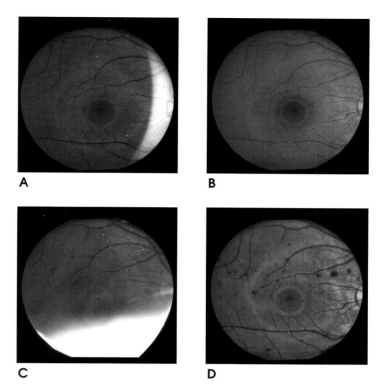

FIGURE 2-42
Typical artifacts. The most common artifacts are related to position errors or interruptions in the imaging path. Crescents can appear on any side of the image and indicate off center camera alignment (A). A light, slightly unsharp area surrounding a fully saturated center indicates incorrect camera to cornea distance (B). Short, light-colored streaks arising from the top or bottom of the frame are stray patient lashes or hair (C). Bright spots indicate dust on the front objective (D).

Electrical energy flows from the electrical outlet to the camera's power pack, where it is stored until a signal is given for its release (*an interruption in any of these circuits is possible*). The photographer properly adjusts the camera to the patient's eye (*incorrect positioning and focusing are possible*). A switch is closed and then stored electrical energy travels to the flash tube where it is transduced into light energy (*a misaligned or nonworking flash tube is possible*). This light energy passes through a series of optical condensers and imaging lenses (*all potentially dirty and/or out of alignment*), out of the camera through the front element (*a literal dust magnet*), and across the air space between the camera lens and cornea (*which can be obstructed by hair, eyelashes, or eyelids*). The projected light passes through the cornea, anterior chamber, lens, and vitreous (*all in various possible states of opacification*) and reflects off the retina (*which may be swollen or hidden from view by hemorrhage*). The reflected light projects back through the vitreous, lens, anterior chamber, and cornea into the front element of the camera lens (*multiplying any previous negative effects*). The light is refracted through another series of lenses toward the camera. Just as the light reaches the camera body, the shutter opens and closes (*the shutter may malfunction or timing may be off*), allowing the light to modify the chemical nature of the film (*assuming the film is correctly manufactured, chosen, and loaded*). Once sensitized, the emulsion is processed (*another complex procedure with its own long list of possible errors*). This image pathway is, of course, dependent on a camera that is aligned correctly with the patient and a patient-photographer relationship that will enable this alignment.

Describing Artifacts

If artifacts are described systematically, we learn about the subtleties of the image and will more likely reason or intuit the artifact's cause. Just as a correct diagnosis from a fluorescein angiogram requires first a

Table 2-4. Descriptors for Fundus Photography Artifacts*

Extent	Full frame	There is no useful information in any part of the frame. The picture may be completely black or white.
	Full image area	The standard fundus image area contains no useful information but black surround (unexposed because of the fundus camera's mask); the film frame numbers are left unaffected.
	Partial image area	The artifact obscures a portion of the retinal image area; the remaining retinal image is of adequate quality.
Character	Location	The artifact can be described as central or peripheral; superior or inferior, or to the right or left.
	Shape	Circular, crescent, or rectangular artifacts with sharp or blurry borders are possible.
	Exposure	The overall photograph may be too light or dark or it may be a double exposure.
	Color	The artifact may be any color: white, yellow, orange, and blue are common. Multicolored artifacts are also seen.
	Sharpness	The full image area may be sharp or unsharp, as can portions thereof.
Distribution		The artifact can be found at the beginning, the middle, or the end of the roll.
Frequency		The artifact may be observed randomly or regularly, throughout a single roll or a single patient, or crossing several rolls or patients. Artifacts can be seen frequently, occasionally, or just once.

*Providing a complete description of fundus photography artifacts helps us reason or intuit their cause. Use the vocabulary from the table above when describing artifacts.

proper description of hypo- or hyperfluorescence, describing artifacts is the first step in determining the cause of fundus photograph errors.

Four essential details should be included in each description of the imperfect fundus photograph: the extent and character of the artifact and the distribution and frequency of the affected slide in relation to other fundus photos in the same or adjacent rolls (Table 2-4). Some common artifacts are illustrated in Figure 2-43. The legends indicate the correct use of descriptors and note the cause of the illustrated artifact.

Managing the Challenging Patient

Successful fundus photography with a cooperative patient who has clear media and widely dilated pupils becomes routine with practice. Not all patients are ideal, however. Patients with glaucoma and diabetes have smaller pupils. Elderly patients often have cataracts. And light-sensitive patients may have difficulty cooperating. In many clinics, fundus photography is performed at the end of the patient's appointment. By the time patients are ready to be photographed, they may be tired and irritable. How can we take successful photographs in difficult clinical situations? Some common problems and their solutions follow.

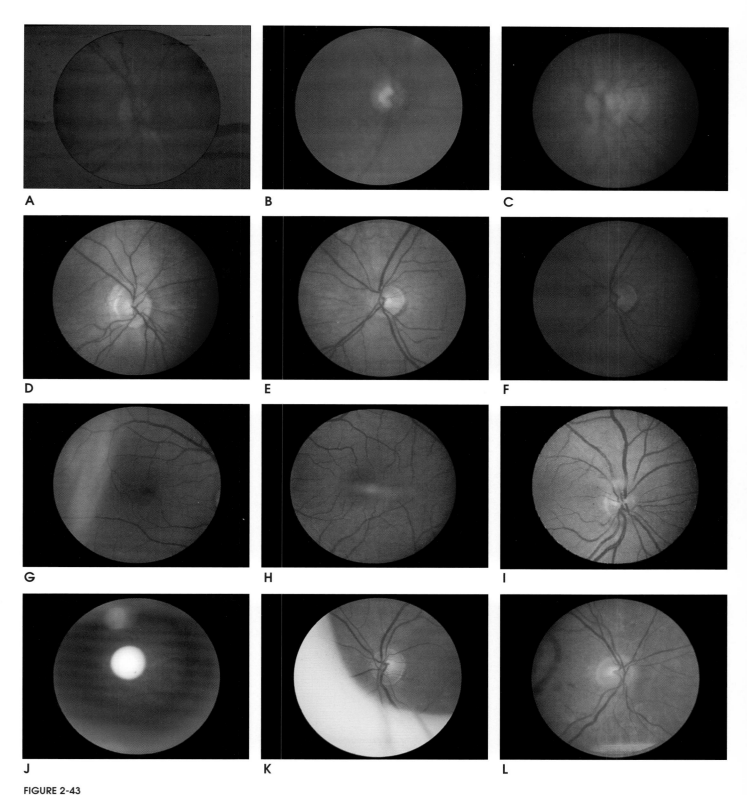

FIGURE 2-43

Describing artifact examples. Extent describes the area the artifact occupies in the photograph. A. This processing error involves the full frame. B. A vitreous hemorrhage would obscure only the full image area, and notably not the black surround. C. "IOL shimmer" fills the frame when off center camera alignment is pursued in a patient whose pupil is larger than the outer diameter of the intraocular lens. D. The same retina is better photographed using central alignment. E. Search for a clear area, shooting around, as opposed to through cataracts (F). G. This multicolored crescent variation is an example of a partial image area artifact. The rest of the fundus photograph is usable.

The character of the artifact is a set of distinguishing features that describe location, shape, color, exposure, and sharpness. H, I. The location of the white artifact (caused by a smudge on the lens) in both these photographs was identical–even with a significant field change. J. Excessive camera-to-cornea distance results in a centrally located spectral reflectance and haze along the periphery of the image area. The crescent shape (K) and linear shape (L) are position-related artifacts. Move the camera in the opposite direction of the artifact to eliminate.

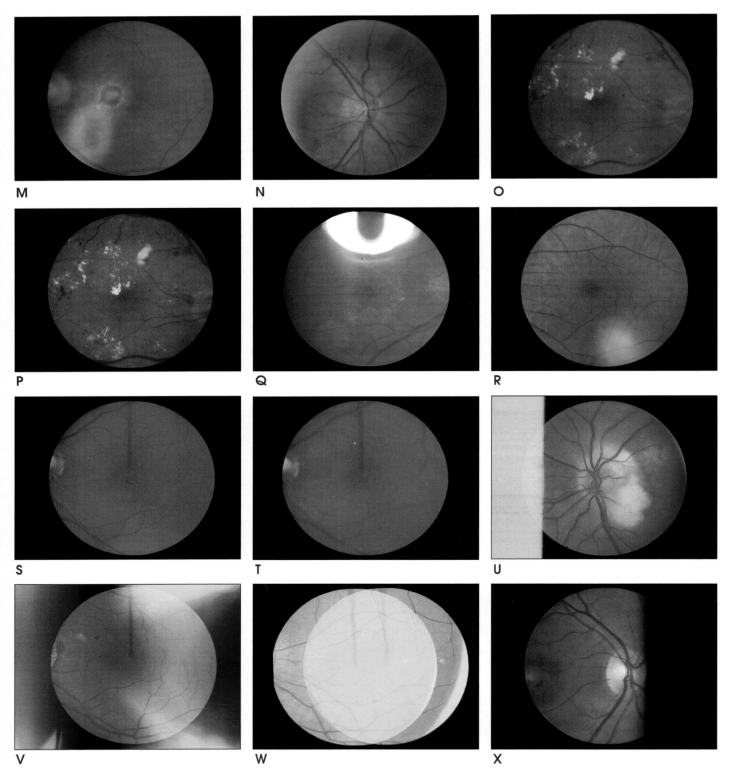

FIGURE 2-43 *(continued)*
M. This irregularly shaped blob was from a blast of freon from "canned air." Artifacts come in all colors. N. This blue haze can be eliminated by changing the objective lens-to-cornea distance. O. Always look for an even, deep color through the viewfinder. An often overlooked artifact is the greenish cast that occurs when color fundus photographs follow an intravenous injection of sodium fluorescein. P. Proper technique requires exposing color photographs before the dye injection. Q. This local overexposure is the result of taking fundus photographs while a patient's glasses are on (it is fine to photograph through contact lenses, however). R. The light area represents a patient's eyelash or hair. Unsharpness can be caused by a number of situations including incorrect eyepiece settings and hazy media. Another setting that has an effect on sharpness is the astigmatism compensation control: correctly (S) and incorrectly (T) set.

Distribution. U. Loading film incorrectly can cause artifacts in the beginning of the roll. V. Opening the camera back will cause a light leak in the middle of the roll. W. A poorly adjusted motor drive can cause double exposures at the end of the roll.

Some artifacts occur with constant frequency. X. When an incorrect shutter speed is set, the shadow of the shutter curtain will obscure a portion of the fundus in each and every succeeding frame until proper sync speed is restored (a faulty camera flash sync may cause intermittent

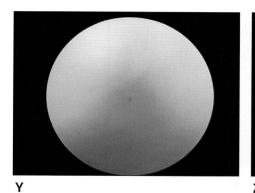

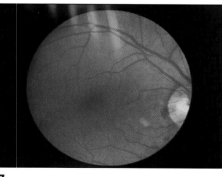

Y

Z

FIGURE 2-43 *(continued)*
problems and indicate the need for service to the camera body). Artifacts may be confined to just one roll or to one patient. Y. A photo-sensitive patient can cause blink artifacts more often than other patients. Z. Light leaks from an unsealed camera will continue throughout fundus photographs regardless of a change in patient or film magazine.

FIGURE 2-44
Dark clouds. If a patient's pupil is significantly smaller than the outer diameter of the illuminating doughnut, a portion of the retina will receive inadequate illumination. The resultant "dark cloud" shifts as the camera's position changes. If you cannot eliminate the underexposed area, minimize its interaction with pathology.

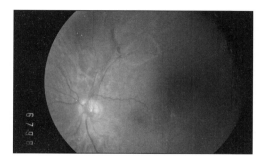

Illumination Problems

Maximum pupil dilation allows the entrance and exit of the fundus camera's illuminating and imaging light rays without interference. Work together with your referring physician to establish a dilating regimen that is safe and provides adequate dilation. Expect widely dilated pupils in young patients who are not taking medications, especially if they have light irises. Expect smaller pupils in older patients, in patients who are diabetic or who are being medicated for glaucoma, and in patients who have dark irides. Less than maximum dilation will make accurate focusing and alignment difficult. Your images may be locally underexposed, especially with wide-angle fundus cameras (Figure 2-44). Decentering the fundus camera may result in better illumination (Figure 2-45).

Unsharp Subjects

The bundle of illuminating and imaging rays must twice pass through the patient's tear film, cornea, anterior chamber, lens, and vitreous. The clarity of the final fundus photograph is directly related to the clarity of each of these layers.

Specific areas of the cornea and lens may affect the passage of light. Maneuver around local areas of unsharpness such as central cataracts, corneal scars, and pterygia. The key to success is positioning the central

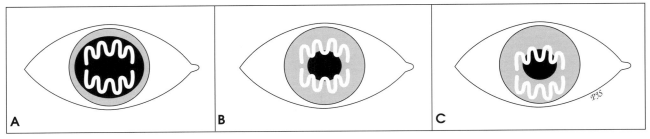

FIGURE 2-45
Decentering the fundus camera may help illuminate the fundus through a small pupil. Normally, the doughnut of the viewing light readily fits within the dilated pupil when centered (A). If the dilated pupil is very small, centering the doughnut may exclude illumination (B). Lowering or raising the camera axis (C) again divides the pupil evenly between viewing illumination and imaging rays. Be sure to increase the exposure to compensate for the smaller amount of illumination.

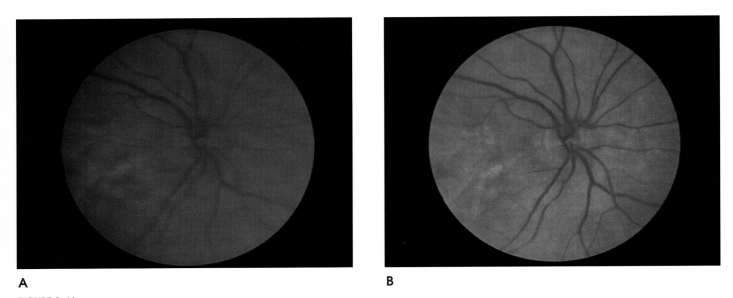

FIGURE 2-46
Look for local areas of sharpness in patients with cataracts. Initial alignment indicates a blurry fundus photograph (A), but careful searching reveals a clear view (B).

imaging light rays through a clear portion of the media (Figure 2-46). Be sure to spend time exploring all possible camera positions.

A dry, swollen, or hazy cornea, asteroid hyalosis, and vitreous hemorrhage represent conditions that can blur the entire fundus photograph. Adequate tear film is essential for corneal clarity and a sharp fundus image. Encourage your patients to blink frequently. Instill artificial tears in the eyes of patients with dry corneas. Topically applying glycerin (under the physician's supervision and with a topical anesthetic) to an edematous cornea may help sharpen the image.[12]

Corneal manipulation diminishes corneal clarity. Applanation tonometry disturbs the corneal epithelium and discolors the cornea with topical fluorescein. Examination by diagnostic contact lenses may cause slight corneal edema and introduce topical methylcellulose. Fundus photography should be performed before any contact lens examination is undertaken. For optimal quality, reschedule patients who have undergone a procedure that involves corneal applanation. If postlaser photographs are requested, multiple rinses with commercially available eyewash preparations may clarify the image.

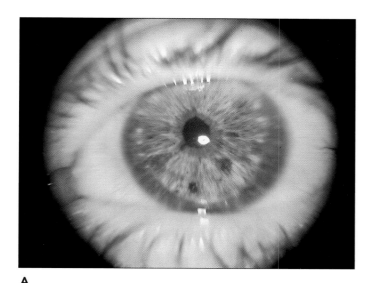

A

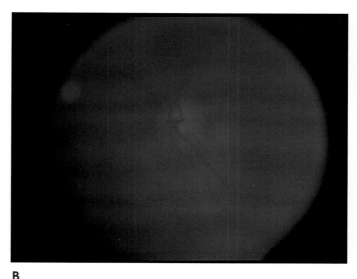

B

FIGURE 2-47
Document compromised media or a small pupil using an external photograph (A). While the resulting fundus photograph may not be a prize winner, it may contain adequate diagnostic information (B).

There is little you can do to sharpen the final photograph if dense asteroid hyalosis, vitreous hemorrhage, or a mature cataract exists. Indeed, obtaining a view of the retina can be a feat in itself. When general haziness is a problem, focusing with a green filter (540–570 nm) may help increase the contrast between the blood vessels and the retina. If blood vessels are indistinguishable, begin by locating the disc: It will look like a bright, blurry circle. Focus as best you can and then, using the disc as your landmark, locate the requested field. Your final photograph will almost always contain retinal details not perceived through the viewfinder (Figure 2-47).

Documenting hazy media or a small pupil will assist in evaluating photographer performance, especially if the question of poor dilation or hazy media versus poor photographic technique arises. Adjust the fundus camera for external photographs by moving the patient's head rest away from the camera's objective lens, inserting the plus diopter setting, and increasing the exposure. Focus should correspond with the level of the opacity. Use the optic disc as a reflector by centering it directly behind the pupil (Figure 2-48).

The Light-Sensitive Patient

Most people have a natural aversion to bright lights. Light-sensitive patients blink and tear excessively when looking in the fundus camera. Avoidance behavior by these patients may make aligning the fundus camera difficult. Younger patients are more often light-sensitive than older patients. Aphakic and pseudophakic patients are generally more light-sensitive, having lost the filtering qualities of their natural lens. Patients with cone dystrophy, albinism, or blepharospasm may be extremely light-sensitive.

Prepare your patient for multiple bright flashes by accurately explaining the procedure. Inform the light-sensitive patient of your progress throughout the photographic session; provide gentle verbal encouragement or praise regularly.

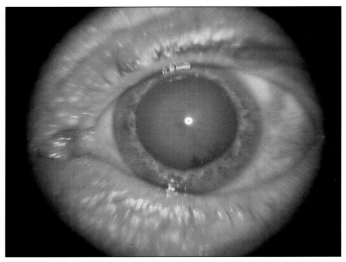
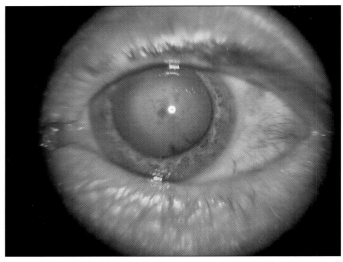

FIGURE 2-48
Using the optic disc as a reflector may help to better identify compromised media.

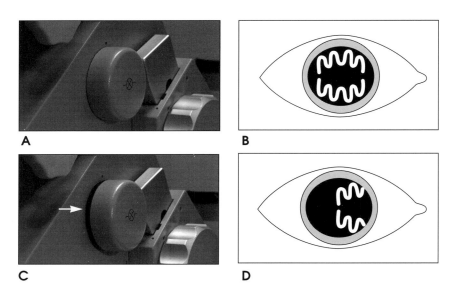

FIGURE 2-49
Dimming the viewing light. If the viewing light has been turned down to its minimum setting and your light-sensitive patient is still uncomfortable, decentering the illumination bulb may provide relief. When the illuminating bulb is correctly mounted (A), the illuminating circle is centered within the dilated pupil (B). Pulling the illuminating housing slightly out (C) decenters the illumination doughnut (D), decreasing the amount of light used to focus. Since the position of the electronic flash tube has not changed, the film image will be correctly exposed.

Many fundus cameras have an illumination intensity knob that adjusts the focusing illumination from virtually nil to very bright. Use the lowest illuminating intensity at which you can clearly distinguish retinal detail. You may find it useful to turn the viewing light up while focusing, then down to a minimal level while shooting. If, at its lowest setting, the illumination still bothers your patient, decentering the illuminating bulb may help (Figure 2-49).

The light-sensitive patient may more easily tolerate focusing when a green filter (540–570 nm) is placed in the illumination path. Be sure to remove this filter just before the exposure.

Be constantly aware of your patient's disposition throughout the procedure. Frequent rest breaks (between, not within stereo pairs) help keep the patient fresh. Tension-relieving techniques, including relaxation breathing, and humor, are useful. Remember that patients are usually trying to do their best—even when it seems that they are not. Use positive

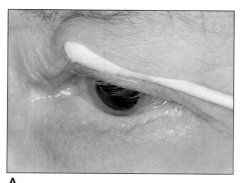
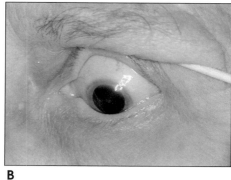
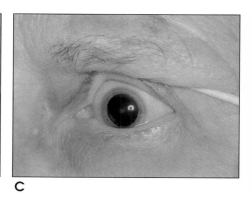

A   B   C

FIGURE 2-50
To retract the upper lids with a cotton-tipped applicator, have the patient look down and place the cotton tip at the lid margin (A). Rotate the applicator (clockwise OD, counterclockwise OS) (B). Instruct the patient to look straight ahead (C) and continue fundus photography.

reinforcement and praise to help your patients work with you, rather than against you.

You must remain in control of your demeanor throughout the procedure. Patients will often adjust their disposition according to your behavioral cues. If you exhibit calmness and patience, your patient will make an effort in that direction. If you become exasperated and exhibit threatening or obnoxious behavior, your patient will often react in a like manner. Don't be afraid to call a time-out if either you or the patient needs some time to regain composure.

Eyelids

A cooperative light-sensitive patient will allow you to lift his or her upper eyelid with a cotton-tipped applicator. An uncooperative light-sensitive patient will require you to depend on an assistant to hold both the upper and lower lids. Use cotton-tipped applicators for all lid manipulation. Place the tip of an applicator at the bottom of the upper lid and rotate up and in to raise the lid (Figure 2-50). Rotate the swab clockwise (as seen temporally) for the right eye and counterclockwise for the left eye. The globe should not be depressed during lid manipulation.

Lid speculum use is not usually recommended: An uncooperative patient may sustain a corneal abrasion. Some photographers suggest the patient hold his or her own eyelids.[13] Be aware that the patient may be more interested in avoiding bright lights than in ensuring that the procedure is successfully completed.

Eyelids may present a mechanical (rather than behavioral) barrier to fundus photography. Lid elevation is necessary for the patient with blepharoptosis. Manage excess eyelid skin with the creative use of tape (Figure 2.51).

Children

Retinal photography challenges quickly mount when the patient is a child. One difficulty is that the equipment is designed for the "average-sized" adult. Specific suggestions for accommodating the smaller bodies of your younger patients are found below.

Good pediatric fundus photography depends on conveying the proper attitude. Successful patient management techniques in the young patient vary with the age of the patient. Infants, toddlers, grade-schoolers, and teenagers all require specific strategies.

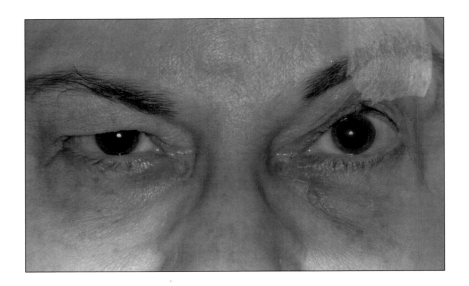

FIGURE 2-51
"Instant lid lifts" with adhesive tape are useful with some ptotic eyelids.

Babies are both the easiest and most difficult patients to photograph. Those who have just nursed are cooperative and sleepy, while those who have missed their naps are invariably cranky and extremely challenging. Patience and good humor are your only means of taming the uncooperative child. Your most emotionally challenging photographic subjects will be the retinas of children who have been abused.

For babies, use a hand-held fundus camera. Alternately, the forehead rest may be removed from the standard-angle fundus camera and your young patients laid on their side.[14] A pediatric speculum provides access to the pupil. Speculum use requires topical anesthesia and a balanced salt solution to keep the cornea moist. A standard mummy wrap with two or three volunteers (for head, torso, and legs) stabilizes the child. Remember to take into account both the decreased pupil size and the shorter axial length in children under 3 years old when setting your flash exposure. Expose several photographs if you can, bracketing toward the lower flash settings.

Verbal communication may be used to your advantage with toddlers and grade-schoolers. Speak directly to the patient, as opposed to communicating through the parent. Introduce yourself to the child with a smile to help establish trust. Remind young children of the special events (such as birthdays or holidays) that are usually associated with picture taking. Explain the intended procedure as just as necessary (using a nod and eye contact to make sure the parents understand). Speak slowly and distinctly. While all patients like to know what to expect, younger children especially fear the unknown. Sharing a frank overview of the process informs children and allays their fears. Let your patient have some fun: Our young patients like to experience photography from the "taking" end. We waste a frame of film but gain their friendship by letting them press the shutter release. An instant film image may be used to elicit a cooperative spirit and creates a great giveaway for show-and-tell.

Difficulties may be encountered during your straightforward attempts at photography. Remember to respect each family's specific disciplinary system. Don't bribe or threaten to punish—other alternatives are available. Games help focus the child's attention on something other than the procedure. The child may *"pretend to be a statue"* or *"find the bunny in the middle of the lens."*

Try setting a mutual goal with the patient. Ask the child to count aloud with you to three. Tell them you will be taking three pictures and have them count each one along with you. You may want to cushion this figure; most children will only allow the negotiated number.

Actively solicit suggestions from the patient. Ask the child *"what can I do to make this easier for you?"* Appeal to his or her friendship with the doctor or parent (*"Dr. ____ thinks these pictures are important. Will you help me get them?"*). If lids need to be held, employ a technician who has previously worked well with the particular child. Above all, remain calm and patient throughout the procedure.

Older children who are difficult may require you to announce, in a firm voice, that *"we are going to take these pictures before you leave. Let's work together to get this over with."* If you feel yourself losing control of the situation, sometimes it is better to leave the room and have the parent and child negotiate the terms of pictures. Be sure to leave with these verbal messages: *"Dr. ___ thinks these picture are important. When I come back, we'll be ready to finish the pictures."* Upon returning to one 6-year-old girl, I discovered that the parent had agreed to pay the child $1.00 for each of three photographs.

It is especially important not to distress the child if you see the patient before the physician has completed the examination. As important as good photographs are, the doctor's examination takes precedence. However, the photographer may be the last health professional to see the child on a particular day. You have the opportunity to make future visits easier by parting with the patient on good terms.

Advanced Techniques

The Periphery

Many retinal diseases (including but not limited to diabetic retinopathy, presumed ocular histoplasmosis syndrome, and retinitis pigmentosa) may manifest changes outside of the posterior pole. Peripheral fundus photography is used to image these areas. The retina described by the standard fields 3–7 is referred to as the midperiphery; retina nearer the ora serrata is termed the far periphery. This section begins by explaining the basics of peripheral photography and concludes by suggesting tips for the experienced photographer.

Two basic techniques allow you to move beyond posterior pole fundus photography: off-center fixation and fundus camera movements. You know that obtaining straight-ahead fixation and centering the illumination doughnut in the patient's pupil will result in a macular photograph. You can visualize the peripheral retina by moving the fixation light off center and then recentering the doughnut of light (usually by looking to the outside of the camera) on the pupil. You can also photograph the peripheral retina by obtaining straight-ahead fixation (using the external fixation device) and then swinging or tilting the fundus camera. Using either one of these techniques results in midperiphery photographs; using both helps you image the far periphery (Figure 2-52).

The "seven standard fields" describe a uniform method of photographing the midperipheral fundus. Standardized field definition was developed to assess the peripheral retina for multicenter studies. It allows the comparison of similar retinal fields, whether they be exposed at your office on different visits, or by ophthalmic photographers in different parts of the world. You should standardize your midperiphery

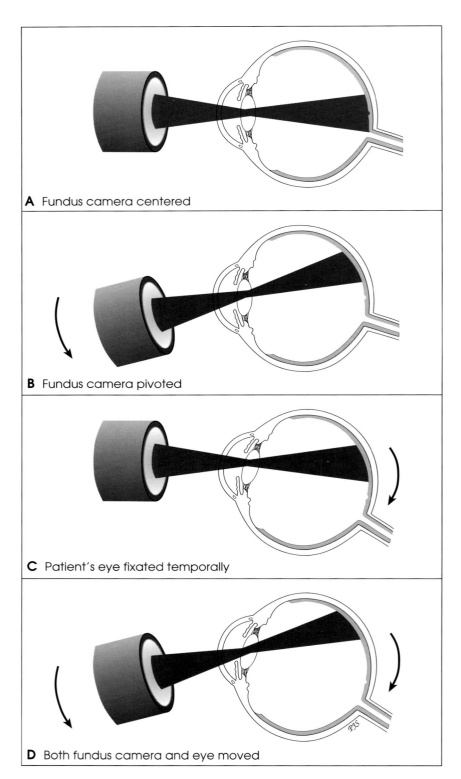

A Fundus camera centered

B Fundus camera pivoted

C Patient's eye fixated temporally

D Both fundus camera and eye moved

FIGURE 2-52
Imaging the periphery. When the fundus camera and the patient's eye are aligned squarely, the macula is centered (A). Swing the camera to one side to photograph the periphery (B), adjusting the distance between the objective lens and the cornea and recentering the doughnut of light on the pupil. Alternately, change patient fixation, rotating the patient's eye up and to the side until the proper field is obtained (C). Use both techniques for far peripheral views (D). A combination of swinging the camera to the side, tilting the camera up or down, and oblique patient fixation may be needed for some peripheral views. Evaluate the need for using the astigmatism compensation control when working in the far periphery.

photographs by learning the anatomic landmarks that define each field (Figure 2-53).

Field 1 is centered on the disc (Figure 2-54). Field 2 is centered on the macula with the disc in the 3:00 (OD) or 9:00 (OS) position. Field 3 is temporal to the macula, including the fovea at the 3:00 (OD) or 9:00 (OS) position. In the right eye, field 4 is superior to the macula and includes

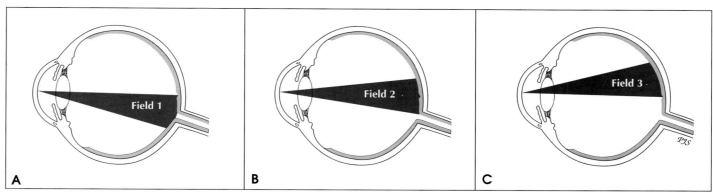

FIGURE 2-53
Seven standard fields. Visualized on a cross section of the eye from above, field 1 is centered on the optic nerve (A). For field 2, the camera is centered on the fovea (B). The nasal edge of field 3 intersects the fovea (C). Field 4 is directly superior to field 2; field 5 is directly inferior. Field 6 is superior-nasal to field 1. Field 7 is inferior-nasal to field 1. Field 8 is a "wild card" field that is assigned to any needed retinal position.

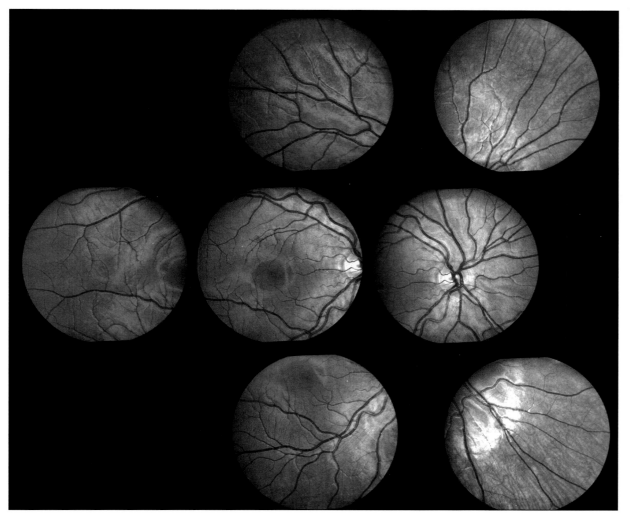

A

FIGURE 2-54
The seven standard fields. These are photographic examples of the seven standard fields in the right (A) and left (B) eyes.

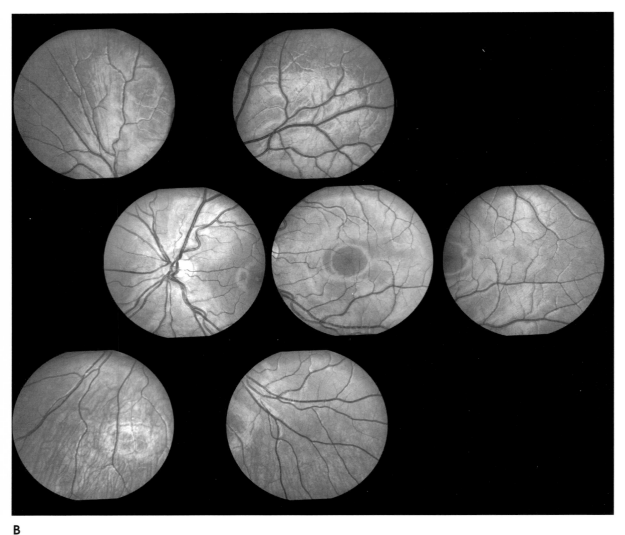

B

FIGURE 2-54 *(continued)*

the 12:00 position of field 2 at its 6:00 position. Field 5 is inferior to the macula and includes the 6:00 position of field 2 at the 12:00 position. Field 6 is superonasal to the disc, including the 1:30 position of field 1 at 7:30. Field 7 is inferonasal to the disc and includes the 4:30 position of field 1 at 10:30. Most photographers image these fields "out of order," proceeding thusly: 2-1-6-4-3-5-7 or 2-1-3-5-7-6-4.

Because practical experience will be your best teacher, begin by photographing the retinal periphery of an office volunteer. Alternatively, expose some peripheral photographs of your patients who need only macula or disc photographs, polishing your skills before you need them.

Obtaining high-quality peripheral fundus photographs can be a challenge. Factors that are optimized for posterior pole photography become mediocre when photographing the far periphery. A circular, widely dilated pupil becomes an ellipse. The retina is imaged through an oblique cross section of the lens. Your camera position, once simple, is now complex. Peripheral fundus photographs may not seem as sharp as your posterior pole photographs. The following practical techniques may help improve their quality.

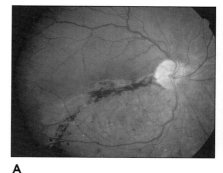 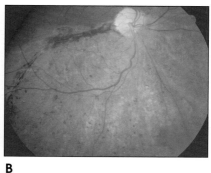

FIGURE 2-55
When photographing the periphery, begin with a macula photograph (A) or include a landmark in your photograph (B).

A   B

1. Begin with an establishing shot. Document the eye (OD or OS) by photographing the posterior pole before you image the periphery or include a landmark (such as the disc) in the photograph (Figure 2-55).

2. Don't limit yourself when positioning the patient's eye or the camera for peripheral fundus photography. Both the internal or external fixation device can be used to obtain fixation. If peripheral photographs are requested of monocular patients, you can use the external fixation device on the eye being photographed. Try verbal instructions if targets do not work; clock hours or simple directions (up, down, right, left) may be helpful. Ask the patient to imagine looking in the center of a square; asking the patient to look to "the upper right hand corner" will result in a superior temporal view (OD). If reliable fixation cannot be obtained, request the patient to look straight ahead (at the wall or at you) and swing or tilt the camera until the proper field is visualized. You may need to stand or crouch when the camera is tilted or swung to its extreme position. If the patient's fixation has reached its limits and you still need to see "just a little bit more," ask the patient to look "beyond the light" to reveal more peripheral retina. A combination of off-center fixation, camera head movement, and patient head tilt extends your range further into the periphery (note: using all three of these options at the same time is possible only with the most widely dilated pupils).

3. Scleral depression (by the photographer or the physician) and extremely wide-angle contact cameras (e.g., the Pomerantzeff or Chromos) can yield photographs that include the ora serrata.

4. Should a normal-angle or a wide-angle camera be used in peripheral photography? Normal-angle cameras always image better in tight spaces. Since the round pupil becomes a narrow ellipse as the eye is rotated, the smaller imaging circle of the normal-angle camera makes it the camera of choice for peripheral photographs in patients with a small or medium-sized pupil. In patients with large pupils, however, an elliptical pupil may still be large enough for a wide-angle camera. These cameras may reveal more of the peripheral retina with their larger angle of view and closer working distance. One wide-angle picture may take the place of several thirty-degree pictures. Attempt peripheral photographs using both fields of view if possible (Figure 2-56).

The astigmatic correction device helps correct the paraxial astigmatism that results from the oblique angles at which the cornea and lens are approached.[15] Use this control visually: Center your subject, then twist and/or rotate the astigmatic correction slowly until a sharper image is

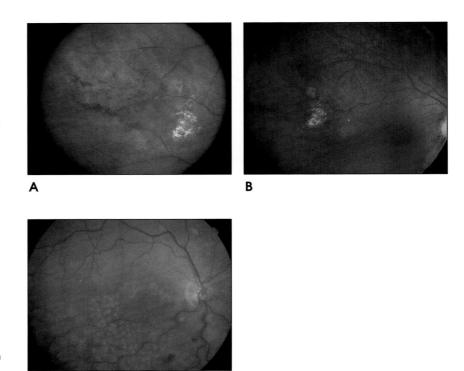

A   B

FIGURE 2-56
Photographing the periphery: wide angle or normal?
The peripheral fundus can be imaged with both
wide-angle and normal-angle fundus cameras.
Choose the angle that best documents the patient's
condition.

FIGURE 2-57
Rinse the cornea with commercially available eyewash
before attempting postlaser fundus photography.

seen. Check the unmodified view before the exposure to be certain that the change is beneficial.

Photographs After Laser Treatment

Fundus photography is often used to document recent laser treatments (Figure 2-57).[16] The overlay function of newer digital imaging systems readily compares the area of treatment with angiographic information, making electronic postlaser photographs clinically advantageous. Unfortunately, the quality of postlaser fundus photographs may be compromised because of the contact lens and lubricant used during the laser procedure. Increase the clarity of your postlaser photos by rinsing the eye thoroughly with commercially available eye wash. We rinse the eye three separate times, asking the patient to blink in between each. Allowing some time (at least 10 minutes) to pass after the treatment helps to resolve corneal edema from the contact lens use.

Fundus Photography with Filters

Two principles enable specific retinal details to be enhanced by using monochromatic filters during fundus photography. First, when used with black and white film, monochromatic filters lighten objects of their own color and darken objects of the complementary color (Figure 2-58). Second, longer and shorter wavelengths of light penetrate the retina to different levels (Figure 2-59). The effects of monochromatic light when photographing the normal and abnormal retina have been described by Delori and Ducrey.[17, 18] In clinical practice, blue, green, and red filters have gained wide usage.

Use your blue fluorescein exciter filter (490 nm) to enhance information from the nerve fiber layer of the retina or vitreoretinal interface (Figure 2-60). Select a slow, fine-grain black and white film such as Kodak Technical Pan or Ilford Pan F film.[19] Focus carefully on the uppermost

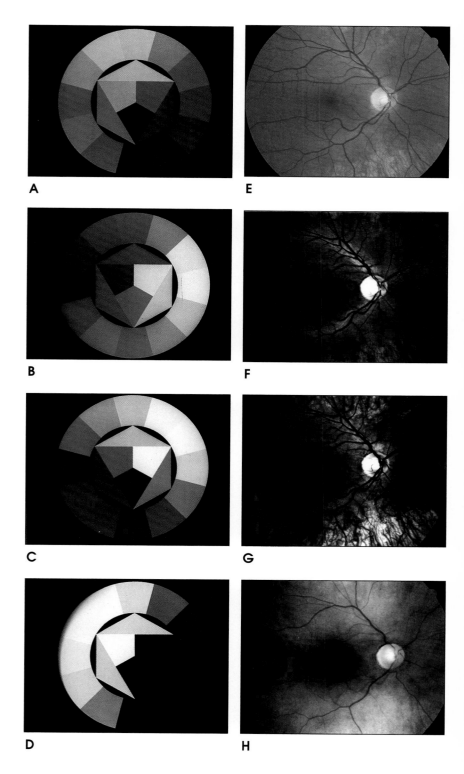

FIGURE 2-58
Black and white tonalities when using colored filters. A 12-hue color wheel was photographed on panchromatic black and white film (A). Yellow is located at 12:00, orange at 2:00, red at 4:00, purple at 6:00, blue at 8:00, and green at 10:00. Blue (B), green (C), and red (D) filters were placed in front of the lens. Note that colored filters lighten the reproduction of similar colors and darken complementary hues. Characteristics of the normal fundus (E) are selectively emphasized using monochromatic filters. A blue, 490-nm filter highlights the nerve fiber layer (F). When a blue filter is used, veins reproduce darker than arteries. The green, 540-nm filter darkens the veins and increases contrast (G). The red, 640-nm filter reveals the choroidal vasculature and lightens the arteries (H). (E–H courtesy of B. Clifton.)

layer of the retina by first focusing on the retinal blood vessels and then moving the focus slightly "up" toward the vitreous. High-contrast development and printing techniques will accentuate the nerve fiber layer.

The monochromatic green filter (often archaically termed a "red-free filter") transmits either 540- or 575-nanometer wavelengths of light. These wavelengths enhance the visualization of the retinal vasculature and hemorrhages by increasing the contrast between the retinal blood vessels and the retinal pigment epithelium (RPE) (Figure 2-61). Using these filters

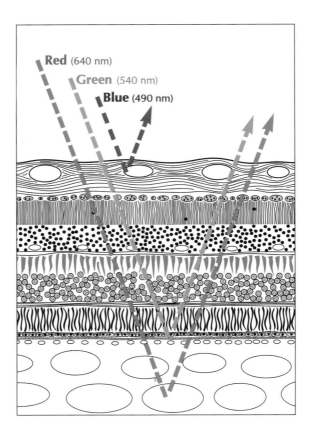

FIGURE 2-59
The wavelength of monochromatic light determines its capacity for retinal penetration. Shorter wavelengths (e.g., blue) scatter more easily and reveal the surface of the retina. Longer wavelengths (e.g., red) scatter less easily, allowing deeper imaging. (Courtesy of B. Clifton.)

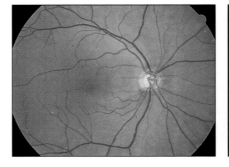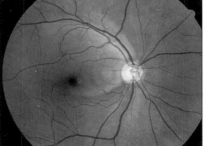

FIGURE 2-60
Your blue exciter filter can highlight changes in the top layer of the retina, as is seen in this example of a nerve fiber layer sector defect. This patient with primary open-angle glaucoma was photographed with Kodak Tech Pan film and a 490-nm filter. (Courtesy of B. Clifton.)

with black and white film results in the best monochromatic representation of the physician's view with an ophthalmoscope. Traditionally, the photographs before a fluorescein angiogram are taken with this filter. Focus on the central retina for vascular studies. Parenthetically, using a green filter when black and white internegatives of color slides are made results in a more pleasing separation between the retinal blood vessels and the choroid.

A red monochromatic filter (640 nm), when coupled with precise focusing, highlights choroidal details (Figure 2-62). This technique can define the borders of pigmented lesions or document choroidal vascular before indocyanine green (ICG) angiography. Focus first on the major retinal blood vessels and then continue focusing slightly "down" toward the choroid.

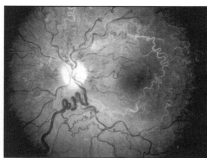
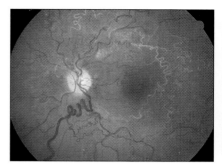

FIGURE 2-61
Your green filter highlights changes in the retinal vasculature by increasing contrast. This arteriovenous malformation was documented using a 540-nm filter. (Courtesy of B. Clifton.)

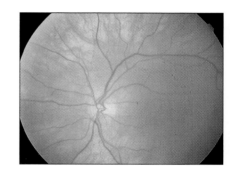
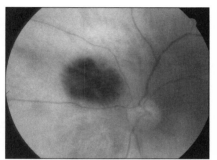

FIGURE 2-62
Your red filter (this photograph used a 640-nm filter) penetrates through the retina to the choroid, in this case documenting a choroidal nevus. (Courtesy of B. Clifton.)

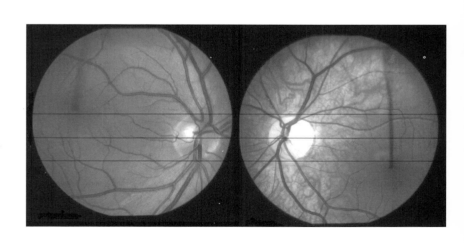

FIGURE 2-63
Document torsion with fundus photography by inserting the internal fixation device and centering the disc within the height of the frame. Compose to include both the macula and disc. The macula in a normal eye will fall slightly below the line that bisects the disc; the macula of the abnormal eye is positioned above (incyclotropia) or below (excyclotropia) this line.

While colored filters may not be useful with every patient, they can selectively highlight specific fundus details in particular cases.

Fundus Photographs for Torsion

Fundus photography can be used to document the objective presence or absence of ocular torsion in patients with torsional strabismus (Figure 2-63).[20] Take extra care to position the patient's head squarely in the head rest for torsion photography. Frame the posterior pole, aligning the center of the disc on the midline of the frame at the 3:00 (OD) or 9:00 (OS) position. Insert and focus the internal fixation device. Double-check that the patient's head has not tilted before exposing the film.

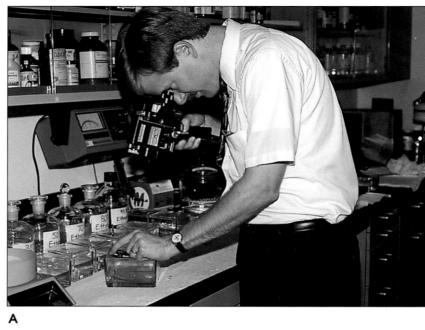

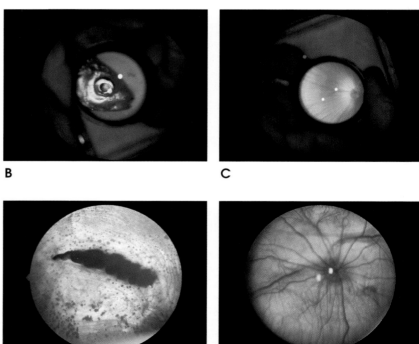

FIGURE 2-64
Fish fundus photography using a hand-held camera and a condensing lens (A). First obtain a red reflex (B), then optimize the distance for fundus imaging (C). An owl retina (D) and rat retina (E) complete this fundus menagerie. (Courtesy of M. Croswell.)

Hand-Held Fundus Cameras

Portable, hand-held fundus cameras are useful in a variety of situations—for babies and small children who are too small for the standard head rest and for supine patients (whether bedridden, undergoing surgery, or being examined under anesthesia) whose condition make standard patient positioning difficult. Animal fundus photography is also often performed using hand-held fundus cameras (Figure 2-64).

Positioning the hand-held fundus camera requires skill and practice. The patient should be stationary (papoose small babies and have one per-

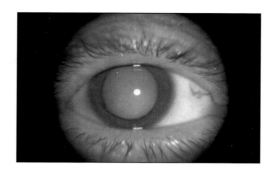

FIGURE 2-65
External photography with the axial illumination of a fundus camera is helpful when documenting leukokoria, or a "white pupil."

son to stabilize the head and one for the feet) and with lids retracted (either by a helper or with a speculum). Hold the camera in your left hand, using your thumb for the shutter release and your right hand for the film advance. Position the front element of the camera about 2 inches away from the cornea. Center on the cornea and focus on a retinal blood vessel or the optic disc. Move the camera closer to the cornea, allowing the fundus to fill the frame. Refocus, optimize color saturation, and minimize the artifacts. Tilt the camera or have your assistant manipulate the eye for disc or peripheral photographs.

Condensing lenses used for indirect ophthalmoscopy may be used with the hand-held fundus camera to alter the field of view or to view through a particularly small pupil. Position these lenses close to the cornea while you view through the fundus camera at arm's length. Increase the exposure to compensate for the greater flash-to-subject distance. Tilt either the lens or the camera until reflection artifacts are minimized.

Not Necessarily the Fundus

If a slit lamp camera is unavailable, your fundus camera may be used to record pathology in the anterior segment. Increase the patient-objective lens distance and dial a plus lens into the diopter compensation setting. Increase the exposure to compensate for the increased distance the light must travel. Focus on the cornea, iris, or lens as appropriate. If the area of interest is translucent, arrange patient fixation to permit the optic disc to act as a reflector. External photographs are useful in documenting patients with compromised media or patients with leukokoria (Figure 2-65).

Auxiliary Lenses at the Photo Slit Lamp

Diagnostic lenses permit fundus photographs to be taken with a photo slit lamp (Figure 2-66). Condensing lenses (e.g., a 60- or 90-diopter lens) help capture a wide-angle peripheral fundus view or slit images of the retina. A Goldmann three-mirror lens is useful for narrow-angle views in the retinal periphery. Slit views of the posterior pole are obtained with the Goldmann fundus lens. The Rodenstock Panfundascope lens is useful for extremely wide-angle views. We encourage you to experiment with the specific lenses available in your office.

The basic technique for using condensing lenses is illustrated in Figure 2-67. Select and clean a lens, recalling that the higher the diopter, the larger the field and smaller the magnification. After seating the patient comfortably at the slit lamp, begin with a wide slit beam at a low or medium magnification. Swing the slit illumination housing slightly off center temporally and de-center the beam in the same direction. Hold the lens about 5 mm from the cornea and adjust the slit lamp to obtain a red reflex. Focus by moving the condensing lens and/or the joystick forward and backward. Select a wide or narrow slit beam as dictated by the subject

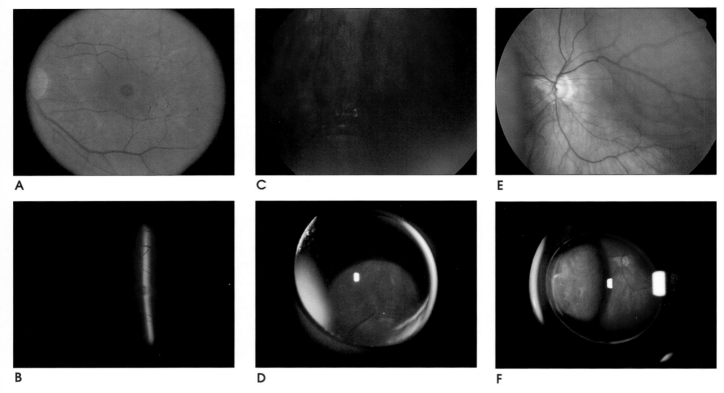

FIGURE 2-66
A photo slit lamp can extend your photographic range. A macular hole (A) is better appreciated with slit illumination (B). This wide-angle fundus photograph (C) does not quite match the reach of a 90-D condensing lens (D) in these photographs of a dislocated IOL. A relatively small portion of the choroidal detachment is documented with a 60-degree view (E). A more comprehensive view is obtained at the photo slit lamp using a wide-angle contact lens (F).

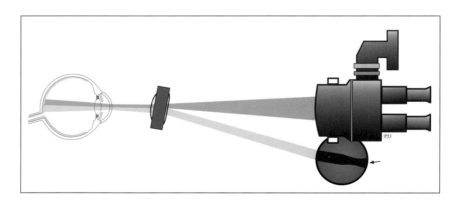

FIGURE 2-67
When imaging the fundus using a condensing lens at the photo slit lamp, direct the illumination slightly off axis. Place the lens about 6-mm from the cornea and tilt as needed to reduce reflections. A lens holder (available from the manufacturer) simplifies the procedure.

matter. Adjust the angle of the auxiliary lens and the angle of illumination to minimize reflections. Change to a medium or high magnification to fill the frame before your exposure. Bracket exposures around your standard slit lamp exposure.

Step-by-step instructions for using diagnostic contact lenses at the slit lamp can be found in slit lamp photography texts.[21] Remember that careless use of diagnostic contact lenses can result in corneal damage. We routinely obtain approval from the attending ophthalmologist before our photographers perform contact lens procedures. Have your physician train you in the proper use of diagnostic contact lenses before attempting to photograph a patient.

Prepare the patient by briefly explaining the procedure. Ensure that the patient is not wearing contact lenses. Apply a topical anesthetic to the patient's cornea and a lubricant (e.g., methylcellulose) to the diagnostic contact lens. After positioning the patient comfortably at the slit lamp, ask the patient to look up and then place the bottom of the lens onto the inferior sclera. Tilt the lens toward the eye until contact is made. Direct the patient to look straight ahead while you center your view, the slit beam, and the pupil under low magnification.

Optimize the location, size, and angle of the slit; the magnification; and the focus for the pathology being photographed. The Goldmann fundus lens requires a medium or high magnification and a slightly decentered slit. Use a slit shape that coincides with the shape of the medium-sized, 67-degree mirror of a Goldmann three-mirror lens for views of the far periphery. A wide, off-center beam and the Panfundascope lens will expose a large retinal area. Bracket your standard exposures at each magnification. Work quickly to avoid any corneal edema that may cloud your photographs. Your sharpest photographs will be obtained during the first 2 minutes.

Fundus photography using a photo slit lamp is not a replacement for standard fundus camera procedures but is an alternative technique to be performed by experienced photographers on specific patients. It is more time consuming than retinal photography using a fundus camera, and the results can be less predictable.

Conclusion

Fundus photography is a challenging but rewarding procedure requiring knowledge, skill, repetition, and patience to master. Although we have focused your attention on technique in this chapter, remember that whether you are a novice or an experienced fundus photographer, you should not lose sight of this most important concept: *The patient is the most important person in your fundus photography room.* Every photographer remembers their first patient, their worst patient, and of course, their greatest fundus photograph. Try this: The next time you sit a patient in front of your fundus camera, take a moment to reflect on the impact your fundus photographs will make on your patient's life and well-being. And then make the pictures as if *your* eyesight depended on it—because the patient's might.

References

1. Wilhelm H, Brower C. *The Permanence and Care of Color Photographs: Traditional and Digital Color Prints, Color Negatives, Slides, and Motion Pictures.* Grinnell, IA: Preservation Publishing, 1993;1.
2. Tyler M. A way to sharper ophthalmic photography through astigmatic correction for the photographer. *J Ophthal Photog* 1981;4:20.
3. Fishman M, Waxler M, Sliney DH, et al. Symposium on light toxicity and its meaning to ophthalmic photographers. *J Ophthal Photog* 1987;10:6.
4. Holladay JT. *Optics, Refraction, and Contact Lenses, Basic and Clinical Science Course.* San Francisco: American Academy of Ophthalmology, 1988;173.
5. Milder B, Rubin M. *The Fine Art of Prescribing Glasses Without Making a Spectacle of Yourself.* Gainesville, FL: Triad Scientific Publishers, 1978;27.
6. Holladay JT. *Optics, Refraction, and Contact Lenses, Basic and Clinical Science Course.* San Francisco: American Academy of Ophthalmology, 1988;109.
7. Ducrey NM, Delori FC, Gragoudas ES. Monochromatic ophthalmoscopy and fundus photography. *Arch Ophthalmol.* 1979;97:288.
8. Blaker A. *Handbook for Scientific Photography.* San Francisco: W.H. Freeman, 1977;97.
9. George TW, D'Anna SA. Comparison of retinal fundus cameras: user's survey results. *Ophthalmology Instrument and Book Supplement* 1983;90(Suppl):80.
10. Kelly MP. A superior method of achieving high myopic retinal focus. *J Ophthal Photog* 1995;17:66.

11. Schatz H, Burton T, Yannuzzi L, Rabb M. *Interpretation of Fundus Fluorescein Angiography*. St. Louis: Mosby, 1978;27.
12. Wong D. *Textbook of Ophthalmic Photography*. New York: Inter-Optics Publications, 1982;67.
13. Coppinger JM, Maio M, Miller K. *Ophthalmic Photography*. Thorofare, NJ: Slack, 1987;89.
14. Szirth BC, Murphee AL, McNamara W. Infant fundus photography. *J Ophthal Photog* 1985;8:30.
15. Busse B, Mittelman D. Use of the astigmatism correction device on the Zeiss fundus camera for peripheral retinal photography. In J Justice Jr (ed), *Ophthalmic Photography*. Boston: Little, Brown, 1982;69.
16. Chamberlin JA, Bressler NM, Bressler SB, et al. The use of fundus photographs and fluorescein angiograms in the identification and treatment of choroidal neovascularization in the macular photocoagulation study. *Ophthalmology* 1989;96:1526.
17. Delori FC, Gragoudas ES, Francisco R, Pruett RC. Monochromatic ophthalmoscopy and fundus photography: the normal fundus. *Arch Ophthalmol* 1977;95:861.
18. Ducrey NM, Delori FC, Gragoudas ES. Monochromatic ophthalmoscopy and fundus photography: the pathological fundus. *Arch Ophthalmol* 1979;97:288.
19. Barry CJ. Retinal nerve fiber layer photography: how widespread is it? *J Ophthal Photog* 1994;16:26.
20. Morton GV, Lucchese N, Kushner BJ. The role of fundoscopy and fundus photography in strabismus diagnosis. *Ophthalmology* 1983;90:1186.
21. Martonyi CL, Bahn CF, Meyer RF. *Clinical Slit Slamp Biomicroscopy and Photo Slit Lamp Biomicrography*. Ann Arbor, MI: Time One Ink, 1985;53.

Chapter 3

Stereo Fundus Photography: Principles and Technique

Marshall E. Tyler

Introduction

A driving force in the advancement of ophthalmic photography is the desire to create the most accurate representation of a patient's condition. The ability of the ophthalmic photographer to record three-dimensional images is one of the most exciting capabilities in our profession. Stereo fundus photography permits clinical examination of the patient's pathology beyond the ordinary two-dimensional view of a conventional photograph. It is fascinating to be able to study a three-dimensional view of an optic nerve, tumor, or retinal detachment, or a fluorescein angiographic image of a subretinal neovascular complex, all without patient movement.

In stereo fundus photography, two images are created photographically and, when viewed, become fused in the brain.[1] When you view the images, your left eye views the left image, your right eye views the right image, and your brain then recreates the depth relationships that were observed at the time of photography. If you have created the stereo photographs by a reproducible technique, they may also permit additional diagnostic interpretation on a follow-up visit.

Many ophthalmic photographers routinely expose all fundus images in stereo. Two exposures are available in case an image is not perfect, and the exposures also provide extra information if the images are a good stereo pair (see the sidebar on terminology). Accept the challenge: Photograph every fundus in stereo and you will find—literally—a new dimension in fundus photography.

In this chapter, the mechanism of stereopsis is discussed first, since how we see in stereo is crucial to understanding how we create excellent stereo images. The history of stereo ophthalmic photography follows. Next, the two methods of stereo fundus photography—*sequential* and *simultaneous*—are discussed, followed by an exploration of stereo viewing techniques and the future of stereo imaging.

Stereo Perception

Timothy J. Martin

The eye, not unlike a camera, is equipped to focus light rays on a light-sensitive substrate. The retina plays the role of the film and is responsible for mapping the formed images. However, the dynamic, interactive characteristics of the living eye, coupled with the complexities of retinal and cortical visual processing, are quite different from the static interpretation offered by even the finest cameras. Even so, the retina and photographic film share a common limitation: They can only provide a two-dimensional map of the three-dimensional world. Photographers, artists, and one-eyed people will be quick to add that there are many depth clues encoded in a single, flat image (Table 3-1), but the most immediate and elaborate sense of depth requires images from two different vantage points (i.e., two eyes) and the neural processing that produces stereopsis.

Stereopsis (from the Greek word *stereos* meaning "solid," hence "solid vision") is the ability of the brain to reconstruct a true sense of depth from the flat images transmitted from the two eyes. The physiology of depth perception is extraordinarily complex. This discussion provides an understanding of the basic physiologic tenets and a foundation for many practical aspects of stereo photography and stereo viewing.

When the eyes are directed at an object in space, the fovea of each eye is trained on that object (Figure 3-1). If the object is at infinity, the visual axes of the two eyes are parallel. For a near object, the eyes (separated horizontally in the adult face by about 65 mm) must turn in, or converge, in order to place the object on each fovea. At the same time, the shape of the lens in each eye must change to produce a shorter focal length (accommodation) to focus the near object. This neural linkage of convergence and accommodation, along with miosis (which is a decrease in the pupillary aperture) make up the *synkinetic near triad*. However, the "effort" required to focus an object provides only a coarse estimate of distance and thus contributes little to stereopsis.

Table 3-1. Monocular Depth Clues

1. Apparent size: The known size of an ordinary object can be compared to its apparent size (if it appears smaller, it must be farther away).
2. Interposition: An object must be in front if it blocks the view of other objects.
3. Aerial perspective: Distant objects appear more hazy, less distinct.
4. Shading: Objects further from the light source may be shaded by those nearer.
5. Geometric perspective: Just as parallel railroad tracks seem to converge to a vanishing point in the distance, spacing appears closer, more crowded in the distance.
6. Relative velocity: Distant objects appear to move more slowly than near objects at the same speed.
7. Motion parallax: Movement of the observer produces greater apparent motion of near, rather than distant, objects.

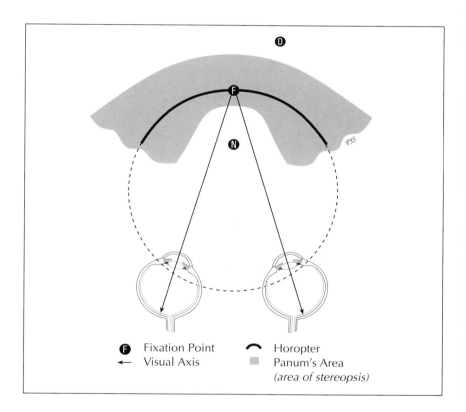

F Fixation Point
← Visual Axis

⌒ Horopter
▨ Panum's Area
   (area of stereopsis)

FIGURE 3-1
Schematic representation of Panum's area and its relationship to important components in the physiology of stereopsis. Physiologic diplopia would be present for objects D and N, both lying outside Panum's area (not to scale).

Through a common fixation point (the intersection of the two visual axes), one can construct a curved surface on which any point would be focused or mapped to precisely corresponding points on the two retinas. This surface is the *horopter*, often simplified as a curved line in the horizontal plane (Figure 3-2). For example, a point 4 degrees to the right of fixation on the horopter would be imaged on each retina precisely four degrees to the left of each fovea (point A in Figure 3-2). Any points lying in front of this surface would not fall on anatomically corresponding points but would be shifted temporally on each retina. Any points beyond the horopter would be shifted nasally, again to noncorresponding retinal points. The further from the horopter, the greater the anatomical retinal disparity. The complex neural circuitry associated with vision is capable of synthesizing depth information from these disparate images, giving the sensation of stereopsis.

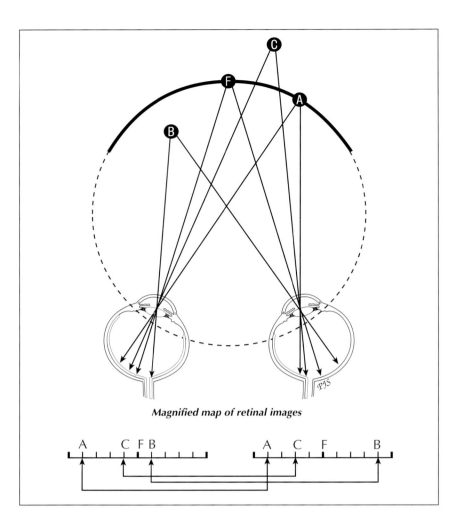

Magnified map of retinal images

FIGURE 3-2
Retinal images of objects on and around the horopter (not to scale). F is the fixation object; lines connecting this object to the fovea of each eye represent the visual axis. The retinal images formed by objects A, B, and C are mapped on a scale to show their position on each retina (relative to the fovea), with the resultant interpretation of retinal disparity as depth. Point A maps precisely to corresponding points on each retina. Thus, A is on the horopter and is the same distance from the observer as the fixation point F. Point B is shifted temporally and thus is perceived as being closer to the observer. Point C also maps to different locations; as it is shifted nasally, it is perceived as being farther away from the observer than F (not to scale).

However, beyond a certain distance on either side of the horopter, the brain cannot cope and an image becomes double rather than being perceived as a single object in three-dimensional space. This limit of stereopsis defines a curved space, represented for simplicity in the horizontal plane as *Panum's area* (see Figure 3-1). The shape and size of the horopter and Panum's area vary with the viewing distance, the distance between the two eyes (or cameras), the firmness of fixation, and an individual's own stereoscopic abilities. Given the constraints of Panum's area, we are subjected to many objects in virtually every view of our environment, which results in "physiologic diplopia." (Physiologic diplopia can be experienced by focusing on the thumb of an outstretched arm, while noticing an object more distant, and vice versa.) Cortical processing is very effective in suppressing the awareness of this ever-present diplopia.[2]

Since this sense of depth is essentially resynthesized from disparate two-dimensional maps from each eye, one can understand how a synthetic sense of depth can be created by appropriately produced two-dimensional images presented simultaneously but independently to each eye. To achieve fusion, there must be enough similarity in the two images for the eyes to "agree" on fixation points. To achieve stereopsis, the disparity of image components must not exceed the limits of Panum's area. Since the parameters of the horopter and Panum's area are dependent on apparent nearness (via the synkinetic triad), the amount of convergence and accommodation required to view these images should also be within the normal physiologic range.

Not everyone can synthesize depth. An obvious example would be the observer who has only one seeing eye. The mechanism responsible for the complex phenomenon of depth perception forms during early childhood and is not always entirely successful. The developing visual system must meet a number of challenges for success: clear, equal vision in both eyes, with both being able to point precisely at the object of regard. Keeping one's eyes properly aligned (orthophoric) requires precise feedback (clear images), as well as intact machinery (working muscles and nerves) to make appropriate adjustments in eye position. Fusion is achieved when the brain can successfully use the images from the two eyes to "lock" the visual axis of each eye onto the object of interest. A poorly seeing eye that cannot achieve fusion has trouble keeping alignment, causing a "sensory" strabismus, since no feedback is available to check the eye's position in space. Poorly seeing eyes tend to drift, often becoming exotropic (turned out). On the other hand, nerve or muscle deficiencies in eye positioning ("motor" strabismus) make fusion difficult and cause two completely different images to be presented to the brain. Since the machinery cannot move the eyes to eliminate this disparity, diplopia and confusion may result. The visual system in young children may overcome this intolerable state by "turning off" one eye. If the inactivation becomes chronic, the neglected eye never develops normal vision and becomes amblyopic.

Profound amblyopia or overt strabismus precludes stereopsis, but stereopsis is not an all-or-none phenomenon. The power of an individual's stereopsis can be estimated by noting the minimal retinal disparity required for that individual to perceive depth. A common clinical assessment uses polarized glasses and the Titmus stereo test (see Figure 3-32). The subject is required to identify which of four circles appears elevated, using nine images of increasing difficulty. Mild amblyopia or small-angle strabismus may allow good fusion, but cripple stereopsis.[3] In short, many people (including some photographers and ophthalmologists) may not be able to appreciate the full sense of the depth conveyed in stereo photographs.

Stereo photography—no matter how cleverly performed—cannot convey the same visual experience as the "real thing." If the photographs are high quality, taken from ideally disparate positions, and viewed with a device that creates the optimal amount of physiologic accommodation and convergence, then what is missing? First, in viewing a real three-dimensional object, the fixation point is not confined to a specific plane as defined by a photograph but is dynamically varied by the viewer in all three dimensions of space. Also, the viewer can vary the viewing distance, which will alter convergence/accommodation factors and dynamically optimize Panum's space, giving additional depth clues. As in monocular parallax, stereopsis may be greatly enhanced by side-to-side movements of the viewer's head, and this full stereo effect can only be approximated photographically with holography. However, despite these shortcomings, creating a stereo photograph often provides visual information of which the sum is far greater than its parts.

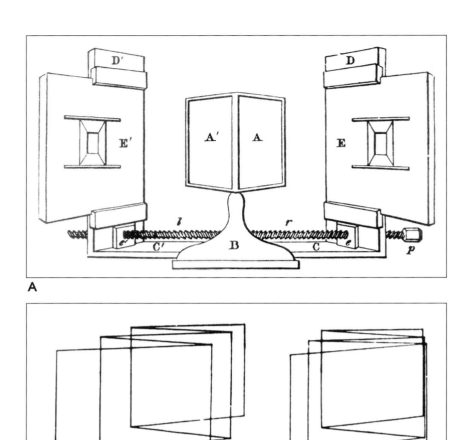

FIGURE 3-3
This diagram of Wheatstone's stereoscope (A) illustrates his use of mirrors to view stereoscopic drawings (B). (Reprinted from J Jones. *Wonders of the Stereoscope.* New York: Knopf, 1976.)

Historical Review of Stereoscopic Fundus Photography

While stereoscopic vision was first described by the Greek mathematician Euclid (280 B.C.), it was not until the 1830s that Charles Wheatstone (inventor of the linear motor and concertina) described a device for the stereoscopic display of visual information (Figure 3-3).[4] Wheatstone's first experiments were limited to drawings, since the photographic media of his time, daguerreotypes, were difficult to illuminate evenly. In 1850, David Brewster developed a more practical stereoscope, one that used lenses for the direct viewing of photographs placed in a darkened box (Figure 3-4).[5] Stereo viewing became a popular parlor pastime in Victorian England after Brewster introduced his lenticular stereoscope at the Great Exhibition of 1851,[6] and it became popular across the Atlantic after Oliver Wendell Holmes, Sr. (physician, poet, and essayist) described (but did not patent) the familiar Holmes stereoscope (Figure 3-5).[4] Among the many types of stereo cards that were published was an elaborate set of fundus paintings in stereo.[7]

Early fundus photography (see Chapter 1) was such a technical challenge that the first stereoscopic photographs (by Thorner[8]) were not published until 23 years later in 1909 (Figure 3-6). Thorner's stereo technique included an elaborate scheme for flipping the camera upside down between exposures. A more practical sequential technique involving side-to-side shifting was described by Metzger in 1926.[9] Better stereoscopic

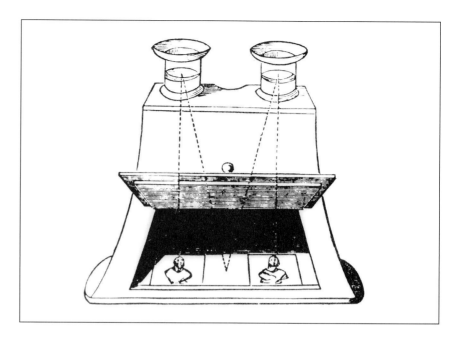

FIGURE 3-4
A variation of Brewster's stereoscope is used daily by ophthalmic photographers on light tables around the world. (Reprinted from J Jones. *Wonders of the Stereoscope.* New York: Knopf, 1976.)

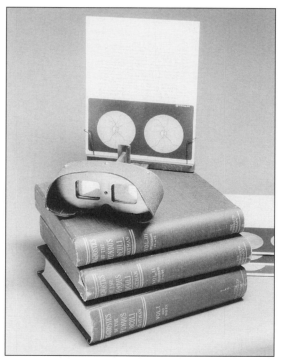

FIGURE 3-5
The inexpensive Holmes stereoscope used "half-lenses" and displayed 80-mm–wide photographs. It is shown here with a card from the collection "Diagnostics of the Fundus Oculi."

fundus photographs (but without technical explanation) are contained in Bedell's 1929 atlas, the first atlas to include stereoscopic images.[10]

In 1939, a physician and a photographer, Louis Bothman, M.D., and Reuel W. Bennett created a fundus atlas, *Stereoscopic Photographs of the Fundus Oculi.*[11] It included 50 stereo cards printed on photographic paper. The images had been taken with the Nordensen fundus camera.

Other methods for sequential stereo imaging were attempted in the early 1960s. Stenstrom described the rotation of the fundus camera about the pivot point,[12] but this technique ignored cornea-induced parallax (which, by itself, optically creates a "convergence view" of the fundus)

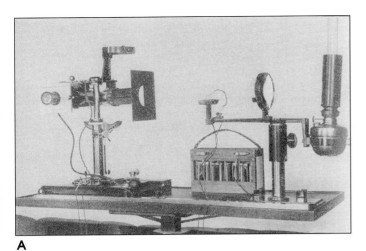

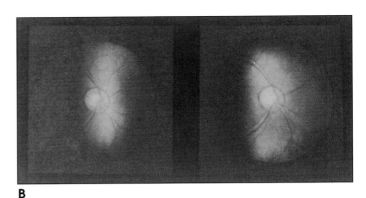

FIGURE 3-6
A. Thorner's sequential stereo fundus camera. Thorner published the first stereoscopic fundus photographs (B) in 1909. Illumination is uneven, as with most Thorner fundus photographs. (Reprinted from W Thorner. Die stereoskopische photographie des augenhintesgrundes. *Klin Monatsbl f Augenh* 1927;78:338.)

and resulted in nonstereo images that were difficult to fuse. Allen used the technique of shifting the fundus camera laterally and later created a stereo separator using a solenoid to control the angling of an optical flat (plano lens): As the glass flipped between two positions, the optical axis of the fundus camera was displaced laterally by a fixed amount.[13] (See the next section for a detailed description for using this device.)

Norton's 1953 fundus camera, based on the indirect ophthalmoscope, introduced simultaneous stereo fundus photography[14, 15] but never became commercially available. In 1964, a more practical design was developed by David Donaldson. Harold Edgerton, an MIT optical engineer and photographer who perfected the modern stroboscope, designed special "end on" flash tubes for this camera. Their stereo fundus camera used two prisms, which split the light from a single front lens element and directed it to two different frames of film[16] (Figure 3-7). Variations of this design remain in use today. Simultaneous stereo imaging is important for visually or electronically comparing and analyzing stereo photographs.

Instrumentation

Basic Stereo Photographic Techniques

Stereo photography creates two images of the same subject taken from two positions—that of the photographer's left eye and that of the photographer's right eye. After being processed, the images are then presented to the appropriate eye for viewing and the viewer's brain recreates the three-dimensional view. The goal of this process is to recreate the image as if the viewer were at the site of the photography. There are both desirable techniques to use and undesirable traps to avoid. This chapter attempts to help you avoid the latter, especially those of image distortion and image convergence.

In stereo photographs, the optical systems are kept parallel to each other and perpendicular to the plane of the subject. This introduces the least amount of distortion in the film image (Figure 3-8), and for the same reason, images should be viewed parallel to the visual plane. The distance between the two optical systems is called the stereo base.

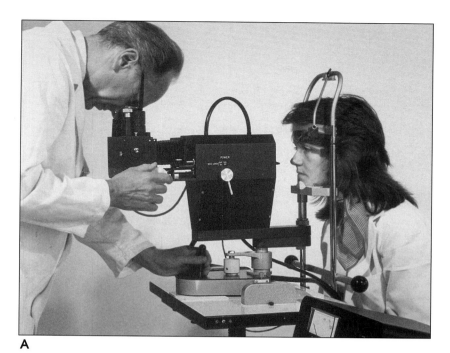

A

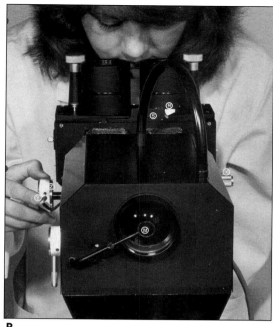

B

FIGURE 3-7
Donaldson's simultaneous stereo fundus camera.
A. Dr. Donaldson with his stereo fundus camera.
B. Front/top view of camera. C. Cross section of
camera optics. (Reprinted from the Operating
Instructions for the Donaldson Simultaneous
Stereoscopic Fundus Camera.)

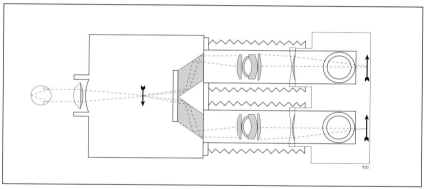

C

Stereo Fundus Photography

Most modern mydriatic fundus cameras are capable of producing sequential stereo images—that is, taking one image of a stereo pair after the other. Precise techniques are used to create clinical stereo image pairs of the highest quality with the least stress to the patient.

The requirements for camera positioning are evaluated from the perspective of the optical systems that are in front of the subject—that is, the cornea, lens, and retina. Understanding the optical systems makes it easier for the photographer to achieve consistent stereo images. Light rays traced from a single point on the human fundus are imaged by the eye's optical components at a distant point, perhaps even at infinity (Figure 3-9). It is this phenomenon that permits cornea-induced stereo photography to work.

Convergence (rotation of the camera viewpoint) around the subject occurs inside the patient's eye, since the optics of the eye are being used when taking the fundus photographs. Convergence is permitted in photomacrography (typical magnification of 1× to 25×) with a subject of a limited depth, such as the eye (see the sidebar on convergence). To create high-quality stereo images, it is important to keep the film plane of the fundus camera parallel to the fundus image.

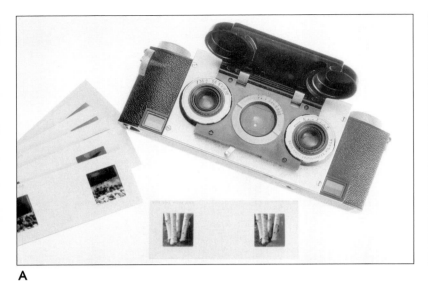

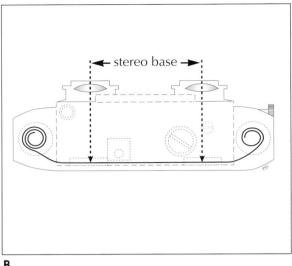

FIGURE 3-8
Nonophthalmic stereo cameras. A. Realist stereo camera. B. Optical system of Realist stereo camera.

Convergence in Stereo Photography

A subject that is relatively flat in elevation is sometimes photographed with cameras in which the lenses and film planes are rotated and aimed at a single point on the subject (see Figure 3-10). This is easily accomplished by using the optics of the human eye. Flatness, or elevation in this case, is the relative distance from the near-point of the subject to the far-point anywhere in the picture. This technique creates image disparity, which makes the image more difficult to view. This disparity can create image viewing difficulties if the subject has too much visual elevation. If a close-up photograph—of a gross specimen, for example—is exposed, the ability to view the stereo image is very different from that ability when a background can be visualized. A sharp background increases the overall stereo depth of the photograph and thus may make the image harder to view because of image disparity. Fortunately, the distortion is made less objectionable with backgrounds without details or the lack of distant far-points as in fundus photography.

Sequential Stereo Fundus Photography

In 1964, Lee Allen[13] described the technique that most ophthalmic photographers now use for achieving sequential stereo fundus photographs. Positioning of the camera for stereo fundus photography starts in the same manner as for monocular fundus photography. The camera is shifted slightly to the left and then to the right of the central position (Figure 3-10), the stereo pair being thus exposed at each position.

There are additional locations where the fundus camera's doughnut of light can be positioned for stereo fundus photography. Factors influencing the choice of positioning include pupillary dilation, the desired stereo base, and media opacities.

Photographers with Zeiss 30-degree cameras have found that another view of the fundus can be seen after going beyond (side-to-side) the area where iris reflections form a crescent-shaped artifact. By sliding the camera further, you can see the bright crescent reflex followed by another clear image. Since the latter image is taken through the peripheral cornea, its quality (sharpness and evenness of illumination) may not be as good as that of the images obtained centrally, but it will permit you to greatly increase the stereo base of your photographs. The peripheral cornea may introduce some astigmatism into the optical system, but this can be compensated for with astigmatic correction.[17] Illumination may also be decreased since part of the illuminating doughnut of light does not enter the pupil (Figure 3-11).

Media opacities in the peripheral lens may limit your stereo base (Figure 3-12). A stereo pair with minimal stereo may still be better than one good monocular image.

If your images are exposed in a consistent order for each patient, then editing will be easier. For a glaucoma patient, a routine photographic sequence might be: right eye: disc-left image, disc-right image, disc-left image, disc-right image, macula-left image, macula-right image; left eye:

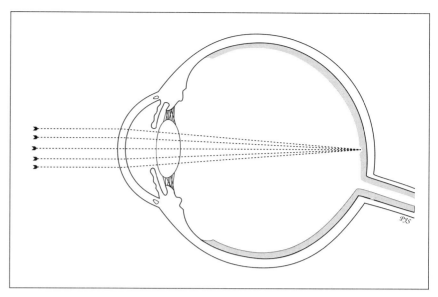

FIGURE 3-9
The eye in cross section showing parallel light (infinity) converging on a single point on the fundus. Imaging rays coming from the patient's fundus will also produce similar parallel rays of light. A fundus camera pointed at any portion of the pupil will record an image of the same part of the fundus. Sliding the camera will simply record the fundus from a different vantage point.

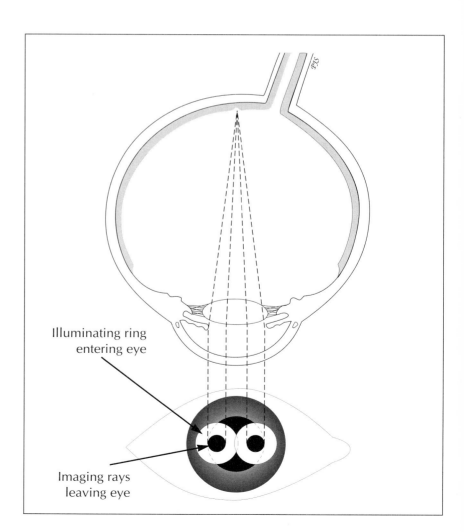

FIGURE 3-10
Stereo fundus imaging. Two fundus photographs are required to make a stereo pair. The diagram shows the pupillary positioning of the two image areas (small dark circles) and the fundus camera's doughnut of illuminating light for stereo fundus photography.

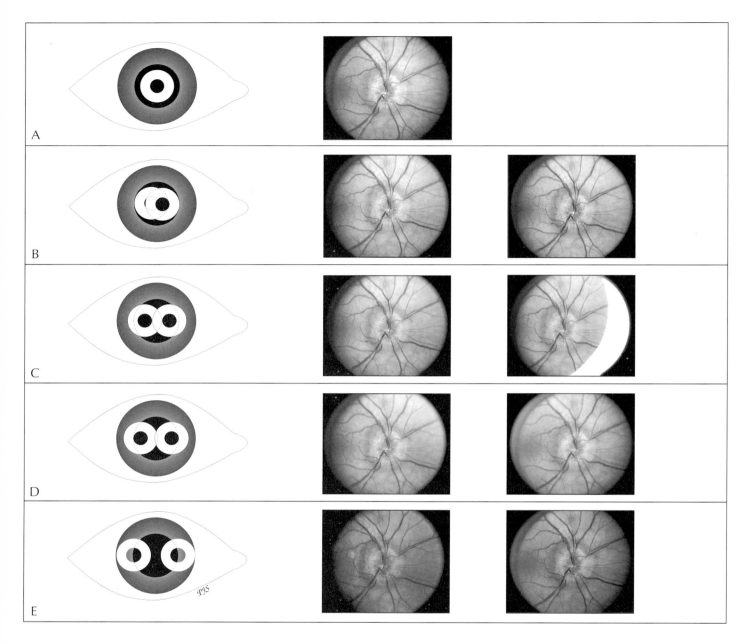

FIGURE 3-11
Illumination positions through a dilated pupil. A monocular photograph results when you center the illuminating ring in the pupil (A). A small stereo separation (B) reproduces a minimal stereo effect (hypostereo) in the final photographs and images will be evenly illuminated. Shifting each view slightly to each respective side (C) creates a crescent-shaped artifact. Further shifting to each side, past the crescent artifact, produces a wide-based stereo pair (D). Notice that the images are unevenly illuminated due to amputation of the illuminating ring. Further sideways camera movement reduces both the illuminating and imaging light rays, resulting in an underexposed image that cannot be used (E).

repeat for left disc and macula. This provides a backup set of stereo disc images in case of a patient blink.

DIAGNOSTIC INTERPRETATION: LIMITATIONS WITH SEQUENTIAL STEREO PHOTOGRAPHY
The stereo base (the separation between the center of the lenses) of sequential stereo frames, and therefore the three-dimensional effect, may be inconsistent between photographic pairs taken at the same session, as well as at different patient visits. When interpreting visit-to-visit photographs, the physician should judge only relative changes in position of various anatomic structures and should not attempt to determine any absolute depth perception information between stereo images. Measurements are also invalid because of potential variability of stereo bases.

ALLEN STEREO SEPARATOR
In an effort to increase the repeatability of the stereo base, Lee Allen[13] developed a solenoid-operated plano-glass lens that is in front of the

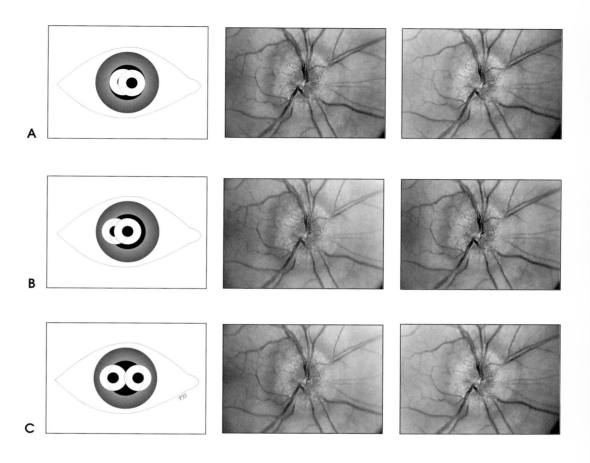

FIGURE 3-12
Three positioning methods for stereo fundus photography. Positioning both illuminating beams inside the dilated pupil results in minimal stereo (A) but may be necessary in patients with peripheral opacities of the media. Central camera placement maximizes image quality: The central and a right or a left partner (B) can create your stereo pair. This choice will provide a minimal stereo base but may permit stereo photography when there is a localized opacity of the media that would interfere with an image pair taken with the desired stereo base (C).

front objective lens of the fundus camera (Figure 3-13A); this attachment is named the Allen Stereo Separator (manufactured by Zeiss). When the angle of the optical flat is changed, the optical position of the fundus camera is slid sideways (Figure 3-13B). The amount of stereo separation (stereo base) is adjustable from 2.25 mm to 3.5 mm. With a foot switch, the photographer alternates the two positions of the separator. To use the Allen Stereo Separator, first line up the left image and then flip the separator and see if the right image is clear. Adjust and repeat until you feel that you have two clear images. Finally, return the separator to the primary position, take the two images, and hope that the patient's eye does not move. The Allen Stereo Separator automatically alternates positions after each photograph is taken.

The quality of the image pairs may be reduced because the predetermined stereo base cannot be optimized for each patient. Additional record keeping is required to note the stereo base for each pair and which pairs were unsuccessful due to poor patient cooperation.

The separator improves the repeatability of the stereo base between stereo pairs, but there is still no guarantee of a consistent stereo base, since there may have been some patient movement when the pairs were taken. Additional issues concern the fact that the glass plate is another

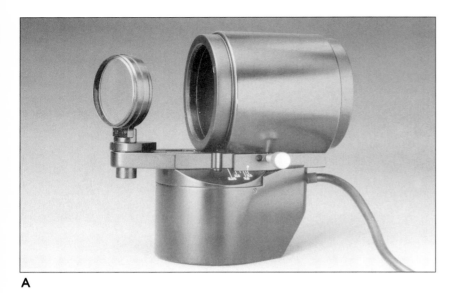

A

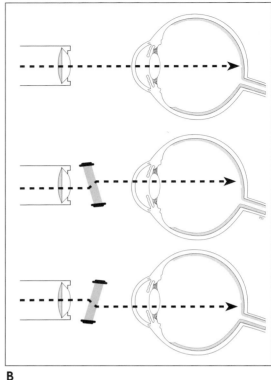

B

FIGURE 3-13
Allen stereo separator. A. Photograph of the solenoid-activated plano glass plate mounted in front of the Zeiss fundus camera. B. Optical path using the Allen stereo separator shows how the camera is optically shifted in front of the patient's eye.

surface for children's fingerprints and adults' nose-prints. Some photographers feel that it is an advantage to have the "lens protector" in place for pediatric patients while others prefer to use a true lens cap whenever the camera is not in use.

Some fundus camera manufacturers have a small locking knob that limits the camera's lateral movement to a stereo base of about 3 mm. The steps needed to take a stereo pair using this method are the same as for any other sequential stereo pair, and the patient movement problems are the same. Only stereo photographs obtained simultaneously can guarantee a repeatable stereo base.

Fluorescein Angiograms in Stereo

SHOOTING ORDER
The same techniques to align the camera in color fundus photography are used in stereo fluorescein angiography (FA). The film in most fundus cameras travels from left to right (photographer's point of view). Film FA studies are usually cut into strips of five or six frames to be placed into negative sleeves. To have the first image at the upper right corner of the contact sheet so that the images are right side up, the first image is to the right of the second image. The right side of the stereo pair must be exposed first: right side, left side, etc. If the order is not correct, then the pairs of images will produce stereo images in which the stereo depth information is reversed (depressions may seem to be elevations and retinal vessels will appear to lie beneath the choroid). Alternatively, if

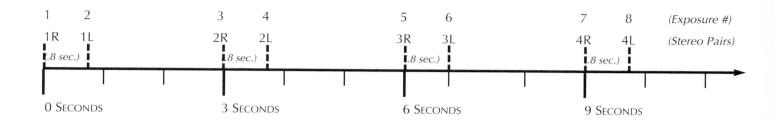

FIGURE 3-14
Optimal timing for stereo pairs during angiography. Visual disparity among stereo pairs reduces the appreciation of stereopsis. Angiography is a dynamic process: The visual representation of blood vessels may change rapidly throughout the process. Expose your stereo pairs with little time between the pictures to reduce the visual differences between the individual pictures in a pair.

negatives are sleeved with the first image in the upper left corner, the image will be upside down but the first image will be on the left. If the negatives are mounted in slide mounts, then the standard left/right stereo technique should be used.

TIMING OF STEREO IMAGES IN ANGIOGRAPHY

The interval between the stereo pairs in angiography is important because the fluorescein sodium dye is moving during the study. Just as it is desirable to have little patient movement between stereo pairs, it is also important to have little movement of dye between the two images that comprise the stereo image. Reducing the time between stereo fluorescein images will reduce the image discrepancy within stereo pairs.[18] A typical sequence would be as follows: Take the right image and pause for 0.8 seconds (the shortest time permitted by most flash power supplies); take the left image and pause for 2.2 seconds; then repeat (Figure 3-14). This timing uses the same amount of film as taking one image every 1.5 seconds but reduces the image disparity by almost one-half. The total time per pair of images remains 3 seconds.

Simultaneous Stereo Fundus Cameras

Alternatives to sequential stereo imaging are available by using simultaneous stereo cameras (Figure 3-15). These cameras have the distinct advantage of providing the physician with images guaranteed to be of constant stereo base. This technique allows both subjective and analytical analysis to be made with a greater degree of repeatability between stereo photographs taken with the same image magnification and stereo base.

Photographing stereo images simultaneously offers other advantages: Patient cooperation is not needed between two sequential photographs—one flash—one stereo pair of images! The disadvantage is the difficulty of simultaneously finding two clear, sharp, and evenly illuminated images through the same potentially small pupil.

The starting point for alignment of simultaneous stereo fundus photography is the same as that for monocular photography; however, you must have two images aligned simultaneously. Aligning these cameras properly requires a modified technique because you are recording two images with a single exposure. Take care to check each image by alternately closing each eye. While all fundus cameras have external fixation

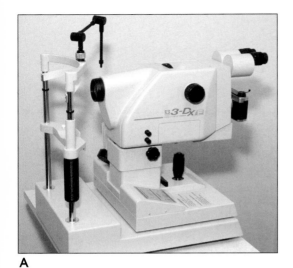

A

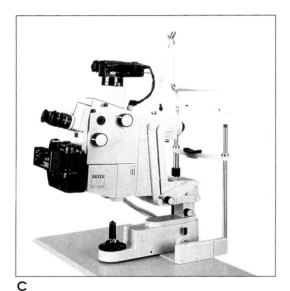

C

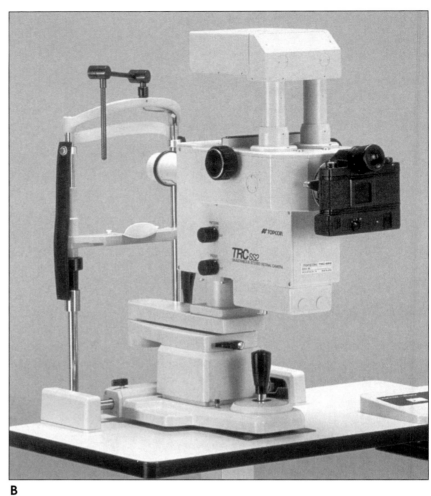

B

FIGURE 3-15
Simultaneous stereo fundus cameras. A. Nidek 3Dx. B. Topcon TRC-SS2. C. Zeiss-Humphrey RC-310. (Courtesy of the manufacturers.)

devices, some stereo cameras have an internal fixation light that, when the patient fixates, attempts to center the optic nerve in the image frame. Keep in mind that these split frame stereo images are vertical, with an image area of 18 mm wide and 24 mm high. The oculars of these cameras are round. If they do not indicate the outside margins of the photographic field, then you will have to estimate what part of the view will be included in your photograph.

While the magnification, and usually the stereo base, of these cameras are fixed, the position of the camera at successive visits may not be identical for each image. Obviously the centering of the subject—the optic nerve, for example—must be achieved with consistency to permit optimal analysis. The optical position of the camera in the pupillary aperture should also be precisely located to achieve greater consistency in visit-to-visit repeatability. If this is not done, the photograph may not be taken from the same viewpoint and therefore image comparison becomes less

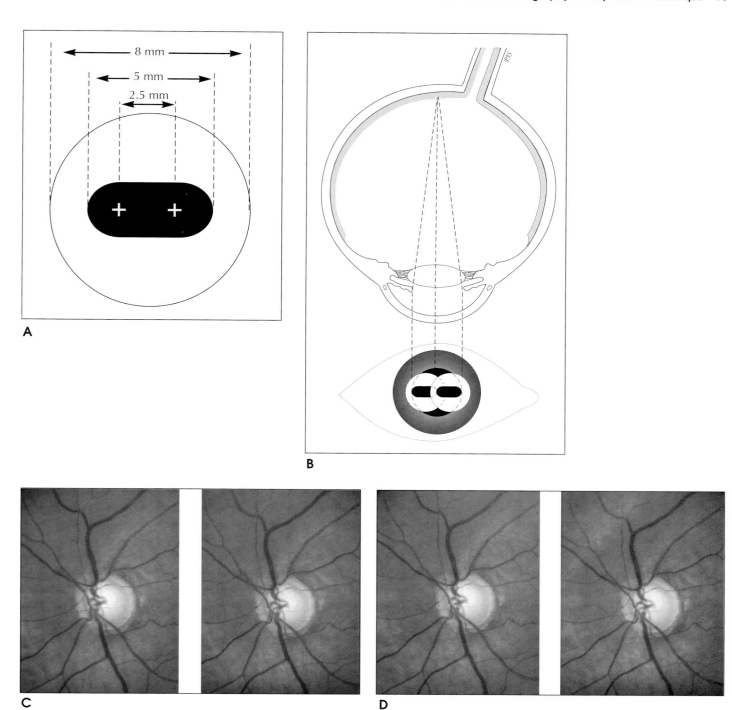

FIGURE 3-16
Variation of simultaneous stereo camera viewpoints. Cross section of eye being photographed with a stereo camera that uses a stereo base of 2.5 mm and an illumination circle that is 1 mm beyond the image aperture. Camera position at the extreme left of the pupil (A) vs. camera position at the extreme right of the pupil (B) shows a maximal change in vantage point of approximately 9 degrees. C. Stereo pair taken from the left side of the pupil and a second stereo pair (D) taken from the right side of the pupil. Note the different viewpoints of the same subject.

useful. Fortunately, because the pupil can only be so large, the maximal potential amount of change in the vantage point is about 9 degrees (Figure 3-16). Use good photographic technique and align the camera on the corneal reflex to reduce this variability. Rotation of the eye is another variable that can compromise stereo consistency. Camera enhancements to improve the ease with which you can maintain optical alignment will make these cameras a more uniform diagnostic tool.

Modifying the stereo base is often not possible with most simultaneous stereo fundus cameras. This may be a limitation if a wider stereo base is required to avoid central lens opacities (e.g., cataracts) or if there is limited dilation (as might be encountered with a patient taking glaucoma medications). Advanced techniques, such as high-low focusing and up-down 90-degree rotation stereo techniques, have not been incorporated into these cameras. Astigmatic adjustments are also unavailable. It also is difficult for the photographer who does not have stereopsis to take full advantage of this technology.

Advanced Techniques

STEREO BASE LIMITATIONS

The stereo base, the distance to the subject, and the relative depth of the subject are all important factors when photographing in stereo. To produce realistic stereo, the stereo base should be about one-thirtieth of the distance from the lens to the near-point of the subject. This rule is founded on the assumption that the photograph has a far point at infinity, but it is not applicable to fundus photography, since the far point in a fundus photograph is only about 25 mm away. Thus, for example, patients with high elevations of neovascular complexes that extend into the vitreous may produce images with relatively distant far-points. Also, retinal detachments are often located anterior to the normal fundus location and therefore you may need to decrease the stereo base to create visually fusible stereo images.

INCREASING DEPTH-OF-FIELD

Ocular pathology may exceed the depth-of-field of fundus cameras. Sequential stereo photography can be used to increase the depth-of-field by combining two images that are focused at slightly different planes of focus[19] (Figure 3-17). This is called high-low (differential) focusing. When working with a subject that is concave, like the cupping of a deep optic nerve, select one view to be focused high and one view to be focused low. Decide whether the right or left image will have the best "view" of the bottom of the optic nerve. That image should be focused deep. The other image should be focused at the rim of the cup. An elevated subject (e.g., tumor) may have a better side to show with the lower focused image.

There is a limit to the amount of image blur that can be fused to create a clear stereo image. Stereo image pairs with an out-of-focus zone between the two images will be difficult to fuse. There must be enough clear common points-of-image information for image fusion to take place.

Once the film is processed and returned, it is very important that you review your work. Unfortunately, during alignment and photography, the brain does a marvelous job of registering even a marginal stereo image, and you may be astonished to find, on occasion, that one-half of your image pair is of low quality. Constantly check your work and refine your technique.

STEREO ORIENTATION

The shape of the pathology is important when determining the appropriate stereo orientation for the photograph. If all of the elevation is in the vertical cross section (Figure 3-18A), little stereo information will be gained if the images are taken with the conventional left/right stereo orientation. For the best stereo view through an indirect ophthalmoscope,

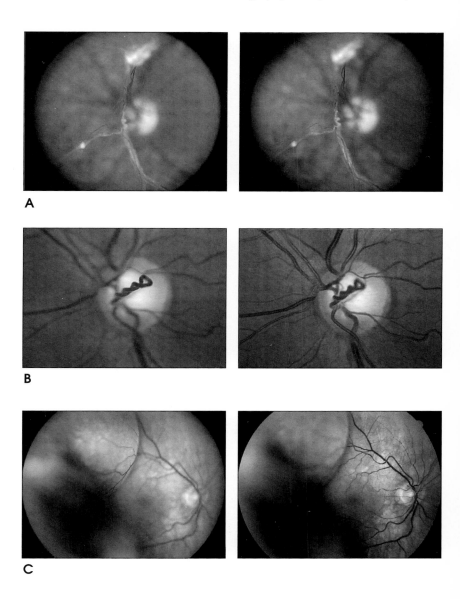

FIGURE 3-17
Differential focusing. Less visual information is conveyed when the focus is adjusted for a single plane (A) than when two different planes are in focus (B). This technique is less effective when the focusing planes are far apart and without commonality (C).

you would need to tilt your head 90 degrees in either direction. This same stereo view can be photographed by modifying your stereo technique.

Rather than shifting the camera laterally, shift it in the up-down direction using the camera elevation control. The resultant photographs can then be rotated 90 degrees and viewed as if you had rotated your head when examining the patient (Figure 3-18C). Slides should be labeled to reflect the photographic method used.

STEREO WITH HIGH MAGNIFICATION AND WIDE-FIELD FUNDUS CAMERAS
High-magnification and wide-field fundus images can be taken in stereo, but the wide-field fundus images may show less depth effect, since the image is recorded at a lower subject-to-film magnification.

The green alignment dots on some Canon wide-field fundus cameras can simplify camera positioning for stereo photography. These dots are located at nine and three o'clock and are normally used for monocular camera alignment. The basic principle is that the green dots replace the

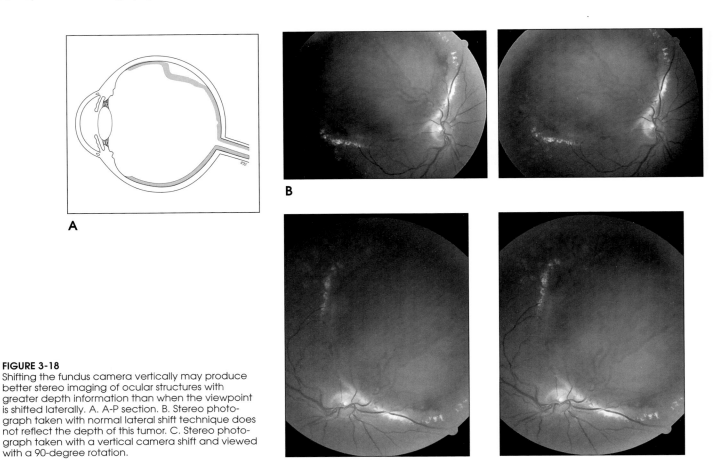

FIGURE 3-18
Shifting the fundus camera vertically may produce better stereo imaging of ocular structures with greater depth information than when the viewpoint is shifted laterally. A. A-P section. B. Stereo photograph taken with normal lateral shift technique does not reflect the depth of this tumor. C. Stereo photograph taken with a vertical camera shift and viewed with a 90-degree rotation.

crescent reflections that are seen on 30-degree cameras. First align the dots for a standard monocular fundus photograph with both dots showing. Move the camera left until the nine o'clock dot disappears and then shoot. Then shift right until you see both dots, continue until you just see the three o'clock dot, and shoot again. This will give the maximal stereo base while maintaining evenly illuminated fields.

Assessing Stereo Images

Once stereo images are exposed and processed, they must be prepared for viewing. This section discusses (1) the different stereo slide formats, (2) the editing process and viewing strategies for the individual, and (3) how stereo images can be viewed by groups of people.

Stereo Slide Formats

In the pictorial stereo photography world, there are many stereo slide formats.[20] Fortunately, only a few transparency (slide) formats are used in ophthalmology. Formats include two full 35-mm frames (two 2 × 2 mounts), split-frame 35 mm (two half-frame images mounted into a single 2 × 2 mount), Realist formats, and Viewmaster disks (Table 3-2 and Figure 3-19). There are many other stereo slide formats, including those for 6- × 7-cm format cameras, but the two 35-mm formats are the ones

Table 3-2. Camera Formats and Some of the Ophthalmic Cameras That Use Them

Format	Image Size (Width × Height)	Fundus Camera
6 perf.	28.5 × 23 mm	Donaldson*
5 perf.	23.5 × 23 mm	Realist
Full-frame 35 mm	36 × 24 mm (22-mm diameter active image)	Zeiss 30-degree
Split-frame 35 mm	18 × 24 mm	Nidek, Topcon, Zeiss

*41 × 101 mm (1⅝ × 4 inches) mounts.

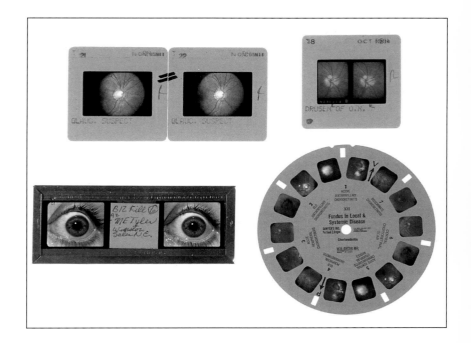

FIGURE 3-19
Photograph of various stereo slide formats: two 2 × 2 35-mm slides, split-frame 35-mm slide mount, Realist stereo slide mount, and Viewmaster disk.

most commonly used in ophthalmology. For more information about other stereo formats, see the manufacturers list in the appendix.[20]

Except for photographic competition entries and specially designed stereo projection systems, we suggest using 2 × 2 mounts to store, view, and project your stereo slides. This choice permits the easy projection of a single monocular frame for conventional (nonstereo) projection. Realist mounts require labor-intensive mounting procedures, and there are no split-frame 35-mm stereo projectors currently being manufactured. Separate 2 × 2 slides are easy to reposition if alignment is not optimal.

The easiest filing solution is to use split-frame stereo pairs mounted in conventional 2 × 2 slide mounts. These are ready-to-go stereo pairs. Make sure that the film processing laboratory understands that these are stereo images and that two similar images are to be mounted in one standard mount. Occasionally a lab will mount 36 stereo images as 72 half-frame 2 × 2 slide mounts. Sending with the unprocessed film a correctly mounted sample slide or explanatory note can help to avoid confusion.

REALIST MOUNTS
Donaldson fundus[16] and anterior segment cameras use a variation of the Realist mounting system. The frame width of the images from the Donaldson stereo fundus camera is less than the 36-mm frame width of standard 35-mm slides, which is 28.5 mm. Realist mounts are known as the "6-P" or "6-perf." format, after the width of the image that was six perforations on the 35-mm film. ANSI Standard PH 1.14-1990 shows a

perf.-to-perf. distance of 4.75 mm. The "standard" Realist mount is a 5-perf. width.

The Donaldson camera images are exposed in groups of two stereo pairs (four images). The film is wound in a shorter distance after the first pair of images than after the second pair. The pairs are laid out in the following order: #2-R, #1-R, #2-L, #1-L (remember the camera inverts the image). These cameras require special 2 × 2 slide mounts, which have a narrower aperture than full-frame 35-mm slides (6-perf., 28.5 mm wide × 23 mm high).

The common 5-perf. size of Realist mount obscures a bit of the left and right sides of the actual image area from a 30-degree Zeiss fundus camera.

VIEWMASTER

A common stereo format from the 1950s was the Viewmaster reel. These disks hold seven stereo pairs of transparencies (10.5 mm × 11.7 mm image area). Handheld viewers are still available in toy stores. They permit viewing one pair of images at a time when you hold the viewer up to a light source. These disks are still used as a distribution format for ophthalmic books that include stereo images.[21, 22]

Editing Stereo Images

Selecting only the best quality images of each view helps maintain a medical record of the highest quality. Selecting appropriate images is easier when stereo images are photographed using a standard sequence, as noted previously. The slides can simply be placed in a standard slide page with the stereo images paired together. All processed stereo images should be checked by the photographer to ensure that the images are properly aligned and the stereo-depth relationships are correct—i.e., the retinal blood vessels are seen in front of the choroid and optic nerve cupping is seen as a depression (not as an elevation). It is important to be familiar with the normal and abnormal retinal pathology because it is relatively easy to trick an inexperienced viewer into perceiving a depression where there is in fact an elevation, or vice versa. Only the best pairs should be saved and labeled as stereo. Adequate monocular images may be kept, but not marked as stereo. A photographer without stereo perception can take excellent stereo photographs with standard monocular cameras since stereo vision is not required to use a monocular camera.

Mounting in Realist Mounts

Stereo slide mounting guides have numerous horizontal lines for checking the vertical placement of the slide frames. They are also useful for checking for any rotation that has occurred between exposures. Note that there are vertical lines for adjusting the stereo window. Place corresponding parts of each slide over the same horizontal line and the vertical lines. Use the far line under the most distant subject in your slides (Figure 3-20).

SORTING STEREO SLIDES WITHOUT STEREO PERCEPTION

There is no substitution for binocular vision when studying stereo images. It is necessary to have two images fused into one for you to actually see in three dimensions. This does not mean, however, that binocular vision is required to shoot stereo, nor to identify stereo pairs. While it is not possible to "see" stereopsis if you have monocular vision, it is possible to predict with some reliability whether two slides will constitute

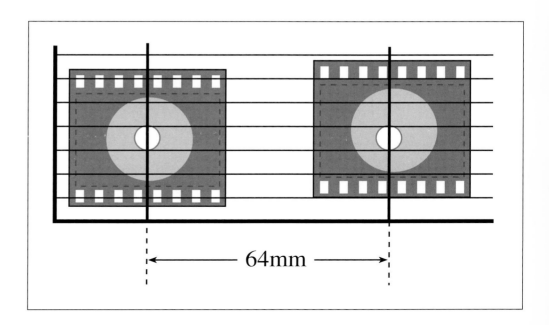

FIGURE 3-20
Grid for aligning stereo images into Realist slide mounts using 64-mm spacing.

a stereo pair. Also, with some knowledge of eye anatomy, the left and right images may be identified. Working at a light box and using a loupe, lay the two slides on top of each other. Look for lateral deviation of structures (typically vessels) in the superimposed images. If there is a deviation, then the two images will form a stereo pair. Usually, the greater the degree of deviation, the greater the stereopsis.

The following procedure is based on a left-to-right stereo technique (shooting the left image first, then shifting laterally to shoot the right image). When using this left-to-right technique, the left image takes the left position and the right image takes the right position in the slide sheet. This technique is not essential, but establishing a routine when shooting stereo adds to the predictability factor and eases the identification process. Also, when superimposing the image by overlaying slides, the slide mounts *must* be lined up precisely over each other without overlap.

First, lay the presumed left image (slide) of an attempted stereo pair on a light box. Take the presumed right image (slide) of the pair and lay it precisely over the left image so that the slide mounts line up exactly on all four sides. Second, using a loupe, carefully observe the superimposed image—see if the top image deviates to the right of the bottom image. When elevation or thickening has been documented, lay the right image (right half of the pair) over the left image (left half of the pair) and look for a deviation of the top image to the right.

When cupping or depression has been documented, the top image should deviate to the left. If you orient the slides so that the right deviating image is the top image and place it in the "right half" position of the slide sheet, the depression or cupping will actually look as if it is coming toward you, instead of falling away! To determine which is the left image, try to identify a structure that is deep (posterior) in the image. This "deep" structure will be laterally to the left on the left slide.

This monocular technique for identifying stereo pairs can be tedious and time consuming. It will, however, enable the photographer who is monocular or unable to see in stereo to orient the slides properly into stereo pairs.

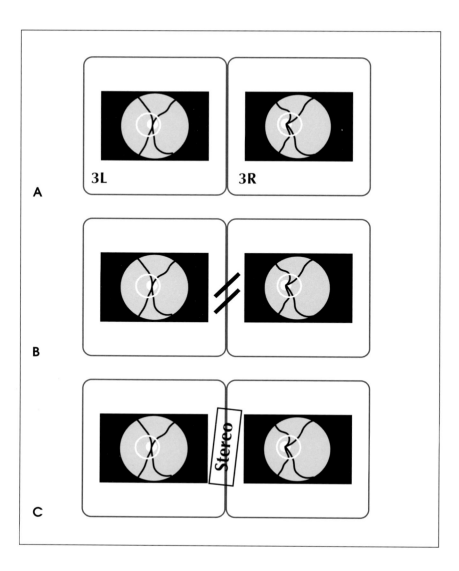

FIGURE 3-21
Labeling conventions for indicating stereo on the pairs of 2 × 2 slides. Slide pairs labeled with sequential pair numbers and L & R (A), a simple set of lines (B), or a rubber stamp with the word stereo (C).

Labeling of Stereo Slides

Stereo slides should be edited, marked, and placed into the chart so that they are easily identifiable. This is very helpful to the clinician.

Marking of the stereo pairs can be accomplished using a variety of methods. Pairs for a particular patient from each visit can be numbered sequentially and identified as to whether the individual image is the left or the right image (Figure 3-21). If the slides are not to be removed from the plastic slide pages, then a simple line[23] or a pair of lines may be used to indicate stereo pairs. The word *stereo* can be written or rubber stamped between the two slides. Avoid time-wasting mix-ups due to not marking your stereo pairs; pick a method and use it consistently.

Viewing Stereo Images

Stereo images may be viewed by an individual or a group. The following section on individual viewing discusses dual 2 × 2 transparencies, split-frame 35-mm transparencies, Realist mounts, Viewmaster transparencies, and lenticular transparencies. Several methods of viewing

FIGURE 3-22
2 × 2 slide viewer. A. Standard 2 × 2 stereo viewers allow you to lay two 35-mm slides side by side on a light table to view them in stereo. B. The best viewers have high-quality, two-element glass lenses, a comfortable PD, and ample space for your nose.

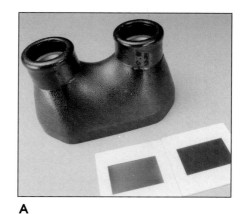

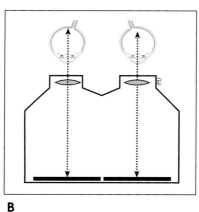

A **B**

paper prints, lenticular prints, and Vect-O-Grams are covered, as is stereo viewing of computer images. The section on group viewing outlines various projection systems and equipment requirements and their use.

Personal Viewing

Personal viewing techniques fall into two categories based on image size: images that are smaller and images that are larger than the average interpupillary distance (PD) of about 60 mm. Of the two techniques that allow you to view stereo images without viewing paraphernalia, parallel viewing requires that you accommodate your focus without converging your eyes, and the other requires that you overconverge your eyes (cross-eye) to achieve stereopsis. All other techniques require optical devices to assist you in seeing the stereo images.[24]

2 × 2 STEREO SLIDES

The most commonly used stereo viewing techniques in ophthalmology are for viewing two full-frame 35-mm stereo slides. The slide that was taken through the left side of the pupil is so positioned in the viewer that it can be viewed by your left eye, and the right image is so positioned that it can be viewed by your right eye. Most stereo slide viewers have a pair of +4 to +12 diopters lenses (see the manufacturers list in Appendix C.) This permits you to relax your accommodation and avoid convergence. A few viewers use compound lenses to reduce distortion and increase sharpness. Once the two images are seen as one, you can adjust the focus with either a focusing adjustment or by physically changing the distance between the slides and the lenses (Figure 3-22). For extensive viewing, you might consider having an optical shop make you some +10 glasses.

If you have a large amount of accommodation and/or are myopic, you may not need a viewer. Simply place the slides, side by side (or with a space between the slide mounts up to 10 mm) on a light table and orient your eyes exactly perpendicular to the center of the slides. Using a sloping light box may make it easier to position your head and eyes properly. Place your face very close to the slides and relax your convergence by imagining that you are looking far into space. Allow both images to overlap and become one image. Do not be concerned about image sharpness at this point. Rather, keep your eyes perpendicular to the two slides and slowly move your head away from the slides to a distance of 6–12 inches, while attempting to focus on the slides without losing the single image and having it become two images. If you see two separate images, you are

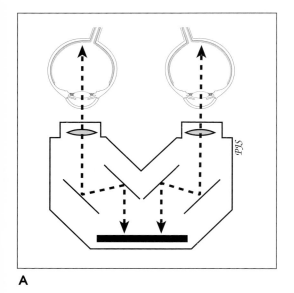

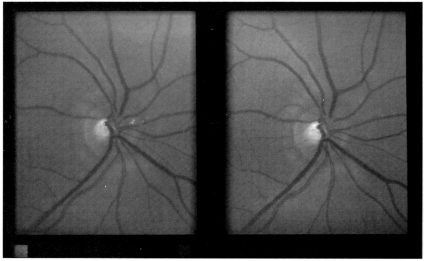

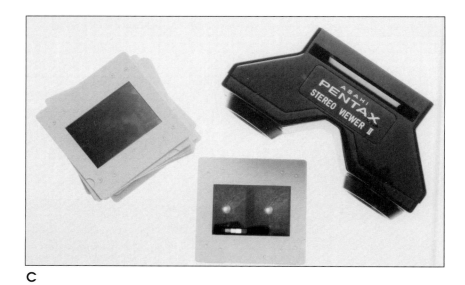

FIGURE 3-23
Split-frame 35-mm stereo slide. A. Schematic drawing showing the optical paths. B. Split-frame stereo slide. C. Photograph of split-frame stereo viewer.

moving back from the slides too quickly and your eyes are converging. Relax and try again. Viewing stereo slides cannot be practiced in a rush! With practice, you may be able to grab a slide page out of a chart, hold it up to a light source, and view the images in stereo. The key phrase is, *with practice*.

SPLIT-FRAME 35-MM STEREO SLIDES

Split-frame (sometimes mistakenly called half-frame) stereo images have two vertical images displayed on a single 35-mm slide frame (Figure 3-23). Most camera systems produce slides with the left image on the left, but a few systems produce slides with the image that is to be viewed with the left eye placed on the right side of the slide. Consequently, there are two types of split-frame stereo viewers. If you get a viewer with the wrong configuration of optics for the slides you are producing, you will get stereoscopically reversed images—e.g., disk cupping will be presented as an elevation.

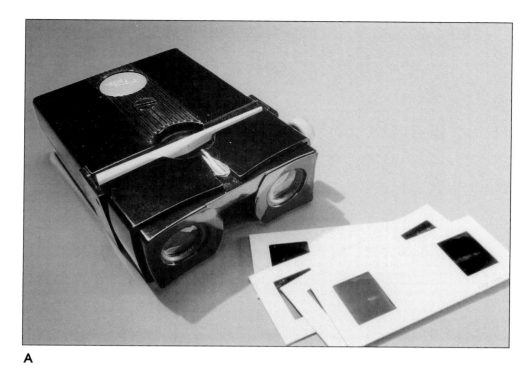

A

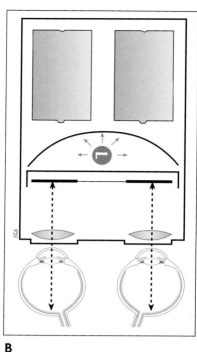

B

FIGURE 3-24
A. Realist battery-operated viewer. B. Schematic drawing of viewer.

REALIST STEREO SLIDES

Realist stereo slide mounts can be viewed with a set of plus lenses, in a single stereo pair viewer (Figure 3-24), or a drum viewer that holds 18 stereo pairs. Currently, these drum viewers are no longer available except on the used market.

VIEWMASTER REELS

Viewmaster reels are often used to illustrate ophthalmic textbooks, usually with foldout viewers. However, purchasing a higher quality viewer is well worth the investment. Even a toystore viewer will out-perform the folding viewers (Figure 3-25).

Computer Images

The dynamic range and color saturation are very good on computer screens. Stereo images can be displayed on the monitor or printed on paper (from the computer image file), the same as for the standard viewing systems as noted above. Side-by-side (small), side-by-side (over 60-mm), and red-blue images are useful viewing methods. Monitor resolution is a limitation, since it is less than one-tenth that of 35-mm slide pairs. Zooming the image on the monitor may help to overcome the limits of screen resolution.

Stereo viewing *hoods* can be used to cover the monitor and provide the appropriate optics to aid in seeing side-by-side images (Figure 3-26). Over-under image pairs are viewed with a different mirror configuration.

Red-blue stereo glasses may bring back memories of comic books and grade-B movies, but in ophthalmic photography, they have some very good applications. Since our angiographic images are usually viewed as monochrome (gray-scale) images, it is possible to color one of the two stereo images red and the other blue, display them on a color computer screen, and view them through red-blue glasses. The left

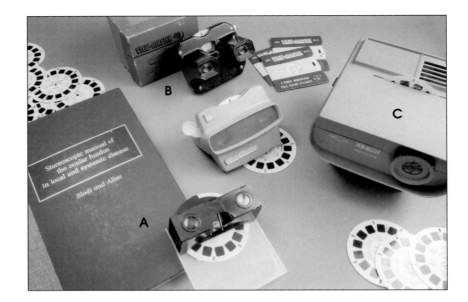

FIGURE 3-25
Viewers for Viewmaster reels showing a foldout-type supplied in textbooks (A), two commercial viewers (B), and a nonstereo projector (C).

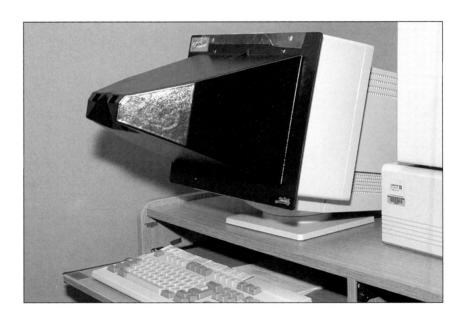

FIGURE 3-26
Stereo viewing hood for a computer monitor.

image is typically colored red and is viewed through a red lens in front of your left eye. The right eye has a blue (and sometimes cyan or even green) filter, and since such a filter does not pass very much red light, your right eye will not see the left image (and vice versa). An advantage of the red-blue system is that your head position (rotation) is not critical. It is also an inexpensive way to view the images.

Color stereo images may be combined into a single color image that is viewed with red-blue glasses. Specialized computer programs (e.g., 3D Maker by Synthonics; see the manufacturers list in Appendix C) make this task easier. While this software works well for angiograms and images that have a full spectrum of colors, the effect on the mostly red fundus images is not as good.

Software that both stores the aligned stereo images and allows their printing on paper or onto slide film is useful.

Computers can use other viewing systems that are not possible with either prints or slides. These techniques require electronically controlled

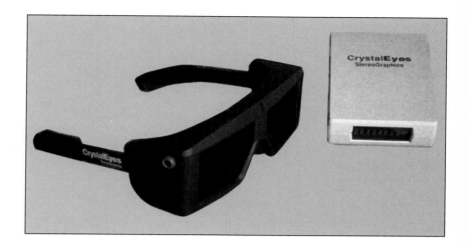

FIGURE 3-27
LCD glasses used with a computer-controlled monitor to display color stereo images. (Courtesy of StereoGraphics, Inc.)

Stereo in Publications

Below are sample instructions that you might use to convey your stereo reproduction needs to the publisher and your explanatory text for the viewer:

INSTRUCTIONS TO THE PUBLISHER:
This figure is a stereo pair. The two images, while they may appear similar, are different. The figure has been submitted to you precisely and correctly aligned so that the readers can view the image in stereo (three-dimension). Exact sizing must be followed in order to have the image viewable by the greatest number of readers. The image must be run at 100%, so that the final images will be reproduced as two 55-mm–wide (2-inch or 12-pica) squares with a 4-mm (⅙-inch or 1-pica) gap between the images. Please include the two black dots that are positioned directly over the exact center of each image. These are important aids to assist readers in viewing this image. *Caution: under no circumstances should you strip the two images separately or reverse their placement, as that will destroy the scientific integrity of the image.*

INSTRUCTIONS TO THE READER:
These two images comprise a stereo pair. When viewed properly you will see a three-dimensional view of the subject. To do this, you must look at the left image with your left eye and the right image with your right eye. The following steps may assist you in viewing this stereo image:

1. Use stereo viewing glasses of +5 to +8 diopters.

2. Situate yourself in a comfortable viewing position with good lighting on the stereo image.

3. With both the print and your eyes level, place the image very close (2 inches) to your face with the left image in front of your left eye and the right image in front of your right eye. You should see a single out-of-focus image.

4. Slowly increase the distance between your eyes and the image until you see a sharp stereo image.

glasses. In one technique, the computer alternately displays the images comprising the stereo pair at a rate of at least 30 images per second, and the image is viewed on a single screen by a person wearing computer-controlled liquid crystal device (LCD) glasses. The stereo images are first processed to create two half-height images, one over the other. An electronic device is inserted between the computer and the monitor and displays the two images alternately. This control box sends out an infrared timing signal to the LCD glasses to control the opacity of the lenses. The LCDs have the ability to turn opacity on and off and therefore permit the two stereo images to be sequentially viewed through the appropriate eye (Figure 3-27).

Another system uses a polarized LCD panel placed over the computer monitor screen while the person viewing it wears standard polarized stereo glasses. With this system, the glasses must be horizontal to create maximal image extinction, the same as for stereo slide projection. The glasses are inexpensive, so this system may be useful if a large audience is involved.

Prints and Publications

While prints are not commonly used to view stereo images in a clinical setting, there are a variety of viewing methods that may be available to see the stereo images found in publications.[25] An understanding of these viewing methods will assist you in selecting the appropriate publishing method for stereo images and will allow you to tell the person reviewing your images how to look at them. It is important to be able to inform the publication's editor and printer of size requirements for easy viewing.

A commonly used stereo printing method involves two images printed just less than 2 inches in width with a small space between them (see the sidebar on stereo in publications). It is important to make sure that the distance between common points on the stereo images is not greater than the average PD of 60 mm. A good working rule is that each of the images should be no wider than 55 mm. If you have a narrow PD or the printer has made the prints too large for convenient viewing, then you can use base-out prisms, one for each eye to assist in viewing (Figure 3-28A).

Some stereo magazines print larger images to increase image sharpness. To assist in viewing, they often include a set of +4.0, 8-D base-out prism viewing glasses with each subscription. These glasses are also useful for viewing stereo images that are each 60- to 90-mm wide.

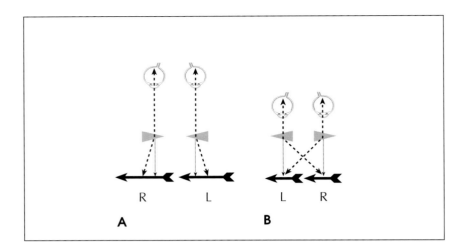

FIGURE 3-28
Print viewing with pairs of prisms. Prisms can be helpful when viewing stereo print pairs. A. Use base-out prisms, 4 diopter, when viewing prints wider than 60 mm. B. Use base-in prisms to assist in cross-eyed viewing.

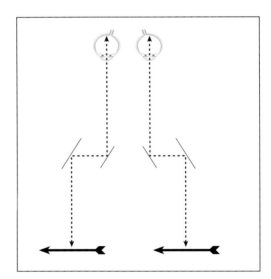

FIGURE 3-29
Schematic drawing of a Brewster stereoscope. Four mirrors are used to increase the viewer's pupillary distance (PD).

Usually the left image is on the left and the right is on the right, but if the images have been printed in reverse, you must cross your eyes to see stereo with the proper depth relationships. The cross-eyed method prohibits the easy use of magnifying lenses and makes it difficult for some individuals to fuse the images. There also is some image distortion, since some parts of the image are farther away from the eye than the center of the image. If you cannot cross your eyes sufficiently for free viewing, try base-in prisms to imitate cross-eyed viewing of large prints (Figure 3-28B).

Larger prints may require an optical device to align your eyes with the images. Base-out prisms are useful only if the images are relatively small (see Figure 3-28A). If the images are larger, try a mirrored viewer (Figure 3-29).

SINGLE-MIRROR VIEWING
A unique printing technique requires just a single mirror to view the stereo image (Figure 3-30). As usual, the image for the left eye is on the left and that for the right eye is on the right, but the right image is printed as a left-right reversed image. Follow this viewing technique: The right image is reversed with a mirror that is placed vertically in front of your nose with the reflecting side toward the right. Look directly at the left image with your left eye and with your right eye also try to view the left image. If the mirror is aligned properly, you will view the reversed

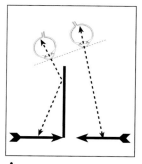
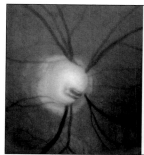
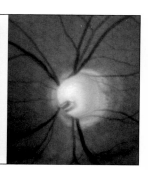

A   B

FIGURE 3-30
A. Use a single, small mirror for viewing an image pair when one of the images is left-right reversed. B. The right image has been printed in a "mirrored" version. For correct viewing of the print, a mirror must be used to interrupt the vision of your right eye.

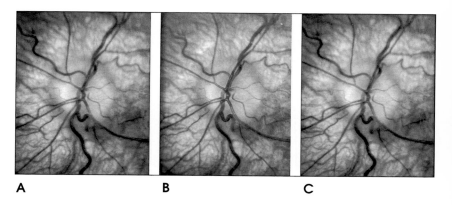

A   B   C

FIGURE 3-31
Set of three images for stereo viewing. Images A and B may be viewed using the parallel technique; images B and C may be viewed using the cross-eyed technique.

right image through the mirror. Fusing these two views reveals a stereo image. The only catch is that either the right image must be printed slightly larger or you must lean your head to the right so that both image paths are the same length.

THREE-IMAGE SET

An interesting approach is to provide three images: L, R, and L. The first two images are paired for "parallel" viewing and the second and third images are paired for cross-eyed viewing (Figure 3-31).

It is important that you purchase the proper equipment to view large-print stereo images (see the manufacturers list in Appendix C). I know of one experienced ophthalmic photographer who prided himself in being able to free-view large prints using the cross-eyed method. He did this for many years and later in life acquired double vision whenever he was tired.

OVER-UNDER PRINTS

The over-under prints method allows you to perceive stereo with two stacked horizontal images. The viewer contains multiple mirrors that are precisely set for a specific print size and a specific stereo separation. If you are interested in this format, obtain the viewer first and then create your images to fit it.

VECTOGRAPHS

Single prints that can be viewed without lenses or mirrors make viewing easier for people who have difficulty fusing images that may not be optimally aligned. The Titmus stereo fly test is an example of the Vectograph viewing system, which uses two superimposed and polarized images viewed through polarized glasses (Figure 3-32).

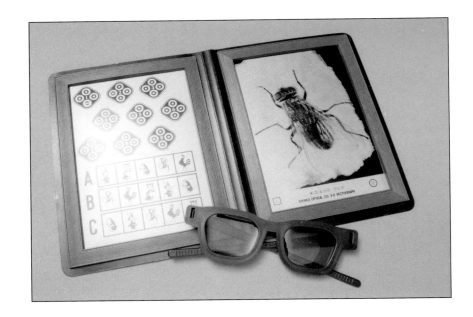

FIGURE 3-32
Vectographs are viewed using polarized glasses. A common vectograph is the Titmus fly test.

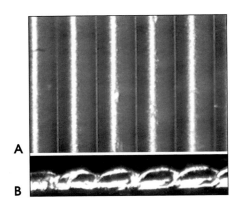

FIGURE 3-33
Photomicrograph (75×) of a lenticular print. A. Front view. B. Cross section.

LENTICULAR PRINTS

Lenticular prints require no viewing aids: no mirrors, lenses, or glasses! The two stereo images are created in alternating thin vertical strips, which are cemented behind a series of lenses. The lenticular lens permits both of your eyes to see the many small vertical slices of an image. Your left eye sees the left image and your right eye sees the right image (Figure 3-33). The width of each individual lenticular lens determines the horizontal resolution of the image. The image resolution on the small lenticular prints is 180 lenses per inch (Lentec—see the manufacturers and suppliers list in Appendix C). Each lens has an image pair behind it. A 4- × 3-inch print of an optic nerve will not provide as much information as a stereo pair of 35-mm slides, due to the resolution limitation of the number of lenses used to create the image.

Lenticular prints and transparencies can be made into poster-size images. One lenticular print has been used on the cover of the *Journal of Ophthalmic Photography*.[26] This image was created using a Nidek 3Dx simultaneous stereo camera, and the split-frame stereo image was reproduced by Lentec, Inc.

RED-BLUE GLASSES

Printing monochromatic stereo images as a single color image lets most viewers perceive stereo image with red-blue glasses (Figure 3-34). The left

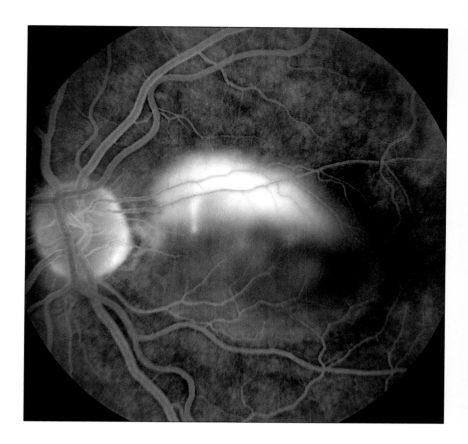

FIGURE 3-34
Bicolor stereo image viewing. A stereo fluorescein angiogram to be viewed with red-blue stereo glasses.

image is printed in red and the right in blue. Red-blue stereo allows images to be printed larger, thus presenting more information than small side-by-side images. Computer programs may also be used to create red-blue images from full-color images (see previous discussion on computer images). This technique is not often used because of the expense of color printing.

Group Viewing

The key principle of stereo projection is the same as other stereo viewing strategies. Each eye must be presented with an individual image. Stereo projection in ophthalmology is most commonly performed with two polarized images projected on a single lenticular screen. Other seldom-used alternatives include projecting two separate side-by-side images or projecting two black-and-white images through red and blue filters.

Slide Mounting

If stereo pairs are projected, you have responsibilities to the audience. The audience members do not have the option of repositioning the slides to permit fusing of the images. For audience comfort and ease of stereo fusion, you should ensure that the images are aligned perfectly in the slide mounts. You do not need to view this in stereo. You will need a light table with a grid for checking similar image points on two images. The grid must have like points under each of the stereo images (see Figure 3-20). Position the mounts so that the slides are aligned on the grid horizontally. Use the grids to ensure that identical points in both images are positioned similarly on the grid. Obviously the two images are slightly different since they are stereo images, but aligning the majority of image points will work well. After the images are aligned, tape the properly positioned slide film in place and finish the slide mounting.

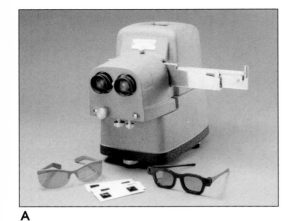

A

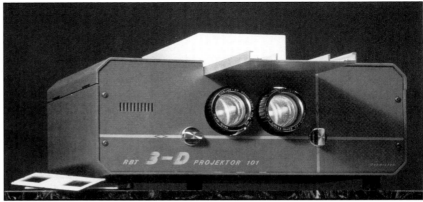

B

FIGURE 3-35
Two stereo slide projectors with internal polarizing filters. A. Realist dual lens projector. B. RBT stereo projector. C. One of the two 35-mm projectors with
external polarizing filters used for stereo projection.

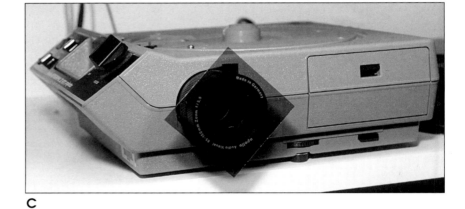

C

EQUIPMENT AND TECHNIQUE FOR POLARIZED STEREO PROJECTION

Polarized image projection can be performed either with specialized
stereo projectors (requiring Realist mounted slides) or with two standard
2×2 slide projectors with polarizing filters over the lenses (Figure 3-35).

Specialized stereo slide projectors use a specialized two-lens configuration and Realist-size stereo slide mounts. The projector permits horizontal and vertical image positioning, as well as focusing adjustments.
The Realist projector is no longer manufactured but is available on the
used market.

Satisfactory stereo projection can be obtained with two standard 2×2
slide projectors, polarizing filters, proper screens, and polarizing glasses.
Polarizing filters reduce the amount of projected light. The light level is
further reduced by the polarizing glasses, making it important to use
bright projectors for stereo projection. We prefer the optics in the Kodak
Ektagraphic projectors, because (1) they deliver more light than the
equivalent Carousel models, (2) modification of their light sources can
further increase the screen brightness, and (3) they precisely align the
slides horizontally, while the Carousel models do not.

Polarizing filters (e.g., Polaroid #HN38) are mounted in front of the
projection lenses of standard 2×2 slide projectors. The rotational orientation of these filters is crucial to successful stereo projection. These filters, like stereo glasses, must be oriented 90 degrees from each other.

The projectors should be positioned next to each other (side-by-side
or stacked) and on axis with the projection screen. Use two identical,

nonstereo slides for preliminary alignment. The edges of the mount should be projected clearly, with an image of a grid of vertical and horizontal lines. A pair of slides of an Amsler grid is an ideal subject. Creating two slides, one photographed through a red filter and the other through a blue filter, will help you keep track of each image while you are aligning the projectors. Align the images on top of each other, adjust the zoom for identical image size, level the slides with the projector feet, fine-tune the vertical and horizontal adjustments, and finally, recheck the magnification.

To align the polarizing filters, first put on a pair of polarized stereo viewing glasses. While projecting the right image on the screen, view the image with your *left* (wrong) eye. The glasses must be placed squarely on your face, and your head should be held level. Why view the right image with the left eye? Because it creates the minimal amount of light for the wrong image to reach an eye. Rotate the filter for maximal extinction. It is important to get maximal reduction of image brightness for the image that is not to be seen. Repeat the procedure for the other filter with the other eye. Doublecheck your work by viewing the right image with your left eye and vice versa. Recheck for maximal extinction. Do not be confused if the filters appear to be set at 45-degree angles, as the filters in the glasses are typically set at 45 degrees to each side of vertical.

The projectionist plays an important role in ensuring that the audience will have a great viewing experience. A good projectionist can make a great session; a poor projectionist can ruin the show. All stereo images are not created equal; camera-subject alignment, camera rotation, and slide mounting are just a few of the variables. The projectionist is like an airplane pilot. The pilot can safely navigate a pleasant trip around a storm, at the same time presenting the passengers with a great view. Or the pilot can fly straight through the storm and hope that not too many people get sick. Poor stereo projection and motion sickness are similar—neither is very pleasant.

The projectionist may need to do some touch-up alignment with each pair of projected images. If the projectors are mounted in multimedia racks, the adjustments will be smooth. Marks on the adjustment knobs will permit you to return the projector to its primary calibrated position while switching to the next stereo image. A good projectionist will remind the audience to take a break for a few seconds between images to permit him or her to check the alignment of the next pair of images.

Remove your stereo glasses when you align the images. You will need to see both images to position one on top of the other. The central portions of the subject should overlap. If mounting is imperfect, ignore the frame edges and adjust the projectors for maximal subject overlap. Vertical alignment is critical. Horizontal alignment can, to a greater degree, be overcome by the audience, so set the vertical first and then bring the images together horizontally.

The horizontal position of the images will place the image in space— that is, at the screen, in front of the screen, or behind the screen. Review the information in the stereo mounting section about positioning the stereo window.

Because the projection screen must not disrupt the orientation of the polarized light from the projectors, silverized screens are used. Lenticular silverized screens reflect brighter images for audience members who are seated to the side of the projection axis (Figure 3-36). Glass-beaded screens, the most common type of projection screen, will reorient the polarized nature of the light from the projectors and thus will not produce stereo images.

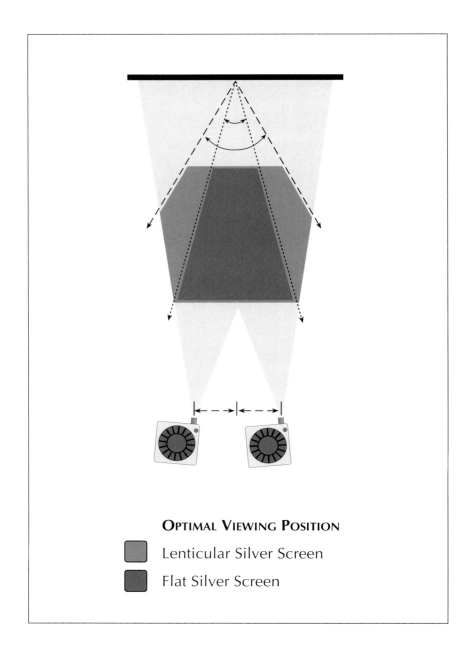

OPTIMAL VIEWING POSITION

Lenticular Silver Screen

Flat Silver Screen

FIGURE 3-36
Viewing angles for stereo projection screens.
Silverized projection screens and their acceptable
viewing angles.

OTHER PROJECTION OPTIONS
Split-frame stereo images could be projected through a specially
equipped "dual lens" 2 × 2 projector. This lens assembly produces two
overlapping images, which are filtered with polarizing filters.

Two images can be projected side by side, either in a split-frame format or by two separate 2 × 2 slide projectors. These are the same techniques used to look at side-by-side images in print or on a computer
screen. Viewing of these images can be accomplished in one of two ways.
If the images are placed with the image for the right eye on the left screen,
and vice versa, then those viewing them must cross their eyes while
maintaining focus in the distance. A pair of base-in prisms helps many
viewers. If the images are oriented with the image for the right eye on the
right and so forth, then base-out prisms are used to assist in viewing the
images. These images are referred to as being for "wall-eyed" viewing.

Future of Stereo Imaging in Ophthalmology

The value of the two images that comprise a stereo pair is truly greater than the sum of the parts. The additional information provided by stereo imaging should not be underestimated. In the changing medical community, the ability of the clinician to obtain medical advice without the consultants having to see the patient will play an important role in future ophthalmic photography. With computer network capabilities, the ability to access a stereo view of the fundus of a patient in a remote location may become an accepted practice.

Simultaneous stereo camera images taken with reproducible stereo techniques permit computer analysis of these images. Through optic nerve analysis, the diagnosis of glaucoma may become possible even before functional field loss is manifested. Thus, the ability to photograph stereo images is a crucial skill. The ophthalmic photographer must have complete understanding and control of the theories and practices of ophthalmic stereo photography in order to ensure the ultimate care for the patient.

References

1. Julesz B. *The Foundations of Cyclopean Perception.* Chicago: The University of Chicago Press, 1971.
2. Tychsen L. Binocular Vision. In W Hart Jr (ed), *Adler's Physiology of the Eye: Clinical Application* (9th ed). St. Louis: Mosby-Year Book, 1992;773.
3. Von Noorden GK. *Binocular Vision and Ocular Motility: Theory and Management of Strabismus* (4th ed). St Louis: Mosby, 1990.
4. Jones J. *Wonders of the Stereoscope.* New York: Knopf, 1976;14.
5. Darrah WC. *The World of Stereographs.* Gettysburg, PA: W. C. Hannah, 1977;2.
6. Morgan H, Symmes D. *Amazing 3D.* Boston: Little, Brown, 1982;10.
7. Oatman EL. *Diagnostics of the Fundus Oculi.* Troy, NY: Southworth, 1913;1.
8. Thorner W. Die stereoskopische photographie des augenhintesgrundes. *Klin Monatsbl f Augenh* 1909;47:481.
9. Metzger E. Die stereophotographie des augenhintesgrundes. *Klin Monatsbl f Augenh* 1927;78:338.
10. Bedell AJ. *Photographs of the Fundus Oculi.* Philadelphia: Davis, 1929;1.
11. Bothman L, Bennett RW. *Fundus Atlas— Stereoscopic Photographs of the Fundus Oculi.* Chicago: Year Book, 1939;1.
12. Stenstrom WJ. A modification of the new Zeiss fundus camera. *Arch Ophthal* 1960;64:935.
13. Allen L. Ocular fundus photography. *Am J Ophthalmol* 1964;57:13.
14. Norton HJ. Absolute three dimensional collared retinal photographs. *Trans Am Acad Ophthalmol* 1953;57:612.
15. Norton HJ. Absolute electronic retinal stereophotography. *Am J Ophthalmol* 1947;40:808.
16. Donaldson D. A new camera for stereoscopic fundus photography. *Trans Am Acad Ophthalmol* 1964;62:429.
17. Bussy BJ, Mittelman D. Use of the astigmatism correction device on the Zeiss fundus camera for peripheral retinal photography. *Int Ophthalmol Clin* 1976;16:2.
18. Tyler ME. Stereo sequence programmer for retinal fluorescein angiography. *J Biol Photographic Assoc* 1977;45:19.
19. Tyler ME. High-low focusing to increase depth of field. OPS annual meeting, 1977.
20. 3D-Web. 3D Frequently Asked Questions, 1996. HTTP://www.3D-web.com/3dfag.htm
21. Blodi FC, Allen L. *Stereoscopic Manual of the Ocular Fundus in Local and Systemic Disease.* St Louis: Mosby, 1964;1.
22. Gass JM. *Stereoscopic Atlas of Macular Diseases: Diagnosis and Treatment* (3rd ed). Vol 1. St. Louis: Mosby, 1987;1.
23. Walker BP. Photographic filing systems. *Int Ophthalmol Clin* 1976;16:2.
24. Merin L. Construction and use of stereo viewers. *J Ophthal Photog* 1981;4:39.
25. Ferwerda JG. *The World of 3-D, A Practical Guide to Stereo Photography.* Borger, The Netherlands: 3-D Book Productions, 1987.
26. Tyler M. Cover: lenticular print of optic disk edema. *J Ophthal Photog* 1993;15:1.

Chapter 4

Fluorescein Sodium and Indocyanine Green: Uses and Side Effects

Paula F. Morris

Introduction

Angiography is a diagnostic tool used to reveal circulation characteristics. Ocular angiography documents certain ocular pathologies using either of the biological stains, fluorescein sodium and indocyanine green. To better understand the different types of ocular angiography, this chapter discusses these two dyes—their origins and mechanisms, how they are used, and the consequences of their use.

Angiography as a Diagnostic Tool

Angiography has had a place in the diagnosis and treatment of pathologies involving circulation since 1919, when Heuser first performed an angiogram on a living person.[1] Before the discovery of x-rays by Wilhelm Roentgen in November 1895, studies of the circulatory system had been done without being able to observe the actual pattern of blood flow. In January 1896, Haschek and Lindenthal performed an angiogram on a cadaver hand by injecting a chalk-like substance into a vein. It took 57 minutes of x-ray exposure to produce the picture.[1]

By injecting a marker (an indicator) into the bloodstream and using appropriate equipment to image it, the presence or absence of blood flow and its pattern can be determined. This is helpful in determining the caliber of vessels, detecting circulation blockage, and observing circulation patterns in ischemia or neovascularization.

As angiography is a study of circulation, it can be performed anywhere there are vessels to be imaged. Fortunately for ophthalmic patients, angiography of the eye is less physically invasive and uses simpler equipment than angiography of the rest of the body, which requires x-rays and radio-opaque agents.

Nonocular Angiography

Usually, nonocular angiography is performed as the patient lies down on a support table, using cardiac monitoring equipment and an *imaging chain*.[2] The imaging chain consists of a generator/cine pulse system, an x-ray tube, an image intensifier, an optical distributor, a 35-mm cine camera, a television camera and monitor, and a gantry. The angiographic room must be large enough to adequately house this equipment. Also, most x-ray imaging room walls must be shielded with 1 mm of lead up to a height of 7 ft and must have windows of lead-treated glass to protect personnel[3] (Figure 4-1).

In contrast, an ocular angiography patient routinely sits on a stool or chair. Retinal angiography requires a fundus camera with a 35-mm film camera back, while choroidal angiography requires a fundus camera with an infra-red digital imaging system. In either case, special shielding of personnel and patient is unnecessary because no x-ray radiation is involved, and the procedures can be performed in any area of reasonable size to accommodate the patient, the camera, and the photographer.

In nonocular angiography, the radio-opaque agents, called *contrast agents*, are based on iodine. Organic iodine is an excellent opaque medium because of its high atomic number and chemical versatility and because it is less toxic than inorganic iodine. Currently, nonionic iodine-based agents with medium osmolality characteristics and low-osmolality contrast materials (LOCMs) are gaining in popularity because they improve patient comfort and lower the incidence of side effects.[4] (Osmolality refers to the number of particles in a given volume of solution, which affects the ability of a solution to permeate through membranes to equalize its concentration.)

Nonocular angiography is accomplished radiologically by generating x-rays and directing them through the area of the body being studied. It exposes patients and operators to the highest radiation levels of any x-ray studies.[5] For this reason, the number of radio-opaque angiograms a patient can receive may be limited. A maximum number of procedures per patient is now being investigated. Most of the incident radiation is absorbed by the patient, with less than 1% of the radiation passing through the body to the image intensifier. The rest of the incident radia-

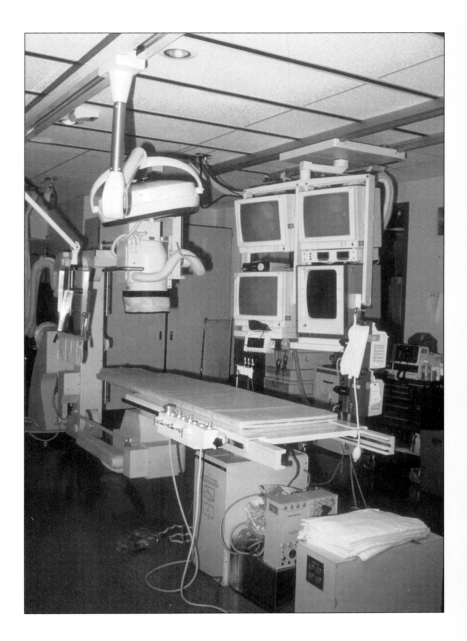

FIGURE 4-1
Nonocular angiography. The imaging chain needed to record nonocular angiographic images consists of a generator/cine pulse system, an x-ray tube, an image intensifier, an optical distributor, a cine camera, a television camera, a monitor, a gantry, and a table. (Courtesy of Michael Palczgnski.)

tion scatters back into the room where the people conducting the test may be exposed. Because the x-ray tube is located beneath the support table, most of the scatter radiation is directed back to the floor. Shielding methods are used to protect parts of the patient's anatomy and to reduce the operator's scatter dose of radiation.

When a radio-opaque agent is present in the bloodstream, it blocks the transmission of the x-rays to the image recording system and provides the contrast that delineates the vessels. Materials that are dense are less transparent, and radio-opaque agents are very dense because of their high molecular weight.

In nonocular angiography, the contrast agent can be introduced to the bloodstream in various ways, depending on what part of the anatomy needs to be studied and the patient's physical condition. Some techniques are more invasive than others, but all involve exposing arteries

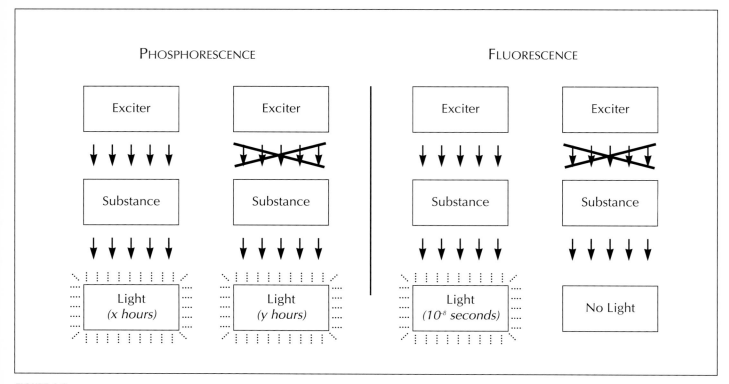

FIGURE 4-2
Types and durations of luminescence. Luminescent materials may be categorized as either phosphorescent or fluorescent. A properly exposed substance with phosphorescent properties will continue to emit light for hours after the exciter is taken away. A properly exposed substance with fluorescent properties will only emit light in the presence of the exciter.

and veins so that catheters can be inserted and the introduction of the contrast agent can be controlled and directed to the study area. The large branches of the circulatory tree—the femoral artery or the brachial artery—are most frequently used.[6]

To produce a nonocular angiogram, a catheter is threaded to the appropriate site and the contrast material is released in a bolus. The agent circulates through the vessels to be studied and then moves on, quickly becoming dilute and losing its ability to be imaged. Many boli of the contrast agent are introduced in the course of a nonocular angiogram, resulting in a large amount of dye being used, sometimes exceeding volumes of 100 ml.

Ocular Angiography

Ocular angiography is accomplished photographically through a dilated pupil, recording fluorescent light waves emitted from the dye present in the bloodstream. Fluorescence is one of two kinds of light emission called luminescence, the other being phosphorescence (Figure 4-2). Photo-luminescence occurs when certain substances are exposed to short-wave electromagnetic radiation and the substances absorb energy. This excites the molecules of the substance to a higher energy state. As the molecules return to their original state, they emit a longer wave length radiation, or they luminesce.[7] Fluorescence is short-lived, occurring during excitation and stopping 10^{-8} seconds after the exciting stimulus is removed. Phosphorescence is a delayed light emission that continues for periods of time after the exciting stimulus is

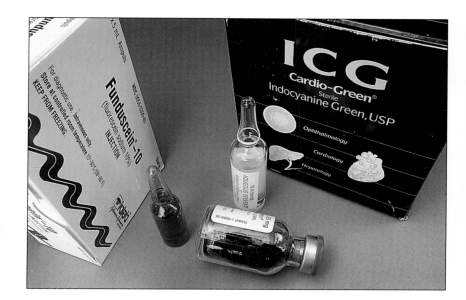

FIGURE 4-3
Types of ocular angiographic dyes. Vials of fluorescein sodium and indocyanine green dye as prepared by the manufacturers. The fluorescein sodium is ready for use, but the indocyanine green must be combined with the accompanying saline solution before injection. Both dyes have fluorescent properties.

removed, as in a child's "glow-in-the-dark" toy. Fluorescein sodium and indocyanine green both have fluorescent properties, and their emissions can be recorded on photographic film or electronic sensors. Excitation is supplied by light from the flash tube passing through excitation filters.

In a normal eye, no tissues obscure the view of the posterior pole vascular system. Because of the unique anatomy of the eye, light from the camera can be directed through the transparent cornea, through the pupil and lens, to shine directly on the retina. The light then travels back along the same pathway to the camera's film plane. The dye can be injected into the bloodstream via any vein and travels along the venous system to the heart, flows through the cardiopulmonary circuit, then up the carotid arteries, to the ophthalmic arteries, where some will circulate through the choroid and some will course through the central retinal artery to the retina.

Dyes Used in Ocular Angiography

Fluorescein sodium and indocyanine green (ICG) are the primary dyes used to perform ocular angiography (Figure 4-3). They do not have similar chemical configurations and are not of the same chemical "families." While they both have fluorescent properties, fluorescein sodium has much stronger fluorescence abilities. ICG contains a small amount of sodium iodide, but it is not radio-opaque and is used in ocular angiography because of its fluorescent properties.

Interestingly, while the retina and choroid of the eye are intimately associated, their circulatory characteristics are very different, as are methods for performing angiography of each. It is not surprising, then, that the dyes used to accomplish these studies are very different as well. Because of these differences, this chapter discusses each of these dyes individually.

Before describing the unique characteristics of these dyes and clearing up some misconceptions, it is valuable to explain some basics about biological stains.

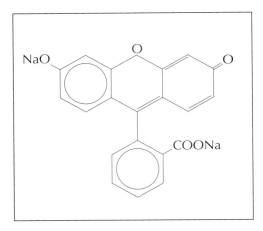

FIGURE 4-4
Molecular diagram of fluorescein sodium.

Biological dyes are colored substances used to help reveal the gross and microscopic structure and nature of plant and animal tissue.[8] Manufacturers of dyes give them two classifications: natural and synthetic. Natural dyes are mineral or plant products. Because of their natural impurities, which cannot be controlled, they are decreasing in use because they cannot be certified for use in drugs and cosmetics. Synthetic dyes are manufactured dyes produced through chemical reactions. The first synthetic dyes were derived from aniline, a derivative of coal tar. Synthetic dyes used in drugs, cosmetics, and food are assigned identifying food, drugs, and cosmetics (F, D, & C) and color index (CI) numbers by the Federal Color Standards Directory.

The color of a dye is determined by its chemical configuration in combination with its *chromophore*. Chromophores are carbon rings with double bonds involving carbon, oxygen, and nitrogen that are associated with color. Dye groups based on their color are classified by similar chemical structure. Chromophores alone do not dictate color, as identical chromophores can be found in all the colors of the rainbow.[9]

Fluorescein Sodium (Resorcinolphthalein Sodium)

Fluorescein sodium ($C_2OH_{10}Na_2O_5$) (Figure 4-4), or resorcinophthalein sodium, is the biological dye used to perform retinal angiography. In drug supply catalogs, it is called uranin or uranine yellow. It is the disodium salt of the biological dye fluorescein ($C_2OH_{12}O_5$), also called eosin.

There are some misconceptions associated with the dye fluorescein (eosin), including the mislabeling of retinal angiography. Fluorescein is *not* the dye used in retinal angiography. We use the salt fluorescein sodium.

According to its chemical structure, fluorescein is in the xanthene dye group. There are three classes of xanthene dyes: fluorenes, rhodols, and fluorones. Fluorones (hydroxyxanthenes) are called the fluorescein derivatives as fluorescein has the simplest chemical structure of the group. Other members of the fluorone group used in medicine are rose bengal and mercurochrome.[10]

Fluorescein was first synthesized by Adolf Baeyer in 1871 as a derivative of the dye gallein.[11] It produced a bright yellow color and was intended for use in dying wool and silk. As fluorescein is *insoluble in* water, benzene, chloroform, and ether, Baeyer used hot alcohol to make the textile dye.

Table 4-1. Comparing Fluorescein and Fluorescein Sodium

	Fluorescein	Fluorescein Sodium
Chemical name	Resorcinolphthalein	Resorcinolphthalein sodium
Common name	Eosine	Uranine yellow
Chemical formula	$C_2OH_{12}O_5$	$C_2OH_{10}Na_2O_5$
Dye description	CI Solvent yellow 94 CI 45340 F, D, & C yellow #7	CI ACID yellow 73 CI 45340 F, D, & C yellow #8
Physical characteristics	Yellowish red to red powder Insoluble in water, benzene, chloroform, ether Soluble in hot alcohol, glacial acetic acid, alkali derivatives	Orange-red powder Freely soluble in water

CI = color index (assigned by the Color Standards Directory); F, D, & C = food, drug, and cosmetic (assigned by the FDA).

Because fluorescein cannot dissolve in water, it cannot be used in a solution that is compatible with injection into the human body. Fluorescein sodium, however, is freely soluble in water—thus, its use in retinal angiography. Because of the practically universal use of the term "fluorescein angiography," it is not reasonable to try to correct the mislabeling, but it is valuable to know that there is a difference (Table 4-1).

WHAT IS FLUORESCEIN SODIUM?

Another misconception about fluorescein sodium is its origin. It has been mistakenly described to patients as a "sugar-based" dye, a vegetable dye, and a seaweed extract, and in some of the ophthalmic literature it is listed as a plant resin.[12, 13] Actually, it comes from a mineral. Its primary component is naphthalene or tar camphor, which is the most abundant component of the carbolic acid fraction of distilled coal tar.[14] Naphthalene's most famous use is as the odor for moth balls! It is also used to manufacture indigo dye, solvents, lamp black, and celluloids. That fluorescein sodium does not occur naturally but is actually a synthetic is reinforced by its assigned F, D, & C, and CI color standard numbers.

To synthesize fluorescein sodium (Figure 4-5), naphthalene is oxidized in the presence of the catalysts mercury sulfate and copper sulfate (used to stabilize the reaction) at 400–500°C to produce phthalic anhydride. Phthalic anhydride is then heated with resorcinol to 200°C to make resorcinolphthalein. Phthalic anhydride is used in producing benzoic acid, phthaleins, synthetic indigo, and artificial resins. Resorcinol is used in manufacturing resins, adhesives, explosives, and cosmetics.

Finally, the yellowish-red powder resorcinolphthalein is dissolved in sodium hydroxide solution, which yields resorcinolphthalein sodium, another name for fluorescein sodium. The drug companies that prepare the fluorescein sodium we use purchase it from chemical supply houses as an orange-red powder that comes in jugs. They purify the powder with heat by autoclaving the jugs with 15 lbs pressure at 250°C. The fluorescein is precipitated out, redissolved in sodium hydroxide solution to make fluorescein sodium, standardized for color and concentration, and adjusted to a pH of 8+, which maximizes its fluorescence.

Several times in the past, manufactured "lots" of intravenous injectable fluorescein sodium have been recalled by drug companies because of contamination by mercury, which can be traced back to improper purification of the fluorescein sodium powder. Remember that the mercury is used

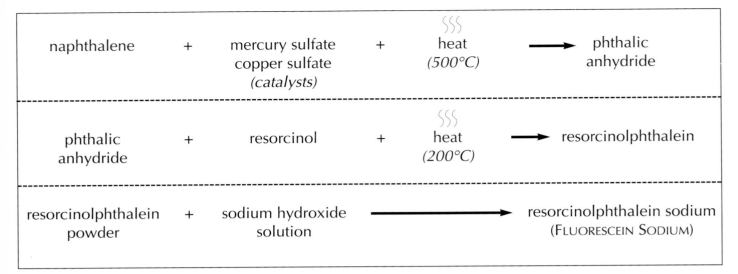

FIGURE 4-5
Fluorescein sodium synthesis.

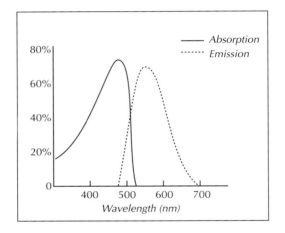

FIGURE 4-6
The absorption and emission spectra of in vitro fluorescein sodium.

in the initial synthesis of phthalic anhydride. Elevated mercury levels in fluorescein are not necessarily an issue in manufacturing industrial products, but they are of critical importance if found in medical supplies.

Fluorescein sodium is highly fluorescent. Its fluorescence is easily visible even in low dilutions. The maximum light absorption and fluorescent excitation of fluorescein sodium is 485–500 nm. Its maximum fluorescence emission is 520–530 nm[15] (Figure 4-6).

When injected into the bloodstream, fluorescein sodium is absorbed by the plasma proteins, particularly the albumins. It is also absorbed by hemoglobin. As this occurs, the intensity of the fluorescence is significantly decreased.[16] The suppression of fluorescence is referred to as *extinction*, and the absorption of fluorescein sodium and resulting loss of fluorescence in the bloodstream is called *extinction by contamination*. This can also occur in the presence of the pyrazolone derivative drugs, such as butazolidin (an anti-inflammatory), and with some iodine compounds.[16] Concentration affects extinction; if a fluorescent material becomes too concentrated, the molecules begin to interact with each

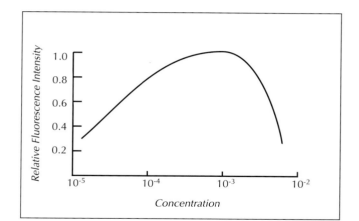

FIGURE 4-7
Fluorescence extinction by concentration. Fluorescence ability can be diminished if too much dye is injected over a short period of time and concentration builds up. (Adapted from A Wessing. Fluoroscein Angiography of the Retina. St. Louis: Mosby, 1969.)

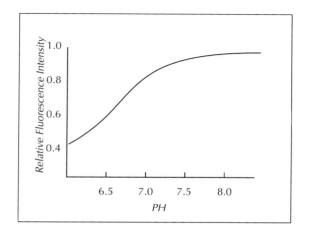

FIGURE 4-8
Fluorescence ability depends on pH value. Fluorescein sodium reaches a maximum fluorescence at pH of 8+. (Adapted from A Wessing. Fluoroscein Angiography of the Retina. St. Louis: Mosby, 1969.)

other, suppressing electron excitation. In fluorescein sodium, increasing the concentration of dye to an excess of 25% results in loss of fluorescence, which is called extinction by concentration[17] (Figure 4-7).

Fluorescence is dependent on pH values. Fortunately, the normal blood pH of 7.38–7.44 allows for almost maximal fluorescence (Figure 4-8).

USES OF FLUORESCEIN SODIUM

The *Merck Index* lists the primary use of fluorescein sodium as examining subterranean waters.[18] It is used to determine the source and volume of springs, to find connections between springs and seas, to detect drinking water contamination sites, and to determine soil contamination by factory waste waters. Fluorescein sodium is the dye used to color the Chicago River green during the annual St. Patrick's Day observance in Chicago (as seen in the 1993 motion picture, "The Fugitive").

Fluorescein sodium has also been approved by the Food and Drug Administration (FDA) for use in manufacturing topical drugs and cosmetics as CI Acid Yellow 73, or D&C Yellow Dye #8. It is used in analytic and clinical reagents for laboratories as a protein label, an immunohistologic stain, and an immunofluorescent label.[18]

Fluorescein sodium was first used in ophthalmology by Erlich in 1881, when he injected the dye into rabbit eyes to observe aqueous

Table 4-2. Fluorescein Sodium Availability and Distribution

Injectable 10%

AK-Fluor (Akorn)	5-ml ampule and vial
Fluorescite (Alcon)	5-ml ampule and syringe
Funduscein-10 (IOLab)	5-ml ampule
Ophthifluor (Deklerht)	5-ml ampule

Injectable 25%

AK-Fluor (Akorn)	2-ml ampule and vial
Fluorescite (Alcon)	2-ml ampule
Funduscein-25 (IOLab)	3-ml ampule

flow.[19] Currently, fluorescein sodium's primary use in ophthalmology is as an external diagnostic aid, combined with topical anesthesia for use in applanation tonometry. It is also used to detect corneal epithelial defects and to assess contact lens fit. Fluorescein sodium for external use is available in a 2% solution form. It is instilled in the cul-de-sac of the lower lid or dried and heat-sterilized on paper strips, which are moistened with sterile water and applied to the conjunctiva in the lower cul-de-sac.[20]

Fluorescein sodium use for retinal angiography is reported last in the frequency of use list. The injectable dye comes in sterile vials or syringes, in concentrations of 10% or 25%. The 10% solution comes in a 5-ml ampule (500 mg), and the 25% solution comes in a 2-ml ampule (250 mg).[21] The dye is not currently available specifically for oral administration. Several pharmaceutical companies prepare fluorescein sodium for ophthalmic use. Table 4-2 lists fluorescein distributors and availability.

Fluorescein Sodium Angiography

Retinal angiography allows the ophthalmologist to study the entire retinal vasculature, not just the larger veins and arteries observable by ophthalmoscopy. The properly filtered fundus camera records fluorescence wherever it is present, including the tiny retinal capillaries. Because the fluorescein sodium reaches the choroidal vasculature (choriocapillaris) approximately 1 second before it reaches the central retinal artery, the field of view brightens or lights up before dye can be seen in the retinal arteries. This effect is known as *choroidal flush*. The fluorescence from the retinal vessels is much brighter than the choroidal fluorescence, which is partially blocked by the retinal pigment epithelium (RPE). In cases in which the RPE is thinned or absent or if something (such as drusen) is present that will transmit choroidal fluorescence to the retina, choroidal fluorescence can be as bright as retinal vessel fluorescence. If retinal vessel fluorescence cannot be seen, either the dye is not present in that area or the fluorescence is being blocked by something between the retina and the camera. The presence of fluorescein sodium can also be documented in vessels in the iris.

To obtain a good retinal angiogram with distinct circulation phases and adequate dye concentration, the dye is injected into the bloodstream in a good bolus (a concentrated mass). The most common injection site is the antecubital space on the medial side (inside) of the arm, in front of the elbow joint. The median cephalic vein, the median basilic vein, and the median cubital veins all run through this area. These are large, superficial veins that are usually visible, palpable, and sufficiently large to handle the injection of a bolus of fluid. A disadvantage of this area is that in some people, the brachial artery may rise just behind the median cephalic vein and run superficially. This increases the possibility of an accidental intra-arterial injection. If it is known ahead of time that the IV line needs to stay in for more than just a few minutes, the antecubital veins should not be used because the patient's arm movement will have to be restricted.

There is a short delay from the time that dye is injected and circulates through the heart and lungs to the time it finally appears in the choroidal and retinal vasculature. This time, referred to as the *arm-to-retina time*, is usually 8–16 seconds, assuming an antecubital injection. Injections made further down the arm or in the hand will take a second or two longer to reach the retina. If the physician is interested in the arm-to-retina time, he or she should be informed of the location of the injection site.

When an antecubital injection is not possible, usually the dorsum (or back) of the hand is the next site considered. The metacarpal veins found there are easily accessible and lie flat on the back of the hand. However, the metacarpal veins are more fragile than the antecubital veins, they may have a smaller caliber, and insertion is more painful because of the large number of nerve endings in the hand.

Another possibility is the accessory cephalic vein, which runs along the radius and is most readily found in close proximity to the bend of the wrist. The vein is usually large and insertion is less painful than in the hand, but it rolls easily and can be hard to stabilize. Also, any movement in the wrist can cause discomfort or cause the needle to be dislodged, which can result in extravasation of dye.

Sometimes an intravenous injection is not possible in the arms or hands, as in patients with impaired circulation, scarring due to burns, damaged vessels due to diabetes, or other extenuating circumstances. Alternate injection sites may include the great saphenous vein of the leg, which is superficial at the internal malleolus (inside ankle bone), or the dorsal veins on the top of the foot. Injection at either site slightly increases the possibility of deep vein thrombosis. Elevating the foot after injection may decrease the delay of dye to the eye if the patient has impaired circulation, but it also may cause undue discomfort to the patient as he or she tries to maintain the position at the camera. Most often, unless the patient is a contortionist, the early phases of the angiogram are sacrificed if the foot is used as an injection site.

Before performing ocular angiography, properly educate your patient about the procedure and also take an appropriate history. Obtaining a history of the patient's previous fluorescein sodium angiographic experiences is of primary importance. Patients who have had previous adverse reactions to fluorescein sodium injections are especially likely to experience them again,[22] and some extra precautions or first aid supplies may be indicated.

Besides reviewing the patient's chart and determining the previous angiographic history, you should ask about general health, drug allergies, and recent episodes of chest pain or respiratory problems. In reference to the impending intravenous injection, questions should include asking the patients if their veins are easy to find, if they have experienced previous difficulty during blood draws, or if they have ever had surgery to their lymphatic system, as happens with a mastectomy. There have been reports of tissue damage when arms without intact lymphatic systems have been injected with fluorescein sodium. Asking the patient to indicate a "favorite" injection site is usually a good idea—the patients know their own history, and it gives them a sense of some control, which lessens their anxiety.

INJECTION TECHNIQUES

Proper injection technique is a learned behavior requiring thorough education. There is controversy in the field of ophthalmic photography over who should inject the fluorescein sodium when performing ocular angiography. Several surveys have been performed, with different results. One survey indicated that of the physicians responding, the majority performed the injections, while others used nurses or other physicians. Few indicated that a photographer performed the injection.[23] However, in a survey of ophthalmic photographers, 24 of 86 respondents reported that they performed the fluorescein sodium injection.[24] In most states it is illegal for anyone who is not a licensed physician or nurse to administer drugs intravenously. In some states it is legal for an unlicensed medical professional to perform venipuncture (insert the needle into the vein) but not push the plunger of the syringe and introduce the dye into the bloodstream.[25] However, some hospitals have policies that are contrary to this finding, and unlicensed personnel are allowed to administer intravenous injections. There are no official universal guidelines that dictate who should perform the injections. Ophthalmic photographers are not licensed as medical professionals and therefore do not meet the specifications stated in the study mentioned above. Some physicians request that their photographers perform intravenous injections anyway. In any scenario, the issue of liability should be considered.

You should find out what the legal ramifications of intravenous injection are in your community and discuss it with your employer. No matter what decision is made, no one should perform venipuncture or intravenous administrations without being IV-certified by a reputable medical education facility. The best scenario allows the photographer to concentrate on the photography while a second person performs the injection and monitors the patient.

The following discussion of IV injection technique is intended to offer basic knowledge of the procedure and not to replace IV certification training. Whether you perform IV injections or not, you should be very familiar with injection protocols and the equipment needed. You should also be knowledgeable about first aid for failed injections, dye side effects, and adverse reactions to the dye. Cardiopulmonary resuscitation (CPR) training is essential for anyone performing ocular angiograms. Ocular angiography is *not* a benign event. It is a very valuable diagnostic procedure but is invasive and carries risks for patients. The risk of possible adverse reactions and complications should be taken seriously by both the physicians ordering the procedure and the photographers performing the study. That the procedure is performed frequently or routinely does not justify a cavalier attitude by the medical personnel involved.

The risks associated with ocular angiography are not limited to the patient. Any time you are exposed to blood or other potentially infectious materials, as in performing venipuncture, you are at risk. The Occupational Safety and Health Administration (OSHA), which is part of the U.S. Department of Labor, is charged with protecting the health and safety of personnel in the workplace. The Occupational Health and Safety Act, Title 29, Chapter XVII, Part 1910, Subpart Z "Toxic and Hazardous Substances", a1910.1030, "Bloodbourne Pathogens" (Dec. 6, 1991), requires that specific precautions be taken to ensure against occupational exposure to and inadequate disposal of potentially infectious materials.[26] This act requires by law that employers provide employees with adequate protection from occupational exposure by providing handwashing facilities, personal protection equipment, engineering controls ("sharps" containers, disposable gloves, etc.), exposure control

Table 4-3. Intravenous Injection Supplies for Fluorescein Angiography

Arm board
To stabilize patient's arm and hand
Tape
For securing needle at injection site
Alcohol swabs
To cleanse the skin around the injection site
3 x 3 gauze pads
To apply to the injection site after the needle is removed or to protect a site that is already prepared
Tourniquet
To restrict venous flow causing veins to become more prominent; a blood pressure cuff may be used instead
Gloves
An OSHA requirement whenever there is potential exposure to blood
Syringe and filter needle/filter straw
To extract fluorescein sodium from vial or ampule
Butterfly infusion set of 21- or 23-gauge needle
To inject fluorescein sodium into vein
3" or 12" tubing connects the needle to the syringe and allows greater flexibility when positioning needle tubing
Less intimidating to patient than a rigid needle/syringe unit
Stopcock
For injecting more than one substance (i.e., fluorescein sodium and indocyanine green or fluorescein sodium and saline)
Sharps container
For proper disposal of needle and syringe; always observe universal precautions
Adhesive bandage
To cover the venipuncture site
Portable lined receptacle
Should a patient become nauseated
Emergency kit
Minimal: oxygen, CPR equipment, antihistamine, smelling salts
Ideal: standard crash cart with above and full complement of injection supplies and emergency medications

plans, employee education, and exposure-incident follow-up. The act also mandates that employees follow strict protocols and methods of compliance for "universal precautions," which include proper hand-washing, proper use and disposal of needles, appropriate use and disposal of gloves and other protective equipment, proper sterile technique, and other precautions in the workplace. Each health care facility, whether a major medical center or private physician's office, must have written procedures for carrying out the OSHA mandates regarding blood-borne pathogens. You should check with your clinic or office manager to get a copy of those procedures and guidelines and then follow them to protect yourself, your coworkers, and your patients.

Injection techniques can vary greatly among facilities, as can the brands and designs of the equipment used. Specific supplies should be dictated by the individual facility, following established IV protocols and procedures. If the facility does not have an existing IV protocol, as may be the case in private offices, state nursing associations or the hospital or surgical center where your ophthalmologist is affiliated can help you obtain copies of IV protocols. In most cases, supplies are chosen by the trained professional performing the injection. In any case, patient safety and comfort should be the first priority in choosing supplies. Table 4-3 lists the supplies needed to perform an efficient, safe IV injection. In thinking through the procedure step-by-step, you can understand the need for each of these items.

As in any medical procedure, sterile technique should be followed. This includes hand washing before assembling the injection supplies, again before donning gloves, and after the procedure is complete. The arm board and the tourniquet or blood pressure cuff that are used should be kept clean as well. All injection supplies should be disposable, and an OSHA-approved sharps container should be within easy reach of the injector for proper disposal of the contaminated needle assembly.

Fluorescein sodium is available in two different concentrations, 500 mg of 10%, and 250 mg of 25%. Which concentration to use is decided by the ophthalmologist and the photographer. The 10% concentration requires that a larger volume of solution be injected, but the dye is more dilute. The 25% solution is a smaller volume, but because the dye is more concentrated, it is theorized that there may be more potential for tissue damage if extravasated. Preparation of the syringe by transferring the dye from the ampule is done when the injection supplies are assembled.

The usual adult dosages are the volumes and concentrations listed above. The usual pediatric dosage is 3.5 mg per lb of body weight, as a 10% solution.[21] Any pediatric dosage should be calculated and approved by a physician or pharmacist.

The chosen syringe should hold 5 ml or greater to accommodate the volume of dye drawn up from the vial. A straight needle of small gauge, a filter needle with a small bevel, or a filter straw should be used to ensure that no small glass shards, which may have fallen into the vial when the neck was broken, will be drawn up into the injection. One pharmaceutical company supplies fluorescein sodium in a specially prepared syringe, ready for injection.[27]

A butterfly infusion set with a needle of 21 or 23 gauge and a cannula of 3 or 12 inches is then attached to the fluorescein sodium syringe. A straight needle or angiocath of the same gauge are alternatives. The size of the needle used depends on the caliber and condition of the patient's veins. You need to take care to protect the patient and avoid extravasation, but also ensure that you will have an adequate bolus for good early phase photographs.

To help ensure that the dye travels through the bloodstream to the ocular circulation in the greatest concentration possible, the bolus of fluorescein sodium can be followed immediately with the injection of 5 ml of normal saline. If this technique is chosen, an IV lock (or stopcock), a sterile adapter which attaches to the butterfly cannula and facilitates additional ports, is used. By using this attachment, several syringes can be added to the line, and several fluids such as fluorescein sodium, saline, or heparin can be injected at different times via the needle inserted in the arm[28] (Figure 4-9). This saves the patient from the discomfort of multiple needlesticks and saves time.

Efficient ocular angiography technique requires that the patient be positioned properly and comfortably at the fundus camera, with the camera and the target eye properly aligned before the needle is inserted. This avoids moving the patient's arm after IV insertion, which may result in dislodging the needle, possibly perforating the vessel. Also, in the case of the Zeiss fundus camera, this eliminates the camera table movement, which may be necessary for proper alignment.

Performing an IV injection is a logical, step-by-step process. First, the injection site is selected and then the site is stabilized using an arm rest. Next, a tourniquet or blood pressure cuff is attached and pressure is applied to restrict the flow of blood from the veins, which makes them more prominent and eases the injection. Sometimes when the veins are small or scarred, they can become more prominent by having the patient make a fist and pump the hand, or hang the arm down by the side and

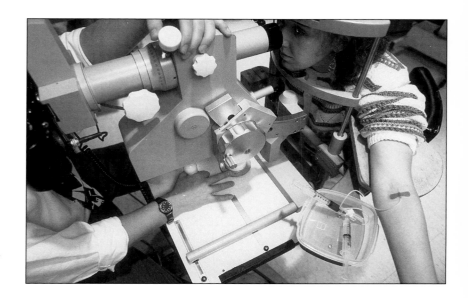

FIGURE 4-9
Multiple-syringe technique. When performing both
retinal and choroidal angiography in the same procedure, syringes of each dye can be connected by
a stopcock, allowing injection of both dyes via one
needle. (Courtesy of William Nyberg.)

swing the arm back and forth. Patting the vein firmly with the fingers
or applying hot packs can assist with vasodilation. These extra efforts
may be helpful or even required when the patient cannot offer an easy
injection target because of diabetes or other circulatory problems. When
the target vein has been chosen, the skin is cleansed with several alcohol preps, using a circular movement around the injection site, which
moves from the center out, or in a "clean skin to dirty skin" pattern.

The needle is then inserted into the target vein with the bevel up, taking care to keep the angle of entry low so the needle does not go completely through the vein. Once the injector feels that the needle is
positioned well within the caliber of the vessel, he or she should draw
back on the syringe plunger gently to look for the presence of blood in
the cannula. Once assured of proper positioning, the blood pressure cuff
or tourniquet pressure is released. Injection should not be attempted until
the pressure is released.

The photographer should signal the start of the injection. The injection
should not begin unless the patient is properly aligned to the camera, or
the early phases of the angiogram may be lost. However, the injection
should start quickly before the needle can be moved accidentally or the
needle bevel clots off. In some patients with poor circulation, as the vessel becomes irritated by the presence of the needle, it may collapse,
resulting in a failed injection. Any attempt to inject fluid into a collapsed
vessel may result in extravasation of dye into the surrounding tissue,
with little dye actually getting into the bloodstream.

In an uncomplicated procedure in which the patient has good target
vessels and no history of previous complications with fluorescein sodium angiography, the needle is removed as soon as the injection is finished. Removing the needle relieves the patient's discomfort and anxiety.
However, if there is a chance that a second IV medication might be needed, such as diphenhydramine (Benadryl) or epinephrine, it is useful to
keep the needle in place to avoid a second needle insertion.

If the needle needs to stay in the vein, the injection of 1 ml of heparin
or a gradual infusion of saline can ensure against the bevel clotting off.
This step is performed when an already in-dwelling IV line is used for
the injection of fluorescein sodium. Using a saline flush will clean
remaining fluorescein sodium out of the in-dwelling line but will not
give the same assurance against clotting that heparin will. Heparin, of

course, should not be used if the patient has clotting problems. The decision to use heparin should be made by a physician before the injection is started.

The speed with which the dye is injected is a source of controversy in the field of ocular angiography. There is little disagreement that the quicker the injection, the more concentrated the dye bolus will be and the better the contrast in the early phases of the study. The differences of opinion lie in whether the speed and pressure of the injection affect the incidence of adverse reactions to the dye. A study indicated that there was a higher incidence of adverse reactions in all fluorescein sodium angiographic patients who receive slower injections (>6 seconds) than with faster injections (2–5 seconds).[29] While this study was not designed specifically to address speed of injection, a formalized, repeatable technique was used by the angiographers participating in the study, and adverse reactions occurred 12 times more frequently with slow injections than with fast injections. Currently, no study has been conducted that specifically addresses all the implications of injection speed. Until such a study has been designed and implemented, the best procedure is to let the patient's physical condition and vessel tolerance dictate the speed of the injection while considering the patient's previous angiographic history and aiming to achieve the best photographic results.

Anecdotally, some angiographers believe that the added volume of the post-dye saline flush may also contribute to nausea. This has not been documented. Others feel that the flush is essential to good dye concentration in the early angiogram phases, since it will flush the dye remaining in the butterfly cannula into the bloodstream. Some feel that it is an unnecessary step that adds expense and time to the procedure. Whether or not the saline flush is used during routine angiography should be a mutual decision between the physician and the angiographer.

Any time the IV line will be used for more than one type of injection, however, a saline flush should be used to clean out the cannula. There has been a case report regarding a potentially serious reaction between two different drugs in an IV cannula.[30] Following injection of fluorescein sodium during an angiogram, the patient rapidly developed hives (urticaria) as an allergic response. Phenergan, an antihistaminic drug, was introduced into the IV syringe, but the remaining fluorescein sodium had not been flushed out. The result was a chemical reaction between the Phenergan, which has an acid pH, and the fluorescein sodium, which has a basic pH. The combination resulted in the precipitation of crystals in the syringe, which blocked the cannula. Fortunately, the crystals were not injected. A new IV line was established at another site to treat the patient's allergic reaction.

Once the injection has been successfully completed and there is no further need for access to the vein, the needle should be removed and the entire injection apparatus immediately discarded into an OSHA-approved sharps container. The needle should be discarded only by the injector to reduce possible exposure of additional personnel to a contaminated needle. Usually an adhesive strip or bandage is all that is necessary to cover the puncture wound. Any excess dye or blood should be wiped off the skin surface. The history taken before the angiogram should alert you to whether the patient is on anticoagulants or has clotting problems. If so, apply pressure to the injection site to aid in clotting and puncture sealing. Any other injection supplies that have been contaminated with blood, such as alcohol preps or gauze sponges, must also be disposed of in an engineering-controlled container such as a sharps container or a doubled, closed disposable bag that complies with the OSHA universal precautions guidelines.

Side Effects and Reactions to Fluorescein Sodium Injections

Drugs and dyes have predictable actions on which we base their use. Fluorescein sodium is used in retinal angiography because of its ability to reveal retinal vasculature with fluorescence and because it is relatively safe to inject into the human body. The fluorescent light emitted by the dye from the retinal and choroidal vessels can be easily documented, then interpreted to determine the presence and possible treatment of ocular pathologies.

Drugs and dyes can have other actions that may not be predictable or desirable. Some of these actions are labeled side effects; some are called adverse reactions. Several studies have been conducted to try to determine the incidence of various adverse reactions to fluorescein sodium, with a wide diversity of results reported. Both retrospective studies, which analyze past occurrences, and prospective studies, which follow a set protocol that looks for specific responses, have been conducted. Because of the difference in their design it is difficult to compare the results of these studies, and it is of little value to state all the percentages reported in each study. What is of value is that all the studies concur in ranking the incidence of these reactions.

SIDE EFFECTS

A drug side effect is a bodily response that is usually predictable and may have a negative impact on the patient. Side effects are transient and do not require follow-up treatment. Fluorescein sodium has several side effects that are very predictable and a few that occur randomly. The product information inserts in each box of fluorescein sodium ampules list common side effects of the drug under the "patient information" heading. As part of the informed consent process, you should educate patients about the predictable side effects of fluorescein sodium.

Some side effects of fluorescein sodium happen 100% of the time. Staining of the skin, sclera, and mucous membranes is the first noticeable side effect. The dye becomes visible as it circulates through the capillaries of those tissues. The discoloration fades within 2–6 hours of the injection and in deeply pigmented individuals may not be very noticeable. Various secretions, including tears and saliva, may also be stained. The patient's urine will be colored orange-yellow and will fluoresce for 24–36 hours after injection. Fluorescein sodium is metabolized in the liver to become fluorescein monoglucuronide, which, along with the excess fluorescein sodium, is excreted exclusively in the urine.[31] Nevertheless, there is no increased frequency of adverse reactions in patients with renal insufficiency or who are on hemodialysis.[31]

The presence of fluorescein sodium in the bloodstream will interfere with some clinical laboratory tests because of its serum concentration.[32] What tests are affected, how long the interference persists, and how to deal with this side effect are discussed later in this chapter.

Other side effects that occur with far less regularity are a "flushing" sensation in the skin, a strong metallic taste in the mouth, tingling of the lips, and sneezing, all of which are transient.

ADVERSE REACTIONS

Adverse reactions are consequences of drug administration that have a negative impact on the patient, may be transient, may require medical intervention, and may lead to death. They have been classified as mild, moderate, severe, and death.[33] These classifications were based on the duration of the reaction, whether medical intervention was required, and whether there were any enduring consequences to the reaction. Also, an attempt was made to determine the frequency of adverse reactions among all patients receiving fluorescein sodium angiography.

Mild Adverse Reactions. Mild adverse reactions include nausea, vomiting, and a vasovagal response resulting in dizziness and lightheadedness. Of all adverse reactions, nausea occurs most frequently. This condition is often accompanied by hypersalivation and gagging, which occurs more frequently than vomiting. The reaction is transient and clears rapidly. It usually begins 30 seconds after the start of the injection and usually only lasts 30–90 seconds. Some photographers instruct their patients to breathe slowly and deeply if they start to feel nauseated, which helps them relax and lessens their anxiety. Some photographers advocate having patients rinse their mouths out with cool water just before the injection. In patients who have experienced more prolonged nausea and/or vomiting with previous fluorescein sodium angiograms, prochlorperazine (Compazine) or promethazine (Phenergan) can be administered either orally or intramuscularly at least 45 minutes before the procedure. In the unusual instance in which nausea is more prolonged, either of the above medications may be helpful.

Vasovagal responses, which are usually evoked by stress or pain, are actions of the vagus nerve that can reduce heart rate and blood pressure. These attacks can respond favorably to the deep breathing technique too. No one knows exactly why nausea occurs, but there is speculation that because fluorescein sodium is very soluble and permeable and has a high pH (8+), it easily crosses the blood-brain barrier and triggers the nausea response through the hypothalamus gland. Some patients who have experienced significant vasovagal response previously may do well with a small dose of diazepam (Valium), given at least 30 minutes before the angiogram. The decision to premedicate patients should be made by the physician, with input from the photographer.

Moderate Adverse Reactions. Moderate adverse reactions include urticaria (hives), syncope (fainting), phlebitis (vascular inflammation), local skin necrosis (death), and localized nerve palsy (paralysis). Urticaria is the second most common adverse reaction, following nausea/vomiting. It is most often a histaminic (allergic) response and should be treated with an antihistamine, such as diphenhydramine (Benadryl) or promethazine. The severity of an allergic reaction is difficult to predict, so medical intervention should be undertaken any time allergic symptoms appear. While it is unusual for a patient to exhibit an allergic response to fluorescein sodium during their first ocular angiogram, some patients may be exposed and become sensitized to the dye when it is used topically during ophthalmic examinations. Any time a patient reports an allergic reaction experienced during a previous fluorescein sodium angiogram, consider medicating with an antihistamine at least 40 minutes before he or she is injected with the dye. Always report a history of fluorescein sodium allergy to the ophthalmologist so he or she can decide what prophylactic measures should be taken to protect the patient, or decide if it is advisable to perform the procedure.

Syncope (fainting) is a strong vasovagal response that is self-limiting and requires first aid, but not necessarily medical intervention. Precautions should be made to protect the patients from injury, lying them in a position that is optimal for good circulation, monitoring their blood pressure, and reassuring them. Depending on their recovery, rescheduling the angiogram for another time when they can be premedicated might be the best option. A physician should assess the patient's general condition before he or she is released from the clinic.

Phlebitis is an inflammation of blood vessels that may occur as a response to the presence of an irritating injection or because the inner wall of the vein has been injured. The symptoms of phlebitis are localized pain at the injection site, redness following the course of the vessel, and pain along the course of the vessel. Phlebitis is usually not diagnosed until at least 24 hours after the injection. Suspicion of phlebitis should be reported to the physician immediately. Phlebitis can be self-limiting, but it also can lead to thrombophlebitis, in which a blood clot is formed in the inflamed vessel. This complication can have far more serious ramifications and requires medical intervention.

Local skin necrosis can occur following extravasation of fluorescein sodium into the skin during an intravenous injection. The high pH of the dye may contribute to the tissue damage. A physician should assess the site any time an extravasation of fluorescein sodium occurs. Have the patient report back the next day after an extravasation so that the condition can be assessed. Any report of edema, redness, or pain should prompt a physical examination of the extravasation site. Medical intervention is required if there is evidence of tissue damage or deterioration.

Nerve palsy can occur if a nerve receives trauma during an intravenous injection. The nerve can be damaged by the needle, or it can be damaged by increased pressure caused by extravasation of dye or blood, resulting in ischemia. Nerve palsies are usually self-limiting, but assessment must be made by a physician about whether medical intervention is indicated.

Severe Adverse Reactions.   Severe adverse reactions involve the respiratory, neurologic, and cardiac systems. All require immediate intervention, all threaten the patient's safety, and all can ultimately result in death. Respiratory reactions include laryngeal edema, bronchospasm, and anaphylaxis. Neurologic reactions are tonic-clonic seizures, and cardiac reactions include circulatory shock, myocardial infarction, and cardiac arrest.

Respiratory reactions may present as difficulty breathing or talking or loss of consciousness. A tonic-clonic seizure is characterized by involuntary movements, heightened muscle tone and muscle spasm, respiratory distress, increased blood pressure, and loss of consciousness. Cardiac symptoms may include chest and radiating arm pain, sweating, increased blood pressure, decreased blood pressure, difficulty breathing, cardiac arrhythmias, loss of consciousness, cessation of breathing, and cardiac arrest.

Although severe adverse reactions are rare, emergency medical supplies, including oxygen, drugs, injection supplies, and CPR equipment should be immediately available anywhere fluorescein sodium angiography is performed (Figure 4-10 and Table 4-4). Everyone performing fluorescein angiography should be trained in basic CPR, and emergency medical personnel should be available immediately. These precautions argue that fluorescein sodium angiography should *not* be performed unless medical personnel are readily available. In a hospital setting, an emergency code should be called in the event of a severe adverse reaction. In a private office that is free-standing from an emergency response facility, strict protocols for how an emergency team can be summoned must be established. You should never perform a fluorescein sodium angiogram unless there are additional people present who can summon help in case you have to perform CPR.

In the classification of adverse reactions, death was attributed to intravenous fluorescein sodium if it occurred within 48 hours of the injection.

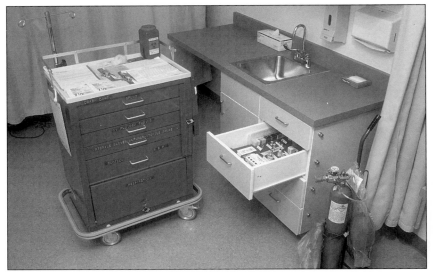

A

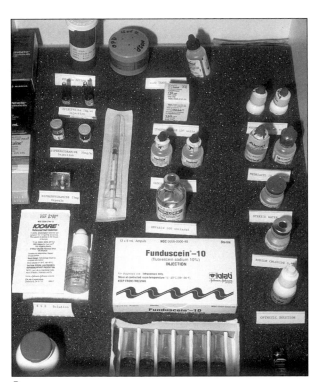

B

FIGURE 4-10
Medical emergency and first aid supplies. Adverse reactions to fluorescein sodium can range from death to severe life-threatening medical emergencies to mild discomfort. A. A "crash cart" containing basic life support supplies should be kept in close proximity to where angiography is performed. B. This drawer containing drugs used in performing ocular photography or first aid has been arranged for easy access and easy identification. (Courtesy of Michael Palczynski.)

The Fluorescein Angiography Complication Survey reported death occurring in 1 of 222,000 ocular angiograms.

COMPLICATIONS OF FAILED INJECTIONS
There are complications arising from failed IV injection attempts that are not considered to be adverse reactions caused by the presence of the dye in the bloodstream. They can occur when proper IV technique is not followed, or if the target vessel is compromised and cannot facilitate the

Table 4-4. Emergency Supplies for Fluorescein Angiography

General medical equipment
  Stethoscope
  Sphygmomanometer (blood pressure cuff)
  Portable oxygen
  Tourniquet
  Alcohol wipes
  Adhesive tape
  Engineering-controlled receptacle (sharps container)
  Ambubag
  Oxygen masks (adult and pediatric)
  Resuscitation mask (cushioned)
  1-cc tuberculin syringes
  5-cc syringes
  Adhesive bandages
  Gloves
Drugs
  Acetaminophen, 500 mg, for analgesia
  Aromatic ammonia inhalants ("smelling salts") for fainting
  Diphenhydramine, 25-mg capsules, and diphenhydramine, 50-mg injection, for allergic reactions
  Epinephrine, 1 mg/ml injection, for allergic reactions
  Promethazine, 25-mg capsules, for nausea
  Nitroglycerin, 0.4 mg (1/150 gr) sublingual tablets, for angina
  Hyaluronidase, 150 units injection, for subcutaneous injections around extravasations
  Heparin, 100 units/ml injection, for maintaining in-dwelling lines
  Sterile water for preparing injections
Food supplies for blood sugar imbalances
  Unsweetened fruit juice
  Graham crackers
  Saltine crackers
  Granulated sugar
  Hard candy

infusion of the injection. In any case, care must be taken to ensure that a failed attempt does not result in a complication.

The most common complication of failed injection is the extravasation of blood or dye out of the vein and into the surrounding tissue. The extravasation of blood can occur when too large a needle is used and it penetrates completely through the vessel, or if compression to the site is not applied after the needle is removed. The resulting hematoma (bruise) can be painful and may also exert pressure on surrounding nerves, causing nerve palsy. Patients taking anticoagulants, including aspirin, or who have clotting problems are at increased risk of hematoma.

A related complication of failed injection is the extravasation of fluorescein sodium. Because of its high pH, the dye is very irritating to surrounding tissues, and, as stated above, can result in skin necrosis. All of the precautions mentioned in the IV injection discussion should be followed. Increased resistance to the plunger of the syringe should signal the injector to stop the infusion and assess the needle position. Although it is helpful for the photographer to have the lights lowered when visualizing the fundus during the early phases of the angiogram, there should be sufficient light to adequately assess how the injection is going. Some offices use "mini" lights or flashlights to illuminate the injection site. When you orient the patient before the injection, tell the patient to inform you immediately if he or she begins to experience any stinging or burning around the injection site. If there is a question of extravasation, needle placement should be assessed, and, most often, the needle should be removed and a new injection site should be selected.

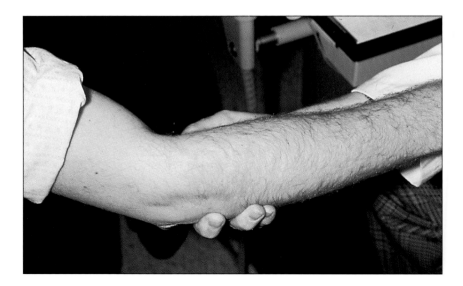

FIGURE 4-11
An intra-arterial injection. Dye has been accidentally injected into an artery and the bolus has flowed away from the heart, into the hand. The dye will stay concentrated in the lower arm and hand, which can result in intense pain. (Courtesy of Csaba Martonyi.)

If the dye is extravasated out of the target vein, the needle should be removed and some of the offending dye may be coaxed out of the needle puncture wound by applying light pressure around the puncture, in much the same way that blood is coaxed out after a digital (finger) blood draw. Although cold packs applied to the extravasation site offer pain relief, warm packs are suggested. The heat may slightly increase the immediate pain, but it will also dilate the capillaries and allow the extravasated dye to diffuse out and become less concentrated. This may be especially important in patients with poor circulation or fragile skin, such as the elderly. The warm packs should be applied for 3–5 minutes. After the dye has diffused out, cold packs can be applied for pain relief. The use of multiple small injections of the enzyme hyaluronidase (Wydase) around the injection site to improve absorption of the dye has also been recommended. Analgesia may be indicated to relieve discomfort. The patient's status should be checked 24 hours after the extravasation.

A less frequent but potentially serious complication of a failed injection attempt is accidental intra-arterial injection.[34] Injection of fluorescein sodium into an artery results in the dye circulating away from the heart, into the distal peripheral capillaries of the arm. This results in increased pressure sensation and, in some patients, intense pain. The arm below the injection site becomes intensely yellow in patches where the undiluted dye has been circulated (Figure 4-11).

Although arteries usually lie deeper in the arm and pulsate, 10–13% of the population have ulnar arteries that are unusually placed and run superficially next to the basilic vein.[35] When a needle has been placed in a vessel, the plunger of the syringe should be drawn back and the blood in the cannula should be checked. Venous blood is dark red in appearance, but arterial blood is bright red because of its oxygen content.

First aid for intra-arterial injection may include plunging the affected area into cold water for pain relief, as well as administering analgesics. A physician should be summoned immediately to assess the patient's condition and determine what analgesia is appropriate. A successful retinal angiogram with concentrated, observable dye in early phases is not possible as the dye has been deposited in tissues fed by the injected artery. The patient should be closely followed for several days after the injection.

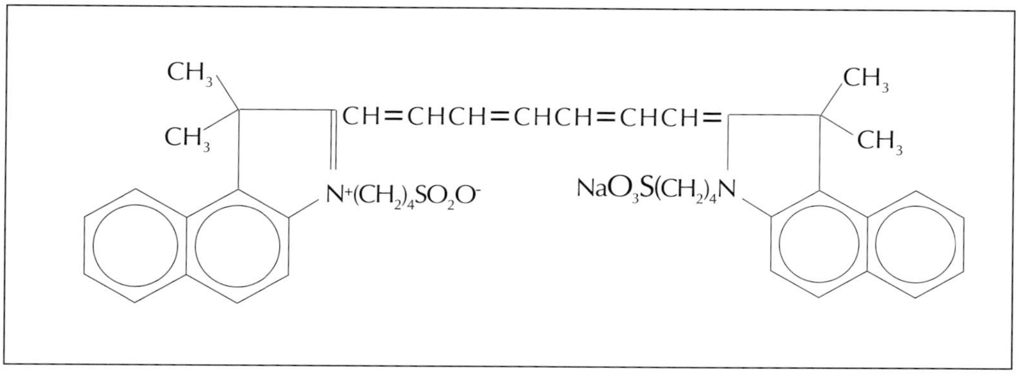

FIGURE 4-12
A molecular diagram of indocyanine green.

SPECIAL CONSIDERATIONS

Patients who require special caution during intravenous injections include elderly patients with senile skin changes (thin skin due to loss of collagen and adipose tissue), patients with impaired circulation such as diabetics, patients with blood abnormalities, patients with impaired or absent lymphatic systems such as mastectomy patients, and patients who are dehydrated or underweight. (An intravenous injection nightmare would be an anorexic, diabetic teenage girl.)

Fluorescein sodium angiography is contraindicated in patients who are pregnant and in juvenile asthmatics and should be used with caution in patients with a previous history of severe adverse reactions to the dye and patients who have a recent history of chest pain or cardiac irregularities. It is not contraindicated in nursing mothers, although the dye has been found in mother's milk, nor is it contraindicated in patients on hemodialysis or in renal failure.

There have been reports of patients developing skin photosensitivity resulting in increased risk of sunburn after injection of fluorescein sodium. This may be a photoallergic reaction enhanced by sunlight.[36] It does not appear to be a common reaction.

Effect of Fluorescein Sodium on Laboratory Tests

Bloom studied the effect of fluorescein sodium with certain serum laboratory tests.[32] Serum and urine samples were checked. No interference was found in the urine samples, but of 27 serum analyte tests, six were affected by the presence of fluorescein sodium in the blood. Those tests affected by fluorescein sodium were levels of creatinine, cortisol, digoxin, quinidine, thyroxine, and total protein. The interference may persist for as long as 24 hours after injection. These tests can be performed on various analytical systems, and not all tests on all systems were affected.

To avoid false test results, when you orient your patients before fluorescein sodium angiography, they should be informed that the dye may affect some test results. If they are scheduled for tests within 24 hours of the angiogram, either they should have their blood drawn before the injection of the dye or you should give them a list of which tests by which analytical system are affected. They can then take the list to the laboratory where alternatives may be found.

Indocyanine Green

ICG ($C_{43}H_{47}N_2NaO_6S_2$) is a tricarbocyanine dye used to perform choroidal angiography (Figure 4-12). According to its chemical structure, it is in the polymethine group of biological stains. It is marketed under the brand name Indocyanine-Green and is also known as Fox Green.

A relatively safe synthetic dye, ICG is the result of a complex synthesis of a derivative of glutaconic aldehyde with an indolium hydroxide compound.[37] Sodium iodide is added as a dipolar ion and is necessary to achieve solubility. There is a misconception that iodine is a major component of ICG, when actually, it is not even part of the empirical chemical formula of the dye. The iodide ion is added to make ICG soluble and safe for human use. The dye comes as a dark green, blue-green, or green-black powder that must be mixed with sterile water to form an aqueous solution for injection.

ICG was first used by the Eastman-Kodak company in the manufacture of Wratten filters and in infrared photography.[35] In the 1950s, after satisfactory treatment by Dr. Fox of the Mayo Clinic, an official of Kodak offered him an array of dyes from their photochemical shelves for possible medical applications; ICG was one of the dyes offered. Eventually, ICG was turned over to the Hynson, Westcott and Dunning pharmaceutical firm for further development for medical use and received FDA approval in 1956. It was determined that ICG was appropriate for use in cardiac output studies, then later proved to be applicable for liver function studies and choroidal angiography.

WHAT IS INDOCYANINE GREEN?

ICG is a very complex synthetic that is soluble in water and methanol but is practically insoluble in other organic solvents. Even when dissolved in sterile saline, it is unstable and the solution must be used within 10 hours.[27] The dye comes as a freeze-dried powder from the manufacturers, which sometimes clumps up or clings to the sides of the vial. This clumping, however, is not indicative of contamination by moisture because water content is very carefully controlled. It is recommended that ICG powder be mixed only with the aqueous solvent that comes with it from the manufacturer, as there have been reports of incompatibility with some other sterile water for injection preparations.[27] Of course, sterile technique should always be used when mixing the solution for injection.

Currently, only one pharmaceutical company is listed in the drug literature as a source of medical-grade ICG, which is known as Cardio-Green. Other pharmaceutical companies package angiography kits that contain vials of ICG, but the dye is manufactured by only one company. The synthesis of the dye is protected by two U.S. patents.

ICG is not as fluorescent as fluorescein sodium. In fact, it has approximately only 1/25 the fluorescence efficiency of fluorescein sodium, and its fluorescence is not seen in the visible spectrum of light.[35] Its peak absorption is 800–810 nm and its emission peak is 835 nm within the infrared spectrum[37] (Figure 4-13). The drug heparin contains sodium bisulfite, which affects the absorption peak of ICG and should not be used in conjunction with injection of the dye. Significant concentrations of heparin in the blood before injection may affect the quality of an ICG study. ICG has a pH of 6 and is mixed with sterile water with a pH of 5.5–6.5.

When injected into the bloodstream, ICG is 98% absorbed by the plasma proteins, especially the albumins.[38] For this reason, the dye does not extravasate freely from retinal vessels or from the highly fenestrated vessels of the choriocapillaris. This characteristic is in sharp contrast to the free-leaking characteristics of fluorescein sodium and makes possible infrared angiography to delineate choroidal vessels. ICG is not metabolized after injection but is taken up completely by the parenchymal cells

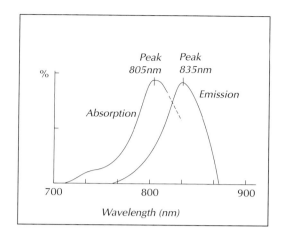

FIGURE 4-13
The absorption and emission spectra of in vitro indocyanine green.

of the liver and excreted in the bile. It is not excreted by the kidneys as is fluorescein sodium. Patients should be informed that the dye does not cause any of the characteristic staining of their mucous membranes and secretions that happens with fluorescein sodium, but their stools will be discolored for several days.

USES OF INDOCYANINE GREEN

As mentioned earlier, ICG was first used medically in cardiac outflow studies. The dye is used as an indicator, and its concentration in arterial blood flow is determined with the use of an oximeter or earpiece densitometer attached to a needle or catheter. The catheter is threaded to the part of the anatomy to be studied, and a specific amount of the dye is delivered in a single bolus.[39] Dye concentration in arterial blood is then sampled, and the efficiency of blood moving through the heart can be calculated.

Since ICG is exclusively excreted in the bile, it is useful in determining liver function and blood flow. Bile duct obstruction will affect the excretion of the dye. To study liver function, blood samples are taken at routine intervals of up to 20 minutes, the samples are centrifuged and coagulated, and densitometry is used to determine the rate of dye retention or dye disappearance in the blood serum.[38] Dye levels exceeding 4% are indicative of impaired hepatic function.[40]

Kogure et al. were the first to use ICG in ophthalmology as ICG absorption angiography of monkey retinas. They performed the procedure in 1970 using a 35-mm fundus camera and color film.[41] In 1971, Hochheimer modified the technique by using black and white infrared film. Then Flower introduced fluorescence angiography using ICG. This new procedure called for improved filters to record the fluorescence with infrared film. Remember that ICG has only 4% of the fluorescence efficiency of fluorescein.

After determining that infrared film was unable to record the presence and location of the poorly fluorescent ICG in the choroidal circulation for long periods of time, Hayashi introduced videography for recording the ICG images. While all of these modifications improved the efficiency of ICG angiography, poor image resolution and the potential for infrared light toxicity and possible increase of retinal temperature because of infrared light exposure hampered the acceptance of ICG angiography as a common clinical diagnostic tool.

In recent years, however, multiple technological advances have modified ICG angiography, resolving many of the previous problems, and the procedure is rapidly growing in clinical use and acceptance. The procedure is done using either a scanning laser ophthalmoscope or an electronic digital imaging system. New digital systems include a fundus camera with an infrared light source, a video camera, possibly several monitors, a personal computer with accompanying customized imaging software, a video cassette recorder, and an optical disk drive for data storage. In addition, the cameras have 35-mm film capabilities with synchronized flash, enlarged apertures to increase the amount of light that can be used for imaging, and appropriate excitatory and barrier filters with special infrared coatings.

Indocyanine Green Angiography

The circulation dynamics of choroidal angiography are the same as in retinal angiography: Dye injected intravenously in the arm flows in the same pattern to reach the choroidal and retinal circulation, as described in the section on retinal angiography. However, the characteristics of the dyes used to document the two separate vascular systems and the imaging systems used to record the circulation patterns are different. ICG is clearly seen in the retinal vasculature as well as in the choroidal vasculature, but because of its almost complete binding to the albumins in the blood, ICG does not "leak" or extravasate out of the choriocapillaris as does fluorescein sodium. Because ICG stays in both the retinal and choroidal vessels, the distinct outlines of the vessels of the choroid can be seen and identified and are not obscured. Since infrared light is much more efficient in penetrating the pigmented layers of the retina, serous exudates, thin layers of subretinal blood, or even medial opacities, ICG can be seen more readily in the choroidal vasculature than can fluorescein sodium despite ocular pathology.

Because ICG angiography is still not widely used and its applications and efficacy are still being investigated, there is some variation in sequencing and technique for performing these studies. Sometimes ICG angiography is performed simultaneously with fluorescein sodium angiography, sometimes sequentially, and sometimes alone.[42] In cases in which ICG angiography is performed solely, a fluorescein sodium angiogram has usually been done within the previous few days, although sometimes ICG angiography is performed specifically because a patient has a known allergy to fluorescein sodium. The two studies are *not* interchangeable, as different information is derived from each, but they are commonly used to complement or enhance each other. Whether fluorescein sodium and ICG angiography should be performed sequentially or simultaneously should be decided by the referring physician and the photographer.

For simultaneous fluorescein sodium and ICG procedures, dosages of the two dyes are combined in the same syringe. The dyes are compatible and can be combined for injection safely. During simultaneous procedures, the early fluorescein sodium phase is recorded, then the infrared filters are put in place and ICG images are captured. Images of the two dyes are taken alternately, switching the camera setting appropriately.

For sequential procedures, one dye or the other is injected first, and the early phase of that study is completed. Then, the second dye is injected after the appropriate filters and flash settings are arranged, and the early phase of that study is completed. As mentioned above in the section on IV injections, a single-needle, two-way stopcock arrangement is easiest on the patient. Remember that heparin contains sodium bisulfite and therefore should *not* be used as an anticoagulant in conjunction with an ICG injection. The sodium bisulfite reduces the absorption peak of

ICG in the blood and diminishes the fluorescence abilities of the dye. Any post-injection flush of the butterfly-syringe set should only be done with normal saline.

The sequencing and time intervals for ICG angiography differ with the pathology to be studied. Images are recorded at about 10 seconds after injection and continue at several-second intervals. These images are recorded even before an image is visible on the monitor. As ICG fills the retinal and choroidal vessels, the image to the camera deteriorates as "blooming" occurs— the dye concentration in both vascular systems is too intense and the image deteriorates. The flash setting is turned down to avoid overexposed images; then, after this initial phase, the flash setting is turned back up. The images are recorded at about 3 minutes, 5–7 minutes, 10–12 minutes, and 25+ minutes. The later phases of an ICG angiogram may yield the most information, depending of the pathology being studied. ICG can remain in neovascular tissue after the dye has left the retinal and choroidal vessels. Sometimes, to assist in photocoagulation of neovascular membranes, reinjection of 1 mg of ICG can help redefine retinal and choroidal vessels, providing landmarks for the physician.[43]

According to the literature, the usual adult dosage for ICG is 40 mg in 2 ml of aqueous solvent.[27] Sometimes a lesser dosage of dye will yield good images, and 25 mg in 3 ml is suggested. In simultaneous fluorescein sodium/ICG injections, 50 mg of ICG in 3 ml is mixed with 2 ml of 25% fluorescein sodium.[42]

Because of its characteristic insolubility, ICG is hard to dissolve and prepare for injection. Even when it appears superficially that the dye is dissolved, great care must be taken to ensure that it is actually in complete solution. Because of its instability in solution form, the liquid should be used within 10 hours. These are the chemical characteristics of ICG and are problems that are not easily solved by its manufacturers. Theoretically, other dipolar ions may make ICG more soluble and stable but may not be safe for human use. The manufacturer's instructions for the dissolving and preparation of ICG should be strictly followed.

Side Effects and Reactions to Indocyanine Green

Unlike fluorescein sodium, ICG does not have multiple side effects and adverse reactions. One possible explanation is that ICG is so bound to the proteins in the blood, it does not extravasate easily out of vessels. The result is that ICG is a relatively benign dye, and patients usually tolerate it well.

The common side effect of ICG is the staining of stools. ICG does not color the skin or the mucous secretions. As it is excreted exclusively by the liver, ICG does not show up in urine. It does not pass to the placenta but has not been proved safe for use in pregnancy.

When adverse reactions occur in a patient during ICG angiography, the first aid and supplies suggested in previous sections of this chapter apply.

MILD ADVERSE REACTIONS
Reported mild adverse reactions include infrequent nausea and vomiting, and lightheadedness. The frequency of mild adverse reactions has been reported as 0.5%.[44]

MODERATE ADVERSE REACTIONS
Moderate adverse reactions reported have included urticaria, fainting, and vasovagal responses. Possibly the vasovagal responses are due to the invasive nature of the injection, not to the dye itself. The frequency rate of moderate reactions has been reported as 0.2%.

Pharmaceutical literature states that anyone with an allergy to iodine should not be injected with ICG. Other literature suggests that patients at risk for allergic reactions are only those with a history of iodide ion allergy.[27] The concentration of sodium iodide in ICG is only 5%. It seems that some patients who report iodine allergy do not experience allergic response reactions to ICG. Some reactions to ICG are pseudoallergic, with a nonimmunologic release of histamine.[45] The University of Paris has reported the synthesis of ICG with a dipolar ion different from sodium iodide, which may not carry the same potential for iodine allergy reactions.[46]

SEVERE ADVERSE REACTIONS

In all the literature, including the cardiac and hepatic specialty literature, there have been 16 severe reactions reported. In each case, the adverse reactions did not seem typical and were not dependent on the dose of ICG. Most of the reactions seemed to be allergic in nature but with no previous histories of allergy. Almost half of the patients experiencing adverse reactions had end-stage renal disease and were on hemodialysis. It may be that patients with uremia respond to ICG with allergic hypersensitivity, but no one is sure of the exact response mechanism. Overall, the adverse reaction rate is 0.05%. Two deaths have been reported in the literature, both due to anaphylaxis followed by cardiac arrest.

COMPLICATIONS OF FAILED INJECTIONS

The proper IV techniques and precautions mentioned earlier apply to injections of ICG. Extravasation of ICG does not seem to cause the same degree of pain caused with extravasated fluorescein sodium, and tissue necrosis has not been reported. This may be due to the lower pH of ICG, and because it is not easily diffused through tissues. ICG is not hyperosmolar, and there is no specific recommendation that hyaluronidase injections be applied around ICG extravasations.

Instances of intra-arterial injections of ICG have not been reported.

SPECIAL CONSIDERATIONS

The same caution used in screening patients for fluorescein sodium angiography should be used for ICG angiography, although fluorescein sodium has a higher adverse reaction rate and the complications with failed injections are also higher. ICG is contraindicated in pregnancy, and it is not known if the dye is excreted in mother's milk. ICG is also contraindicated in patients who have had a previous allergic reaction to it. It seems that allergy to iodine does not always result in an allergic reaction to ICG, but great caution should be taken when using the dye on these patients. First aid and emergency supplies should be immediately available. Nothing has been reported to suggest that juvenile asthmatics are at risk with ICG as they are with fluorescein sodium. There is evidence that patients with uremia on hemodialysis are at increased risk of allergic reaction to ICG.

ICG is also contraindicated in diabetic patients taking the oral antihyperglycemic drug metformin HCL (Glucophage). Because ICG contains an iodide ion, it is an iodinated material that can contribute to acute renal failure and acidosis. Diabetic patients who are taking metformin HCL should stop the drug 48 hours before choroidal angiography and not start again for 48 hours after the ICG injection. A test to evaluate renal function should be done and normal function established before the drug is re-instituted.[47]

Effect of Indocyanine Green on Laboratory Tests

Because of the presence on iodine in ICG, radioactive iodine uptake studies and results can be affected by the dye. As a result, iodine uptake studies should not be performed for at least a week after the injection of ICG.[48]

References

1. Miller S. *Cardiac Angiography*. Boston: Little, Brown, 1984;4.
2. Grossman W, Baim D. *Cardiac Catheterization and Intervention*. Philadelphia: Lea & Febiger, 1991;15.
3. Grossman W, Baim D. *Cardiac Catheterization and Intervention*. Philadelphia: Lea & Febiger, 1991;16.
4. Grossman W, Baim D. *Cardiac Catheterization and Intervention*. Philadelphia: Lea & Febiger, 1991;26.
5. Grossman W, Baim D. *Cardiac Catheterization and Intervention*. Philadelphia: Lea & Febiger, 1991;23.
6. Friesinger GC, Adams DF, Bourassa MG, et al. Optimal resources for examination of the heart and lungs. *Circulation* 1983;68:893A.
7. Wong D. *Textbook of Ophthalmic Photography*. New York: Inter-optics Publications, 1982;83.
8. Lillie RD. *HJ Conn's Biological Stains: A Handbook on the Nature and Uses of the Dyes Employed in the Biological Library*. Baltimore: Williams & Wilkins, 1977;19.
9. Lillie RD. *HJ Conn's Biological Stains: A Handbook on the Nature and Uses of the Dyes Employed in the Biological Library*. Baltimore: Williams & Wilkins, 1977;21.
10. Lillie RD. *HJ Conn's Biological Stains: A Handbook on the Nature and Uses of the Dyes Employed in the Biological Library*. Baltimore: Williams & Wilkins, 1977;335.
11. Baeyer A. Ueber einen neue klasse von farbstoffen. *Ber Dtch Chem Gzellshaft* 1871;4:555.
12. Federman J, Maguire J. Intravenous Fluorescein Angiography. In W Tasman (ed), *Duane's Clinical Ophthalmology*. Philadelphia: Harper & Row, 1991;1.
13. Anand R. Fluorescein angiography. Part 1. Technique and normal study. *J Ophthal Nursing Technol* 1989;8:50.
14. Budavari S (ed). *The Merck Index: An Encyclopedia of Chemicals, Drugs and Biologicals* (11th ed). Rahway, NJ: Merck & Co, 1989;6287.
15. Wessing A. *Fluorescein Angiography of the Retina*. St. Louis: Mosby, 1969;12.
16. Wessing A. *Fluorescein Angiography of the Retina*. St. Louis: Mosby, 1969;14.
17. Wessing A. *Fluorescein Angiography of the Retina*. St. Louis: Mosby, 1969;13.
18. Budavari S (ed). *The Merck Index: An Encyclopedia of Chemicals, Drugs and Biologicals* (11th ed). Rahway, NJ: Merck & Co, 1989;651.
19. Erlich P. Ueber provocirte fluorescenzerscheinungen am augen. *Dtsch Med Wochenschr* 1882;8:21.
20. Gennaro A (ed). *Remington's Pharmaceutical Sciences*. Easton, PA: Mack Publishing, 1990;1275.
21. Olin BR (ed). *Drug Facts and Comparisons*. St. Louis: Facts & Comparisons, 1993;514.
22. Kwiterovitch K, Maguire M, Murphy R, et al. Frequency of adverse reactions after fluorescein angiography. *Ophthalmology* 1991;98:1142.
23. Yanuzzi L, Rohrer K, Tindel L, et al. Fluorescein angiography complication survey. *Ophthalmology* 1986;93:613.
24. Szirth B, Wong D, Bate R, Bartlett D. Legal ramifications of intravenous administration of sodium fluorescein. *J Ophthal Photography* 1989;11:70.
25. Szirth B, Wong D, Bate R, Bartlett D. Legal ramifications of intravenous administration of sodium fluorescein. *J Ophthal Photography* 1989;11:77.
26. U.S. Government. The occupational health and safety act. *Federal Register* 1991;56(235):64175.
27. Olin BR (ed). *Drug Facts and Comparisons*. St. Louis: Facts & Comparisons, 1993;515.
28. Bullock JD, Fezza AJ. A double syringe and three-way stopcock for fluorescein injection. *Am J Ophthalmol* 1974;77:270.
29. Kwiterovich K, Maguire M, Murphy R, et al. Frequency of adverse reactions after fluorescein angiography. *Ophthalmology* 1991;98:1141.
30. Myers P. Case report: a potentially serious reaction between sodium fluorescein and promethazine solutions: flush the cannula before injecting. *Arch Ophthalmol* 1994;112:734.
31. Chahal PS, Neal MJ, Kohner EM. Metabolism of fluorescein after intravenous injection. *Invest Ophthalmol Vis Sci* 1985;26:764.

32. Bloom J, Herman D, Elin R, et al. Intravenous fluorescein interference with clinical laboratory tests. *Am J Ophthalmol* 1989;108:375.
33. Yanuzzi L, Rohrer K, Tindel L, et al. Fluorescein angiography complication survey. *Ophthalmology* 1986;93:612.
34. Cohen S. Accidental intra-arterial injection of drugs. *Lancet* 1948;2:361, 409.
35. Budavari S (ed). *The Merck Index: An Encyclopedia of Chemicals, Drugs and Biologicals* (11th ed). Rahway, NJ: Merck & Co, 1989;786.
36. Hochsattel R, Gall H, Weber L, Kaufmann R. Photoallergic reactions to fluorescein. *Contact Dermatitis* 1990;22:42.
37. *Cardio-Green.* Cockeysville, MD: Becton Dickinson Microbiology Systems, 1990;6.
38. *Cardio-Green.* Cockeysville, MD: Becton Dickinson Microbiology Systems, 1990;5.
39. *Indocyanine Green: History, Chemistry, Pharmacology, Indications, Adverse Reactions, Investigations and Prognosis—An Investigator's Brochure.* Hunt Valley, MD: Becton Dickinson & Co., 1994;6.
40. Gennaro A (ed). *Remington's Pharmaceutical Sciences.* Easton, PA: Mack Publishing , 1990;1271.
41. Yannuzzi L, Slakter J, Sorenson J, et al. Digital indocyanine green videoangiography and choroidal neovascularization. *Retina* 1992;12:199.
42. Miller K. Protocols for the efficacious use of indocyanine green/sodium fluorescein angiography. *J Ophthal Photography* 1993;15:63.
43. Nyberg W. Re-injection technique for establishing landmarks in late phase ICG angiography. *J Ophthal Photography* 1993;15:66.
44. Hope-Ross M, Yanuzzi L, Gragoudas E, et al. Adverse reactions due to indocyanine green. *Ophthalmology* 1994;101:530.
45. Hope-Ross M, Yanuzzi L, Gragoudas E, et al. Adverse reactions due to indocyanine green. *Ophthalmology* 1994;101:531.
46. Cohen SY, Quentel G, Coscas G, et al. Safety of a dye without iodine for indocyanine green angiography. *Invest Ophthalmol Vis Sci* 1995;36:S248.
47. Olin BR (ed). *Drug Facts and Comparisons.* St. Louis: Facts and Comparisons, 1996;577, 582.
48. Young DS. *Effects of Drugs on Clinical Lab Tests.* Philadelphia: American Association for Clinical Chemistry Press, 1990.

Chapter 5

Fluorescein Angiography: Instrumentation and Technique

Patrick J. Saine

Introduction

The view is challenging through the dark blue exciter filter. You appreciate little contrast between the blood vessels and the fundus as you squint through the tiny viewfinder in the darkened room. The injection site is being prepared for the administration of fluorescein dye. On your signal, a syringe filled with a bright red fluid is emptied into your patient's antecubital vein. Quickly, you start the timer and insert the barrier filter—completely obscuring your view of the retina. Then suddenly, magically, your patient's retinal blood vessels fill with glowing sodium fluorescein and you are witnessing bright yellow-green fireworks! Your urge is to stop taking pictures and stare at the show. You are transfixed by the natural beauty of a unique event to which only you and the camera are witnesses. You are performing your first fluorescein angiogram.

Fluorescein angiography is a diagnostic test that documents the dynamic flow of fluorescein dye in the blood vessels of the eye. After sodium fluorescein has been injected into the patient's vascular system, a rapid sequence of photographs records the dye as it flows through both the choroidal and retinal blood vessels. Fluorescein acts as a marker, detailing precise areas of vascular leakage, or conversely, the absence of dye in blood vessels. The ophthalmologist uses these photographs both for diagnosis and as a guide to patient treatment.

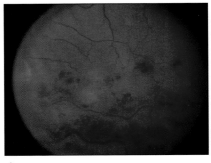 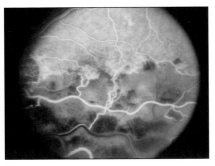

A   B

FIGURE 5-1
Both fundus photography (A) and fluorescein angiography (B) use a fundus camera to obtain retinal images. However, each reveals very different visual information.

This chapter describes the instrumentation and procedure for fluorescein angiography. It includes practical advice about common problems and advanced techniques.

The following essential topics are discussed elsewhere in this book:

• Fundus photography technique (Chapter 2)
• Preparation for a sodium fluorescein injection (Chapter 4)
• Normal side effects and potential complications associated with the injection of sodium fluorescein (Chapter 4)

Fundus photography and fluorescein angiography are both similar and, at the same time, quite different procedures (Figure 5-1). Both use a fundus camera and its requisite alignment and focusing techniques. Fluorescein angiography adds the requirements of an exciter/barrier filter set and specific timing.

Time is an important aspect of both procedures, but for different reasons. Fundus photography documents the retina at a specific moment in time. Retinal changes are followed over days, weeks, months, or years. Fluorescein angiography records, usually in still pictures, the dynamic process of dye flowing through and leaking from retinal blood vessels. Significant changes occur over fractions of seconds. During fluorescein angiography, the pace of photography is faster and the timing of the photographs is more critical.

Successful fluorescein angiography is contingent upon your mastery of fundus photography. If you are comfortable taking color photographs of the retina, then fluorescein angiography will be simple to learn. One way to think of fluorescein angiography is as rapid-sequence fundus photography using colored filters.

Instrumentation

Almost any type of mydriatic fundus camera may be adapted for fluorescein angiography: narrow-angle, wide-angle, handheld, film-based, or digital. Most modern fundus cameras are supplied as ready for angiography by the manufacturer, although a few are not.

Use separate 35-mm camera bodies for color and black and white to reduce both film waste and barrier filter mishandling. This arrangement also adds a measure of security to the fundus photography system: A spare film back should always be available in the event of a breakdown. The camera bodies should be motorized and capable of triggering an electronic flash sequentially for at least 30 seconds at a rate of at least one frame per second.

What is a Filter?

A filter is a device used to separate items. An everyday example is the filter in your furnace. Dirty air is drawn into your furnace through a filter. The filter separates the clean air from the dirt particles by trapping the dust in the fibers of the filter. Clean air then exits the furnace through the vents. Optical filters separate light into different wavelengths in much the same way. White light strikes a blue filter, and blue light exits: The blue light is separated from the white light. Actually, one of two very different mechanisms is at work.

Optical filters can be divided into two categories: absorption filters and interference filters. Most standard photographic filters are absorption filters. They absorb the unwanted wavelengths of light in the same way that the furnace filter traps the dirt from the circulating air. Available in glass (sturdy but not optically neutral) or gelatin (easily scratched but more optically neutral) and in a wide variety of colors, absorption filters are relatively inexpensive to manufacture. Absorption filters are both less efficient and less precise than interference filters (Figure 5-2). The Kodak publication *Filters for Scientific Uses* is a useful guide to absorption filters.[2]

Interference filters reflect rather than absorb unwanted wavelengths of light, allowing sharper wavelength cut-off and greater efficiency. Although they are more expensive to manufacture, their performance is closer to the ideal.

Novotny and Alvis used commercially available absorption filters (KW47 for excitation and KW58 coated with copper for the barrier) in their early fluorescein work.[3] Haining and Lancaster suggested narrow-band interference filters in 1968.[4] Delori et al. described an improved set in 1976.[5] Standard fluorescein filters sets are now almost exclusively interference filters.

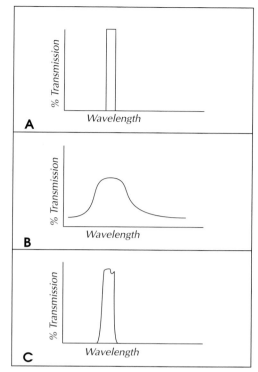

FIGURE 5-2
The transmission curve of an ideal filter is represented with a steep, vertical slope that represents the sharp separation of wavelengths (A). Its efficiency is evidenced by the 100% transmission of the desired wavelengths. The transmission curve of an absorption filter (B) has a gradually sloping curve and a lower level of transmission. Monochromatic interference filters (C) exhibit the best real-world separation of wavelengths and efficient transmission levels.

Fluorescein angiography requires a fluorescein filter set, consisting of an *exciter* and a *barrier* filter (see the sidebar on *What is a filter?*).[1] Sodium fluorescein molecules absorb blue light between 485 and 500 nanometers, become excited, and consequently emit green light between 520 and 530 nanometers (Figure 5-3).[6] In a fluorescein angiogram, the filters optimize the illuminating wavelengths and discriminate between the illuminating wavelengths and the emitted wavelengths.

The exciter filter is blue in color, having a peak transmission of 490 nanometers. It is placed in the optical pathway in front of the light source for fluorescein angiography. This ensures that the retinal illumination is only within the wavelength range that maximally excites sodium fluorescein circulating in the eye.

When this blue light is projected into a normal patient's eye after a sodium fluorescein injection, it is absorbed or reflected by either the circulating sodium fluorescein or by the structures of the eye. If the blue light is absorbed by the circulating sodium fluorescein, then the fluorescein molecules become excited and emit a green light. If the blue light is reflected by areas not containing sodium fluorescein, it reflects unaltered blue light toward the film. After being illuminated by blue light, the returning wavelengths of both green and blue light exit the pupil and continue toward the film.

The fluorescent green light contains important diagnostic information; it tells us where in the retina the sodium fluorescein has traveled. The blue light does not contain important diagnostic information; its task of exciting the sodium fluorescein is complete. We discriminate between the

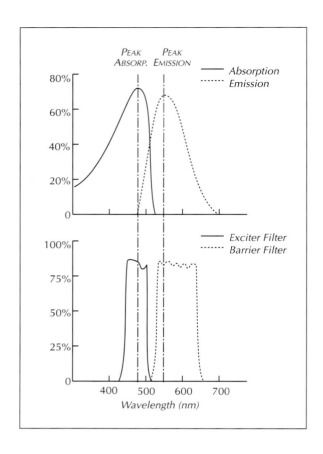

FIGURE 5-3
The absorption and emission spectra of in vitro sodium fluorescein.

two wavelengths of light by placing a barrier filter in the optical pathway between the subject and the film plane. This filter (peak transmission: 525 nanometers) allows only the green light to continue on toward the film (Figure 5-4).

Exciter filters are routinely placed in the optical pathway after the flashtube and viewing light (Figure 5-5). The barrier filter can be situated either in front of the eyepiece and film or just before the film plane. If it is placed in front of the eyepiece and film, you will view directly through this filter during fluorescein angiography. This makes camera positioning more difficult during the initial phases of the angiogram because you see virtually nothing through the viewfinder (note: you can check your alignment by quickly sliding one of the two filters in and out). On the other hand, it allows a clearer view of the circulating sodium fluorescein once the dye has reached the retina.

If the filter is placed directly in front of the film plane, you will view the circulating fluorescein without the benefit of the barrier filter. It may be more difficult to detect the presence of fluorescein in the eye; however, you will have the advantage of more easily appreciating the standard crescent and haze positioning artifacts during angiography. Check your manual to ascertain the precise location of the filters in your particular fundus camera.

The perfect position for a barrier filter has often been debated among veteran ophthalmic photographers. The topic has cooled with the introduction of solenoid-activated barrier filters, which pop in and out of position when activated by a manual switch or the shutter release. This mechanism allows you to choose your view, with or without the barrier filter in place. The manual option is important because the exciter filter may also be used for nerve fiber layer photography.

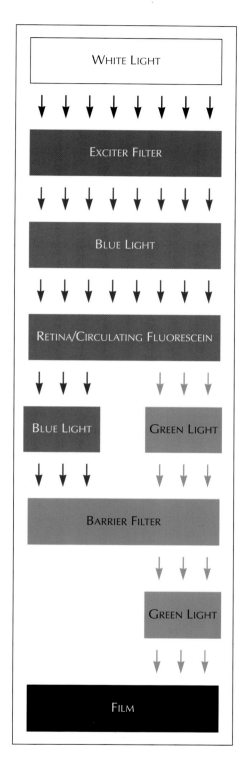

FIGURE 5-4
The exciter and barrier filter. White light enters the exciter filter, which transmits only the blue portion of the light. The blue light enters the eye where it is either absorbed by the fluorescein or reflected by the retina. The light absorbed by the fluorescein is emitted as green light. The green excited light and the reflected blue light leave the eye. The blue light is rejected by the barrier filter, while the green light passes through the barrier filter and is recorded on film.

Like all colored objects, fluorescein filters will eventually degrade (Figure 5-6). Age, exposure to light, and high humidity are some of the factors that contribute to filter failure. Increased pseudofluorescence (see the section on Pseudofluorescence and Autofluorescence) is a sign of worn out filters.

Fluorescein filters should always be replaced as a matched pair to ensure efficiency. In busy offices in warm, humid climates, filters may

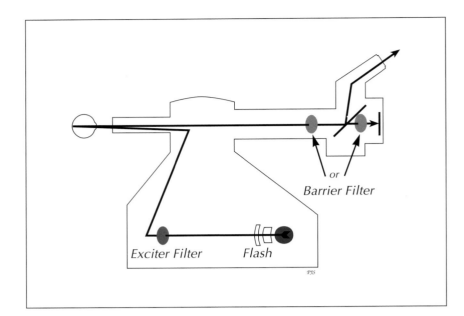

FIGURE 5-5
Filter location. The exciter filter is located after the light source but before the light enters the patient's eye. The barrier filter can be placed in one of two positions: either in front of or behind the single lens reflex mirror. The photographer views through the barrier filter during angiography if the filter is placed in front of the mirror and does not if it is placed behind the mirror.

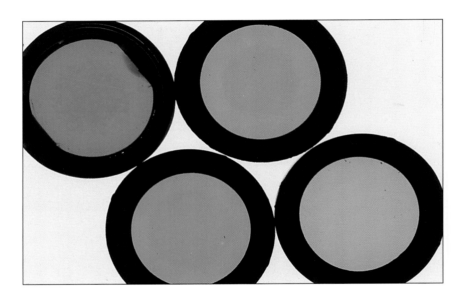

FIGURE 5-6
Note the peripheral discoloration of these barrier filters. Have you inspected your filters lately?

need to be replaced each year. Smaller practices in cooler climates may need to change their filters every 3 years. *When were your fluorescein filters last changed?*

Procedure

This section describes a step-by-step procedure for performing fluorescein angiography (Table 5-1). The nomenclature used in this chapter primarily describes fluorescein angiography using film. The procedure is very similar when capturing images electronically, with the proviso that you are interacting with a computer and monitor as opposed to film cassettes and a darkroom. Learning fluorescein angiography is like driving a car: Once you become comfortable with the process, you can drive any car using your accelerating, braking, and steering skills. In the same way,

Table 5-1. Fluorescein Angiography: Step by Step*

Prepare and position	Prepare the room
	Plan the procedure
Patient contact time ⟶	Perform color fundus photography
	Switch cameras and filter
	Photograph name tag and green filter
	Expose a control photograph
	Re-educate your patient
	Double-check everything
	Solicit injection
Expose	Signal injector
	Begin series—shoot "earlies"
	Shoot pictures at 1, 3, 5, 10 minutes
	Close the session
Follow-up	Process and edit the images
	Deliver the finished product
	Review your work

*Review these steps before or during the procedure to help establish your routine. Post a copy of these steps near your fundus camera for reference.

Table 5-2. Fluorescein Angiography Supply Checklist

Filled syringe	10-cc syringe with 5 cc 10% sodium fluorescein
	5-cc syringe with 2.5 cc 25% sodium fluorescein
Needle	20-gauge straight needle
	23-gauge butterfly, 12-inch tube, ¾-inch needle
	23-gauge catheter
Wound cover	Adhesive bandage
	Gauze or cotton ball with tape
Tourniquet	¾-inch tubing
Cleansing aid	Alcohol pads
Personal protection	Gloves, mask, and safety clothing as needed
	Syringe disposal unit
Miscellaneous	Emergency supplies
	Emesis basin

different brands of cameras or different recording media (film vs. electronic) pose few difficulties for the experienced angiographer.

Prepare and Position

1. *Prepare the room.* Tidy the room. Complete all billing and paperwork. Adjust the stool height and the fundus camera's mechanical controls to their approximate midpoints. Load both camera backs with film—one with color slide film and one with fast black and white negative film. Confirm that the illumination and flash settings, the filter wheel, and the diopter compensation control are in their standard positions. Set your reticle. Prepare the sodium fluorescein injection and injection supplies (Table 5-2).

2. *Plan the procedure.* Have a photographic plan in mind before you escort the patient into the room. Review the photo request form and examine any prior photographs. Note the patient's visual acuity and working diagnosis. Determine the fields to photograph. Select your camera and angle of view, the areas of the patient's retina you intend to document (Table 5-3), and the timing of your photographs (Figure 5-7). If multiple angles of view are selected, be certain that each variation is shot both in color and as an angiographic frame. Ask pertinent questions: On which retinal level should you focus?

Table 5-3. Disease-Specific Fluorescein Angiograms*

Disease	Primary Views ("Earlies")	Angle of View (Degrees)	Recirculation Phase ("Lates")
Macular diseases (e.g., ARMD,CME, CSR, POHS)	Macula	30	Macula (CME: 15-minute lates)
Occlusive diseases (e.g., CRVO, BRVO, CRAO, BRAO)	Macula	30 or 45	Macula and periphery as needed
Systemic diseases (e.g., diabetic retinopathy)	Macula	30 or 45	Macula and 7 standard fields
Site-specific diseases (e.g., tumor, macroaneurysm)	Area of lesion	30 or 45	Area of lesion; include borders

*See Table 8-5 for advanced, disease-specific angiography plan.

How to Determine the Proper Exposure

Begin with the manufacturer's exposure recommendations found in the owner's manual. Tweak this setting by performing a sequence of exposures during the recirculation phase (between 1 and 3 minutes) of a fluorescein angiogram in which you are most interested in the late photographs (for minimal impact on patient care). If no recommendations are available, then use the green filter and take one picture at each flash setting. Choose the best exposure and increase it by two or three exposure steps for your initial fluorescein exposure.

Judge your exposure from original negatives, not from contact sheets. Look for a full range of densities from clear film to dense blacks. The negative image of the control photograph (assuming efficient filters and a young, clear-eyed patient) should be completely clear. The "earlies" should progress from clear to grays to rich blacks. "Lates" will be gray.

A good negative will yield a fine print, given proper darkroom technique. Of course, the instant feedback of electronic imaging shortens this testing process.

Remember that your exposure is a balance between actual film speed (film sensitivity plus exposure plus development) and patient comfort. Fine-grain photographs with full tonality are useless if the required flash setting is too much for the patient to tolerate.

Indications for increased exposure during fundus photography may or may not suggest exposure compensation during angiography. If fundus photography exposure was increased to compensate for a smaller pupil, it is wise to increase the angiography flash setting. On the other hand, if the flash increase in fundus photography is due to darker patient pigmentation, do not increase the angiography flash setting. In general, fundus photography is exposed for the pigment in the retinal pigment epithelium and fluorescein angiography is exposed for circulating dye in the blood vessels (which do not contain pigment).

Should the periphery be scanned during the recirculation phase? Should the iris be documented for signs of rubeosis?

3. *Perform color fundus photography.* The physician compares color fundus photographs with the fluorescein angiogram frames when reading an angiogram. Take color slides at the same session as the fluorescein dye test and before the dye is injected (Figure 5-8).[7]

4. *Switch from the color camera body to the black and white camera body.* Exchange the camera bodies, making sure to flip the camera selection switch if necessary. Check the diopter setting if the camera backs include the eyepiece. If you use a single camera body, load the appropriate film and check that the barrier filter is in place.

5. *Photograph a name tag.* Using the green filter and a low flash setting, photograph a name tag. This identifies the patient's images throughout processing, editing, and filing. You will probably need to increase the viewing light's intensity to focus clearly while the colored filters are in place.

6. *Photograph the fundus using a green filter.* Select the angle of view and focus you will be using during the fluorescein angiogram. Insert a green filter and select a low flash setting to photograph first the nonaffected eye, and then the affected eye. Imaging the affected eye last positions the camera for the early photographs. (Note: the barrier filter located at the film plane will not affect these photographs.)

This is a good time to practice stereo shifts and to determine the best camera placement in eyes with a compromised view. Focus carefully, because this focus will remain unchanged throughout the angiogram (at least until you are more experienced).

7. *Expose a control photograph.* Set the flash for the fluorescein setting (see sidebar: *How to determine the proper exposure*), remove the green filter, and insert both the exciter and the barrier filter. Take a photograph. This will be your control photograph. The section on Pseudofluorescence and Autofluorescence explains how examining this frame can help you determine the integrity of your filters. Reset your timer to zero.

8. *Re-educate the patient.* Remind the patient about the common side effects of the dye injection and prepare him or her for the upcoming test. The patient should have been adequately informed by the physician (who also obtains a signed consent form that details potential complications), so a lengthy discussion is probably not needed. Here's what we tell patients: "What I am going to do now is to go get Dr. _____, who will make a dye injection into your arm. Then I'm going to take a lot of blue pictures of the dye while it is flowing through the blood vessels in the back of your eyes. Two

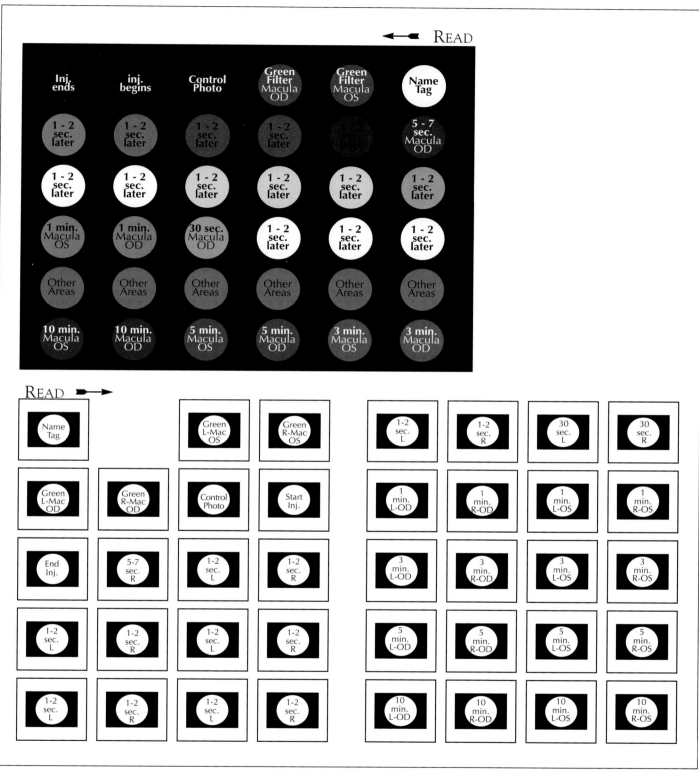

FIGURE 5-7
Timing fluorescein frames. Examples of common strategies used in timing fluorescein angiograms are shown. A contact-printed 36-exposure film of mono-fluorescein exposures is represented at the top. The slots in the fifth row of images may also be dedicated to stereo. A stereo angiogram composed of original negatives mounted as 35-mm slides is shown at the bottom. Adopting a standard angiogram pattern streamlines routine angiography. The experienced photographer departs from the standard when interesting patients require more photographs or when difficult patients limit the amount of photography.

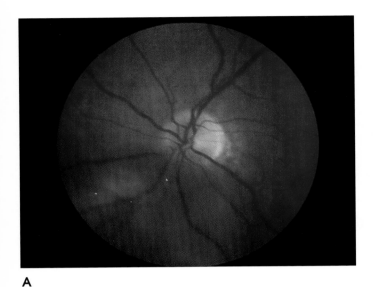

A

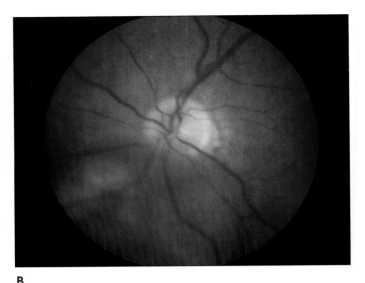

B

FIGURE 5-8
Standard color fundus photographs exposed after a fluorescein injection convey an adulterated coloration of the retina. When performing fluorescein angiography, expose colors before the injection (A) rather than after (B).

things you'll notice from the dye are that your skin will be a little yellow for the next 8 hours, and your urine will be a bright yellow-orange for the next day and a half. Don't worry about either of these things; it's just the dye leaving your body. Do you have any questions?" Strive to make eye contact during the explanation with both the patient and any companions. A reassuring tone is important. A light touch on the patient's hand is optional. Some photographers spend considerable time discussing potential reactions just before the test. In other offices, the physician or nurse thoroughly discusses complications with the patient before the patient visits the photographer.

If you are photographing a light-sensitive or otherwise difficult patient, you may want to insert a "pep talk" here, hoping that it will help the patient cooperate during the early, rapid-sequence photographs. Try this: "I'll be taking a lot of blue pictures right after Dr. _____ makes the injection. These are some of the most important pictures that we'll take today. I'm going to need your help in holding extra still during these pictures. They won't be as bright as the first pictures we took, but there will be a lot of them. Let's try and get some good photographs for Dr. _____, OK?"

If the patient is a less than optimal candidate for intravenous injections (as some large, diabetic, or frail patients are), have the patient hang his or her arms down at the side and suggest that he or she clench and release a fist a few times while you summon the health care worker who will perform the injection.

Before leaving the room:

9. *Double-check everything.* Develop the habit of reviewing major variables just before the test. Make sure that film is loaded in the camera and check the flash setting. Check that the fluorescein injection and supplies are readily available. Confirm your angiographic plan. Have a stopwatch ready (a watch with a second hand will do).

10. *Solicit help for the injection.* Depending on your specific office procedures and your state's laws, ask the attending physician or a registered nurse to perform the injection.[8] Better-quality angiograms

result when someone other than the photographer performs the injection, especially when the photographer is inexperienced. As the photographer, you should concentrate on just one task—obtaining the best retinal photographs. In addition to performing the injection, the other person should monitor the patient for potential reactions, hold lids as needed, and be trained in emergency health care.

Expose

11. *Begin the test.* While the injection site is being prepared, realign the patient, viewing first with the green filter (checking your focus) and then switching to the blue exciter filter. Confirm your alignment by monitoring saturation and crescent artifacts. If you are shooting stereo, perform some practice shifts. Recall your angiographic plan. Take a (quiet) deep breath and feel confident!

    When you are ready for the injection to begin, signal the injector with an "OK" or a thumbs-up sign (you risk losing important early photographs if they begin injecting before you let them know you are ready). In turn, they should signal you with an "OK" or "injection started" as soon as the injection begins. For a good bolus of dye, the injection should last 1–3 seconds. Simultaneously start the camera timer and/or stopwatch and insert the barrier filter into the optical pathway. Take a photograph when the injection is completed to record the injection duration.

    If the barrier filter is placed at the film plane, your view of the blue retina will remain the same. If you view through the barrier filter during angiography, your view will become black as soon as the barrier filter is inserted. Do not panic. Until this point, you had been viewing the fundus with the blue exciter filter. With the barrier filter now in place and no fluorescein dye yet in the retina, there is no light reaching the eyepiece. Your view of the retina will return when the fluorescein dye fills the blood vessels.

12. *Begin taking pictures almost immediately.* Count to five and begin taking photographs at a rate of one image every 2 seconds—even if you do not see anything in the viewfinder. It is important to record the progress of the dye as it fills the choroid. This happens *before* you can clearly perceive the dye through the viewfinder. Your first few pictures may be blank, but you can edit these out later. This timing technique assures you of excellent early-phase photographs—photographs that are critical in diagnoses such as macular degeneration. If you are photographing the angiogram in stereo, remember to shift the camera for each picture.

13. *Increase your picture-taking rate.* Begin taking pictures at a rate of one image per second as soon as you see dye in the blood vessels or approximately 10 seconds after the injection (whichever comes first). These initial photographs (commonly referred to as the "earlies") document the rapid initial dynamics of the fluorescein dye in the choroid and retina. The dye first flows into the choroidal vessels, fills the retinal arteries, and then empties through the retinal veins. It may be difficult to appreciate these changes through the viewfinder, but they will be easy to see in your photographs. The earlies will be among your brightest and sharpest fluorescein frames.

14. *Pause picture taking at about 30 seconds.* This flurry of photographs can continue only so long. Stop taking pictures when 30 seconds are up, when you run out of film or computer space, or when you can no longer appreciate any changes in the dye. With more experience,

you will better appreciate the flow of the dye and develop your own unique shooting rhythms.

Allow patients to take a short break by asking them to close their eyes but keep their head in the headrest. Reassure them that the test is going well. We let them know that "the hard part is over with—there are no more injections, just some more pictures." This is also a good time to evaluate the need to reload film or send electronic images to the hard drive.

If the patient is going to have a reaction to fluorescein, it will most likely occur between 30 seconds and 2 minutes after the injection. Practical suggestions for managing patient reactions are offered later in this chapter.

The person injecting should check the injection site and apply a bandage. (We use bright adhesive bandage strips decorated with popular animated characters. Patients always smile when they discover their—or their grandchild's—favorite cartoon character at the injection site.)

15. *Take recirculation and late photographs.* Photographs taken after the injection at regular time intervals will reveal the extent to which the sodium fluorescein did or did not leak. There is no specific standard for the timing of these photographs; intervals vary both by office and by disease. The minimum acceptable timing of "lates" is 3- and 5- to 7-minute pictures. A complete series would contain 1-, 3-, 5-, 10- or 15-minute—and perhaps even 30-minute—photographs. We routinely expose stereo pairs of both eyes at 1, 3, 5, and 10 minutes after the injection, taking later pictures as requested by the physician and in cases of suspected cystoid macular edema or optic nerve head drusen.

Complete requested peripheral photographs, or scan the periphery per Table 5-2. Advanced fundus photography techniques such as scleral depression and auxiliary lenses may also be pursued.

16. *Close the session.* Let the patient know that he or she did well (even if it's not true) and that you obtained the needed photographs (which you should have). Remind the patient that the colors they are seeing are from the bright flashes. Reassure them that these spots will go away soon. Release patients with a smile, making sure that they feel fine and know where their next clinic stop is. Complete all paperwork, including signing the chart. An uncharted procedure is an incomplete procedure. Finish completely with one patient before beginning another.

Follow-Up

17. *Process the film or save the digital images.* Follow the instructions for developing film found in Chapter 6 or save your digital images as described in your owner's manual. Edit your raw images before presenting them to the physician. Only show the images that are clinically significant and represent your best work. The most complete stereo film fluorescein angiogram contains the following stereo pairs both properly exposed and well composed:

- Monochromatic green stereo fundus photographs of both eyes
- A preinjection control photograph documenting any pseudo- or autofluorescence
- At least one blank frame taken immediately before the fluorescein dye is present in the choroid
- Choroidal filling of the affected eye in stereo at a rate of 1 frame per second

- Arterial and venous filling phases in stereo of the affected eye at a rate of 1 frame per second
- Recirculation (arteriovenous) phase stereo photographs of both eyes (including stereo photographs of the periphery as needed)
- Late stereo photographs of both eyes (at 3, 5, and 10 minutes).

Of course, not every fluorescein procedure will contain the large set of photographs described above. Patients may not cooperate, you may begin taking pictures too late, or your office may have a different routine for late photographs. Electronic fluoresceins routinely contain fewer images to minimize electronic storage space. On the other hand, if you appreciate a very complete test, you can make informed decisions about routine fluorescein angiography at your office.

Always take some time during the editing process to review your work with an eye toward quality control. Ask yourself how this particular angiogram could have been made better.

18. *Deliver the finished product.* Deliver the patient's photographs and chart to the referring physician in a timely manner. In a busy retina practice, angiograms may be requested "stat," or immediately. Many of these stat patients are scheduled for laser treatment the same day. It is up to you to provide the results quickly without compromising quality. Film images usually take 25 minutes to 1 hour to cycle through a complete development process. Electronic images can be made available to the physician in a matter of minutes.

19. *Review your work.* You should endeavor to not only understand pertinent photographic principles but also to appreciate the various disease processes and their effects on the eye. Learn to look at fluorescein studies from the physician's point of view. Schedule regular conferences or ask impromptu questions, but routinely review your fluorescein angiograms with your physician.

Troubleshooting

What a wonderful world it would be if all of our angiograms were perfect! Unfortunately, filters may not work properly, our timing can be off, and patients can be...patients. This section suggests practical solutions for common angiographic problems. The technical problems of filters and timing may be followed by a discussion of managing patients and reactions.

Pseudofluorescence and Autofluorescence

Pseudofluorescence indicates an inefficient fluorescein filter system. *Autofluorescence* describes the "glowing" phenomena of certain entities found within the eye. Both can be detected by examining a control photograph.

The control photograph (step 7 above) is part of every complete fluorescein angiogram. It is exposed with both the barrier and the exciter filters in place and before sodium fluorescein is injected. In a normal patient photographed with efficient, well-matched filters, the control photograph is completely blank (Figure 5-9). This indicates that the barrier filter is properly excluding blue illuminating light and that there is no sodium fluorescein (or anything else) emitting fluorescent light.

Both barrier and excited filter transmission curves overlap slightly (Figure 5-10). If ideal filters—those with extremely sharp transmission

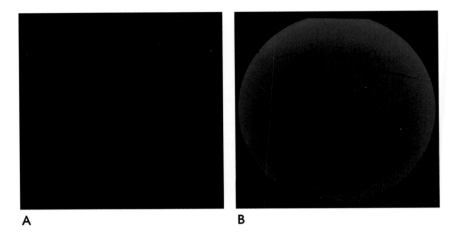

FIGURE 5-9
When an efficient set of fluorescein filters is in place, the control photograph will be devoid of retinal details (A). If the control photograph reveals retinal details (B), then the filter set is either poorly matched or faded.

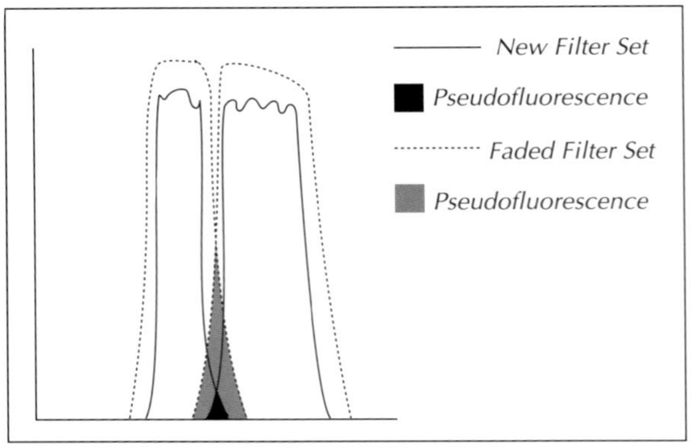

A   B

FIGURE 5-10
Pseudofluorescence. New fluorescein filter sets (solid line) exhibit a minor amount of filter overlap or pseudofluorescence (black triangle). As filters age, they transmit greater amounts of light (dotted line), creating more pseudofluorescence (gray triangle).

curves—were used, then this overlap would not exist. In the real world, however, even new filters exhibit some crossover. Furthermore, as filters age, their transmission characteristics become less discriminatory. Factors that degrade filters include age, high humidity, and exposure to light. As each filter in the pair deteriorates, it begins to pass more wavelengths that overlap with the other. As this supplementary light increases, it crosses the exposure threshold and is recorded on film. This additional light is called *pseudofluorescence*—literally, false fluorescence. Pseudofluorescence contributes to the overall exposure. It masks fine retinal details by overexposing highlights (the fluorescent areas) and decreasing overall contrast (Figure 5-11).

Autofluorescence also causes identifiable retinal details in a control photograph. This happens when structures in the eye act like sodium fluorescein: They absorb blue light and emit green light. Autofluorescent properties have been documented in the cataractous lens, optic nerve head drusen, and astrocytic harmatoma (Figure 5-12). In the second two instances, the autofluorescent images can help the physician determine the appropriate diagnosis.

Fluorescein Timing

A crucial difference between fundus photography and fluorescein angiography is the rate at which the pictures are exposed. It is easy to get to know the patient during fundus photography. The changes you are

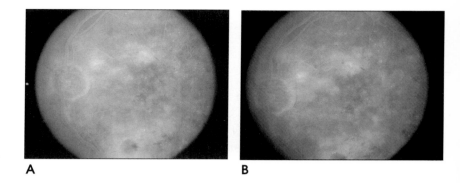

FIGURE 5-11
An efficient fluorescein filter set (A) is compared with a mismatched set (B). Pseudofluorescence masks fine details by effectively overexposing the highlights.

A   B

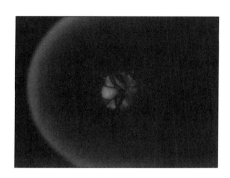

FIGURE 5-12
Using both a barrier and exciter filter—but no sodium fluorescein—when photographing these optic nerve head drusen and astrocytic harmatoma illustrates autofluorescence. You would expect no retinal details in a normal patient's control photograph with a well-matched set of filters.

documenting usually occur between visits, allowing images to be exposed at a more leisurely pace. Alternately, the "earlies" are a very important phase of fluorescein angiography that come and go within 30 seconds. Timing is clearly of the essence.

Begin shooting before you see any dye within the blood vessels. Once the dye has filled the blood vessels, sodium fluorescein's rate of visual change is measured in minutes rather than seconds. Inexperienced photographers may get caught up in the moment and continue to shoot rapidly after the dye has progressed through its initial changes. Remember that the most important images occur as the dye is filling the blood vessels. If you have missed these pictures for some reason (perhaps the patient moved or you forgot to insert the barrier filter), taking a rapid sequence of photos after the dye has filled the blood vessels is of little consequence.

Consistent timing is important during the late phases of the angiogram. Leaking sodium fluorescein is an important clinical finding. Similar timing of late photographs in two fluorescein tests from different dates allows better comparison of the relative activity of a lesion.

When You Can't See the Dye

Particularly unsettling to the inexperienced angiographer are the instances when no fluorescein dye can be seen in the blood vessels after the dye injection. Keep your head and remember that this can be the result of a number of circumstances. Check first with the person injecting: Was there infiltration, extravasation, or an arterial injection?

The patient may have circulation problems. If you don't see dye by 20 seconds after the injection, continue to shoot—but shoot more slowly (1 frame every 2–3 seconds). Admittedly unusual, I have performed angiograms in which the earlies have begun as late as 90 seconds after

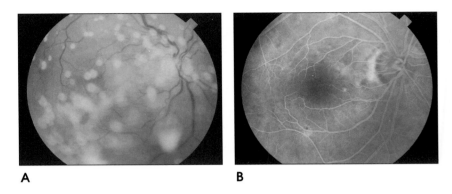

A   B

FIGURE 5-13
Asteroid hyalosis. A green filter (A) shows the extent of these vitreal calcium-lipid deposits, which disappear upon angiography (B). (Courtesy of Peter Hay.)

the injection. Anecdotal experiences have described muscular or overweight patients who, upon straightening and raising their arm, release a "blocked" bolus of dye.

It is often difficult to distinguish dye flowing through the retinal blood vessels of high myopes with clear media and in many patients with small pupils and hazy media. If the injection was successful and you are confident of your alignment and filter selection, the final images almost always will look better than your view through the finder. If your view is compromised, pay special attention to crescent and haze artifacts for alignment, flip to your green filter for viewing, and use standardized timing. More often than not, you will be rewarded by a readable angiogram.

Dense asteroid hyalosis is a good example of a condition that offers a poor view but results in an adequate angiogram. Because these vitreous deposits are not stained with circulating sodium fluorescein, they are rendered invisible using the exciter/barrier filter system (Figure 5.13).[9]

Be aware of potential exposure problems. A poor view through small pupils in clear eyes may yield a better angiogram with an increased flash setting. Brunescent cataracts can act as an additional barrier filter. Their reddish-brown color blocks the blue exciting light and transmits little of the fluorescent green. Turn up the flash power to compensate.

Reactions to Sodium Fluorescein

Fluorescein angiography's relatively low adverse reaction rate is balanced by the very real possibility of severe adverse events.[10] Review the contraindications, the type and frequency of reactions, and the standard emergency kit as described in Chapter 4. This section deals with the practical aspects of managing these situations.

All angiography locations should have a written emergency plan. Specific responsibilities, a list of emergency supplies (see Table 4-4) and their locations, and multiple scenarios—from mild reactions (nausea) to moderate reactions (urticaria) and severe reactions (vasovagal reactions)—should be addressed. Involve all photographers, the individuals responsible for injections, the physician, and the risk manager in the process of writing the emergency plan. Review the plan regularly with all staff involved in day-to-day angiography and make it required reading for new employees.

Nausea and vomiting are the most common adverse reactions to injected sodium fluorescein; these usually occur within the first minute after the injection. Clinical experience indicates that this reaction occurs more often in agitated or nervous patients (and when the photographer is agitated or nervous!), in younger patients, and when the temperature of the room increases.

If a patient becomes nauseated, remain calm, ask him or her to sit back and take slow deep breaths through the mouth with eyes open. A reassuring attitude is important. We suggest to the patient that "the nausea usually passes as quickly as it comes" in low, calming tones. Try humor (*"Not many people react to this dye—you are one of the lucky 2%"*) or distraction (*"The pictures are timed—do you think we can take some more now?"*). Nausea does not always lead to vomiting. If it does, offer your patient an appropriate container. A plastic lined wastebasket is more useful than the often too small emesis basin.

Most minor reactions do not need medical intervention. If you think that the reaction may be more severe, stay with the patient and dispatch another person for a physician or registered nurse (a reminder: the person injecting should remain in the room for at least 1 minute after the injection). Signs of a more severe reaction include lightheadedness, difficulty breathing, fainting, and tightness in the chest.

Moderate adverse reactions to sodium fluorescein include urticaria (hives), which may occur 3–10 minutes after the injection. Urticaria is the result of an allergic reaction that releases histamine. The physician may prescribe an injectable or oral antihistamine to abate the problem. The patient should be monitored until all itching has stopped.

Both vasovagal and more severe reactions require decisive action. Obtain trained medical help immediately. Do not leave the room; rather, make the patient comfortable, perhaps helping him or her to lie on a stretcher or the floor and loosening any clothing around the neck. Locate the emergency supplies and assist emergency personnel. Help with transporting the patient or performing cardiopulmonary resuscitation as needed.

Keep in mind that your patients may be sick or fragile. The population that is likely to have fluorescein angiography includes the elderly as well patients with diabetes. Learn about the special needs of these patients as well as the reactions specific to this test.

Advanced Angiography Techniques

Oral Fluorescein Angiography

Intravenous injection of sodium fluorescein is the administration method of choice. In patients who are unable to receive an injection, it may be advantageous to administer the sodium fluorescein orally.[11] Photographing the injected dye reveals a full range of phases: choroidal, arterial, arteriovenous, and "lates." Oral fluorescein photographs disclose only the late phase of angiography. Oral administration is useful for determining the status of late leaking retinal conditions such as clinically significant macular edema or cystoid macular edema.

Double the intravenous dosage of sodium fluorescein and dissolve it in cold tomato or vegetable juice, or milk for children. Tomato juice masks some of the taste and most of the color. Staining of the patient's teeth can be reduced by using a straw. Powdered sodium fluorescein in capsules is available in Great Britain and Japan but not currently in the United States. Normal side effects, including staining of the skin and urine, are present. Expose a control photograph and record the dye at 5, 10, 15–20, and 30–40 minutes postingestion. This timing allows comparison of any leakage sites at multiple time intervals.

Angiography in Children

As with any medical procedure designed for adults, special considerations must be made for children. The dosage of sodium fluorescein should be

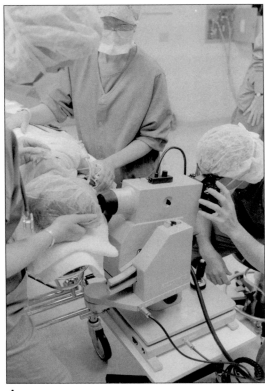

A

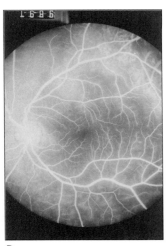

B

FIGURE 5-14
Angiography during examination under anesthesia (EUA). Fluorescein angiography may be performed in the operating room EUA. Use a hand-held fundus camera capable of angiography. Alternately, lay the patient on his or her side and use a standard fundus camera (A). Rotate the photographs 90 degrees for proper viewing (B).

adjusted specifically for the child's weight using the manufacturer's recommendations in the package insert. For example, if a package insert for a 500-mg (5-ml) ampule of 10% fluorescein sodium lists the children's dosage as 3.5 mg/lb, then a 50-lb child should receive 1.75 ml. The mathematics, using ratios with labeled units and two equations, would look like this:

$$50 \text{ lb} \times 3.5 \text{ mg/lb} = 175 \text{ mg}$$
$$175 \text{ mg} \times 5 \text{ ml}/500 \text{ mg} = 1.75 \text{ ml}$$

How many milliliters would the same child receive if a 750-mg (3-ml) ampule of 25% sodium fluorescein (recommended dosage: 5 mg/lb) were used? (The answer is found at the end of this section.)

This reduced dosage also holds true for smaller adults. We use the "100-lb rule"; if the patient weighs less than 100 lb, we calculate a lesser dosage. Larger than normal patients do not need their dosage increased because their greater bulk rarely reflects a larger vascular volume.

Excellent patient management skills are essential when working with children. Explain the procedure fully (using appropriate vocabulary) to both the child and the parents. Reassure them of the safety of the procedure and the importance of taking multiple photographs. Talk the patient and parents through the procedure, encouraging them and keeping their attention focused. Expose a minimal number of fundus photographs, keeping the patient fresh for the fluorescein series. A flawless injection technique is crucial. Consider using an anesthesiologist who may first numb the injection site topically. Shoot for quality, not quantity.

We have successfully performed office fluorescein angiography on patients as young as 3 years. For younger children, consider performing the test during an examination under anesthesia (EUA) (Figure 5-14).

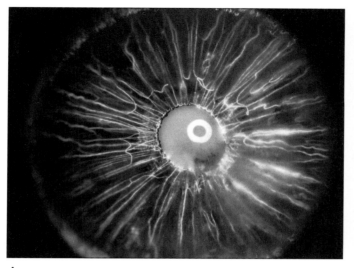

A

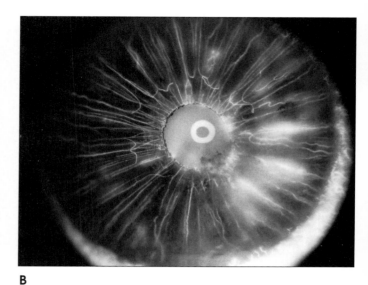

B

FIGURE 5-15
Anterior segment angiography. Angiograms of the cornea or iris may reveal important vascularization information. These early (A) and late (B) iris angiograms were photographed by Dennis Cain.

Table 5-4. Anterior Segment Angiography

Camera	Illumination System
Fundus camera	Standard
Photo-slit lamp	"Coffee can" attachment
35-mm single lens reflex mounted to fundus camera lens barrel	Fundus camera

(The answer to the dosage question above: 50 lb × 5 mg/lb = 250 mg; 250 mg × 3 ml/750 mg = 1 ml)

Anterior Segment Angiography

Abnormal blood vessels in the conjunctiva, cornea, or iris may be the subject of fluorescein angiography (Figure 5-15).[12, 13] Multiple strategies for recording anterior segment angiography have evolved: a 35-mm camera equipped with a macro lens has been mounted along the barrel of a standard fundus camera, a rapid recycling flash (affectionately dubbed the "coffee can attachment") for the Zeiss photo slit lamp has been marketed, and a 25-mm microscope lens has been mounted in front of a 30-degree fundus camera objective (Table 5-4).[14]

Whichever imaging system you use, choose your plane of focus carefully. The focal plane and the specific instrumentation are the major departures from the standard fluorescein procedure. The flash exposure is usually at least two steps higher and should be based on prior empirical exposure tests. Since a dark iris may block fluorescence, the most successful iris angiograms are of patients with light irises.

Color Fluorescein Angiography

High-speed color film may be substituted for black and white film during fluorescein angiography; however, the result is little different than what is seen through the viewfinder. A technique to record retinal fluorescence on a normally colored fundus photograph was developed by

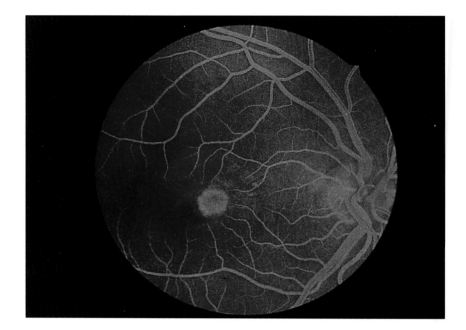

FIGURE 5-16
Color fluorescein angiography highlights fluorescence while representing the fundus in close to realistic color. (From S Shikano, K Shimizu. *Atlas of Fluorescence Fundus Angiography*. Philadelphia: Saunders, 1968;9.)

Matsui in the late 1960s (Figure 5-16).[15, 16] A magenta excitation filter (Wratten number 31 or 34) and a yellow (Wratten number 12) barrier filter were used with a medium-speed color film.[17] The resulting photographs document the circulating fluorescein with the fundus in natural color. Alternate methods include exposing color film using just the exciter or barrier filter. While suitable for the occasional teaching slide, color fluorescein angiography has not gained wide acceptance as a clinically useful technique.

References

1. Wolfe DR. Fluorescein angiography basic science and engineering. *Ophthalmology* 1986;93:1617.
2. Eastman Kodak Company. *Kodak Filter for Scientific and Technical Uses*. Rochester, NY: Eastman Kodak, 1981.
3. Novotny HR, Alvis DL. A method of photographing fluorescence in circulating blood in the human retina. *Circulation* 1961;24:82.
4. Haining WM, Lancaster RC. Advanced techniques for fluorescein angiography. *Arch Ophthalmol* 1968;79:10.
5. Delori F, Ben-Sira I, Trempe C. Fluorescein angiography with an optimized filter combination. *Am J Ophthalmol* 1976;82:559.
6. Emmart EW. Observations on the absorption spectra of fluorescein, fluorescein derivatives, and conjugates. *Arch Biochem Biophys* 1958;73:1.
7. Saine PJ, Bovino JA, Marcus DF, Nelson PT. Timing of color fundus photographs and intravenous fluorescein angiography. *Am J Ophthalmol* 1984;97:783.
8. Szirth BC, Wong GD, Bate R, Bartlett DA. Legal ramifications of administration of sodium fluorescein. *J Ophthal Photography* 1989;11:66.
9. Hampton GR, Nelsen PT, Hay PB. Viewing through the asteroids. *Ophthalmology* 1981;88:669.
10. Yannuzzi LA, Rohrer KT, Tindel LJ, et al. Fluorescein angiography complication survey. *Ophthalmology* 1986;93:611.
11. Kelley JS, Kincaid M. Retinal fluorography using oral fluorescein. *Arch Ophthalmol* 1979;97:2331.
12. Fetkenhour CL, Choromokos E. Anterior segment fluorescein angiography with a retinal fundus camera. *Arch Ophthalmol* 1978;96:711.

13. Brancato R, Bandello F, Lattanzio R. *Atlas Iris Fluorescein Angiography*. Milan, Italy: Kugler & Ghendini, 1995;1.
14. D'Anna SA, Hocheimer BF, Joondeph HC. Fluorescein angiography of the heavily pigmented iris and new dyes for iris angiography. *Arch Ophthalmol* 1983;101:289.
15. Schatz H, George T, Liu J, et al. Color fluorescein angiography: its clinical role. *Trans Am Acad Ophthalmol Otolaryngol* 1973;77:254.
16. Matsui K, Oka Y, Matsui T. Fluorescein fundus angiography in color. *Acta Soc Ophth Jap* 1969;73:653.
17. Shikano S, Shimizu K. *Atlas of Fluorescence Fundus Angiography*. Philadelphia: Saunders, 1968;9.

Chapter 6

The Ophthalmic Darkroom: Processing and Printing Fluorescein Angiograms

Lawrence M. Merin

Introduction

In one of his famous paintings, the surrealist artist Magritte painted an image of a pipe with the caption, "Ceci n'est pas une pipe" (This is not a pipe). Similarly, a fluorescein angiogram is obviously not dye in the retina and choroid, but rather a two-dimensional monochromatic representation of that reality. In this case, the painter and the ophthalmic photographer have the same challenges and opportunities: to ensure that their images communicate effectively.

Ophthalmic photographs use commonly accepted characteristics to convey information. Line, form, and especially tonal gradation are all essential components of the image and represent the physical attributes of the subject. Photographers must carefully choose their materials and master the processes that will reveal these qualities and thus imbue their photographs with veracity and eloquence.

For many, the craft of black and white film processing and printing is an enormously satisfying pursuit. In a world where more and more tasks may be accomplished by the computer and results appear through a sequence of button pushing, exposing film and processing it yourself is an intensely personal and human experience. There is also a magical quality to this activity. I confess that I often still feel a thrill as an image gradually appears on a plain sheet of paper in the developing tray, just as I did when I made my first print in my uncle's basement darkroom three decades ago. That amazement is certainly in keeping with the almost miraculous detail provided in fluorescein angiography. If you pause to linger over a properly exposed and processed fluorescein angiogram, you may find yourself enchanted by the magnificent detail and delicacy in the image.

The materials and processes of black and white photography have distinct capabilities for the reproduction of shades of gray, black, and white. In conventional fluorescein angiography, these attributes are of paramount importance, since film and paper materials are the only way to share the clinical information that the photographer witnesses privately through the camera eyepiece.

This chapter introduces you to the ophthalmic darkroom. The chapter offers a little of the theory and quite a bit about the practice of film development and touches on the methods of viewing and storing the angiographic negatives. Positive printouts in transparency and print formats are often generated from these negatives, and specific recommendations for fine-tuning this process are provided. Printing for exhibition or publication requires the highest level of technical skill, and I offer several suggestions to maximize the aesthetic as well as the informational qualities of the fine photographic print.

Each photographic procedure presents the photographer with choices. The first choice to be made is which camera and film to use to photograph the patient. The proper flash setting is then chosen to produce the correct exposure. Next, you must select a film developer, along with the time and temperature needed to produce proper negative contrast. If a positive version of the original negative is required, you must again choose the positive film or paper and its dedicated processing parameters. The place where the processing occurs, the ophthalmic darkroom, contains hardware and supplies chosen to facilitate the production of informative clinical images.

A note of caution: just reading this chapter will not be enough to master film processing and printing. If you want to become proficient, you must work with and refine the techniques yourself. This chapter provides enough theory to help you understand why things happen and suggests practical measures to help you understand the capabilities and limitations of photographic materials and processes. By reading and experimenting, you should learn how to make photographic choices confidently and enhance your skills as a capable scientific communicator.

The Darkroom

Designing the Ophthalmic Darkroom

The darkroom has been typecast as a gloomy and claustrophobic place where mechanical, boring, or otherwise distasteful tasks occur. By adopting modern design features, however, your darkroom can be a cheerful venue that is conducive to the creation of high-quality ophthalmic images.

As with other design projects, the first step in designing an efficient new ophthalmic darkroom (or renovating an older one) is to assess your specific needs. You should consider such things as the present and potential volume of the photographic service, the number of employees who may need to work in the darkroom simultaneously, whether the facility will process black and white materials exclusively or whether color film and prints will also be processed, and the degree of automation you may

Chromogenic Film

The image that is formed on conventional black and white negative film is composed of metallic silver. There are many different processes available for processing such materials, and that variety means that there is no "universal" method to achieve standardized results. Professional photographers test extensively and use their own custom processing parameters to achieve the results they desire.

Ilford's XP-2 film initially captures the image using silver halides but, during processing, replaces the silver with semitransparent color dye clouds to form a "black and white" photograph. This film is designed to be processed in color negative processing solutions (process C-41), commonly found in automated mini-lab facilities associated with amateur film photoprocessing. Portraiture is the most common subject matter for amateur photographers, and flesh tones in these snapshots can be printed accurately only through tight processing control. For this reason, C-41 chemistry is designed to be used within very narrow limits of time and temperature. Conveniently, this also provides a consistent processing standard for fluorescein angiograms.

XP-2 has a film sensitivity of ISO 400 and thus is similar to conventional films used for fluorescein angiography. It is panchromatic and responds accurately to the specific wavelengths of light used during the study. Its image structure and resolution compare favorably with its silver counterparts, and the film's granularity is actually much finer than that of conventional black and white 400-speed emulsions. The image seen in XP-2 negatives has a magenta cast rather than the gray typically seen in conventional film media but is nonetheless eminently readable.

Most mini-labs routinely produce 3.5" × 5" or 4" × 6" prints, and XP-2 angiograms can be machine printed the same way. These angiographic prints may appear to have a sepia cast, but this will not obscure diagnostic information. The total turnaround time for negatives and prints from such a facility is approximately 1 hour. If specialized printouts are required, such as contact sheets or exhibition prints, XP-2 negatives can be used the same way as conventional black and white negatives. Because of these attributes, XP-2 can be a useful alternative to setting up a dedicated darkroom for small-volume practices.

Table 6-1. Three Styles of Ophthalmic Darkrooms

Minimal	Standard	Advanced
Negative processing	Negative processing Contact prints	Negative processing Contact prints Enlargements

desire. The answers to these service-related questions will logically suggest hardware and physical plant decisions and, in turn, will help determine the budget for the project.

Obviously, the first question is whether a darkroom is a necessary feature of a particular photographic service. For many practices, concerns about quality control, cost-effectiveness, and immediate availability of processing can best be addressed when the darkroom is located within the office or institution. To maximize quality, you can alter film processing at will, to adjust for unusual pathology or physical characteristics of the subject. Consistent quality results from careful attention to detail, and this comes from having all the processing parameters under your control.

Probably the most important aspect of providing your own processing service comes from rapid availability of the photograph. No outside processor can provide angiographic results as quickly as in-house film processing, a crucial benefit for patients requiring urgent treatment for vision-threatening disorders.

The direct costs of in-house processing are typically less than those paid to send the film out. Consumables, such as the cost of processing chemicals, usually come to under $1 per roll. If you factor in indirect costs (space, equipment, labor, and benefits) you may still save money, particularly if you process several angiograms simultaneously.

For an extremely low-volume practice or one in which there is no space for a darkroom, using a professional extramural service for conventional film processing may be a logical choice. Alternately, such a practice might consider using a chromogenic film (see the sidebar on chromogenic film) for expedient processing in the same locality. Of course, practices that acquire digital angiographic equipment may not require a conventional darkroom at all. However, the theories of tonal reproduction included in this chapter are equally applicable to electronic imaging, even though electronic, rather than chemical, means are used to obtain and modify the angiographic information.

Color slide processing for fundus photography and the printing of such slides are outside the scope of this chapter. However, only the busiest ophthalmic practices have the volume that would make color film processing cost-effective, considering supply and labor costs.

Black and white processing, on the other hand, can be either simple or complex, depending on the sophistication required of the service. Three levels of technology are typically encountered in ophthalmic darkrooms: minimal (film only), standard (film and contact sheets), and advanced (film, contact sheets, and paper enlargements). Each category has specific requirements for space, hardware, and supplies (Table 6-1).

What is a darkroom? First, it is a dedicated space designed to control ambient illumination when processing light-sensitive materials. Such a place needs to incorporate three different lighting situations: (1) white light, typically provided by fluorescent or tungsten light fixtures and used for chemical mixing, setting up hardware for processing tasks, and

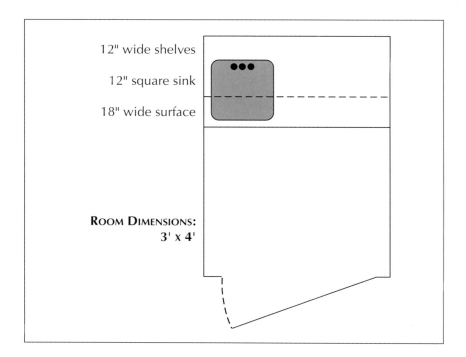

12" wide shelves

12" square sink

18" wide surface

ROOM DIMENSIONS:
3' x 4'

FIGURE 6-1
Plan and elevation of the minimal darkroom. In a space of only 12 square feet, angiographic negatives can be developed, washed, and dried.

general maintenance; (2) total darkness, for loading film into processing tanks; and (3) "safe light" illumination of a specific color (typically amber or red) for paper and sheet film processing. Although other parameters (such as plumbing, ventilation, access, and total area) are all important, the defining character of the darkroom is light control.

Regardless of size and space, a major consideration in designing a darkroom is the division between wet and dry work areas. Because sensitive materials (i.e., unprocessed film and paper) are particularly susceptible to contamination from water, processing solution splashes, and chemical dust, they must be protected from such accidents. Design the darkroom work space so that a physical barrier separates the processing sink and chemical storage area (wet side) from the film-loading area, paper storage areas, and the enlarger (dry side). That barrier might be either an aisle or a partition, depending on the configuration of the room. If floor space does not permit such a division, then the dry "side" may simply be a secure cabinet above the sink.

When planning space for the darkroom, you must anticipate the required square footage for the specific processes you will perform there. For film processing only, a spartan facility as small as 12 square feet is sufficient (Figure 6-1). For a facility to process film and a tray line for contact sheet and print production, a minimum of 36 square feet allows adequate space (Figure 6-2). An even larger space permits other nonclinical photographic tasks (i.e., copy work) to be performed (Figure 6-3).

Because film used for angiography is extremely sensitive to light, the darkroom must be totally light-proof so no stray illumination can strike the film while it is being loaded onto the processing reels. The most common sources for stray light include the gap between the door and its frame, spaces between tiles in acoustical or "drop" ceilings, and holes through which plumbing fixtures enter the darkroom. Apply flexible rubber weather-stripping material (available at hardware or home improvement stores) to the edges of doors to prevent light leakage. Rubber flanges designed to prevent air drafts are also useful to seal the

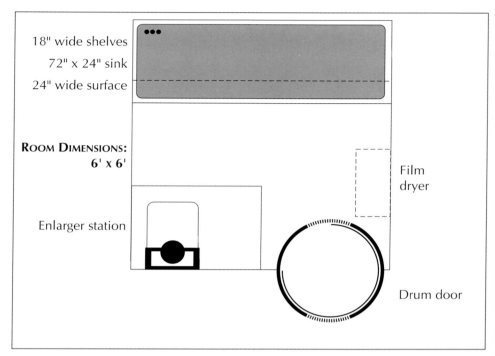

FIGURE 6-2
Plan of standard ophthalmic darkroom. If you have a 36-square foot space, both negative processing and positive printout production may be handled.

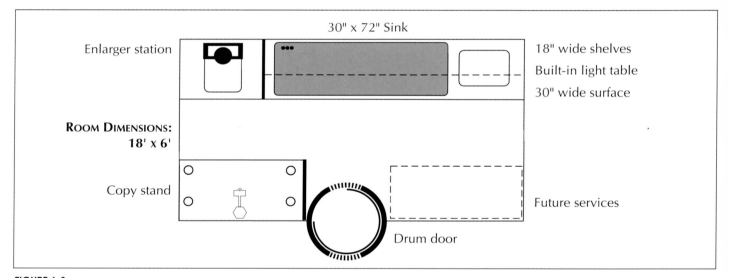

FIGURE 6-3
Diagram of an advanced darkroom. This plan of the Jones Eye Institute darkroom indicates the space allocation for enlarging, processing, drying, and ancillary production activities required to support an academic department of ophthalmology.

bottoms of doors from errant light. Drop ceilings should incorporate tight-fitting tiles to prevent stray light from distant fixtures or adjacent rooms from entering the darkroom.

The best way to detect problems with light leakage is to simply stand in the darkroom for 15–20 minutes after all lights have been turned off inside the room, but with all lights illuminated in adjacent rooms and hallways. This allows you to adapt to the dark and permits even small points of light to be seen. Using opaque black photographic tape, block

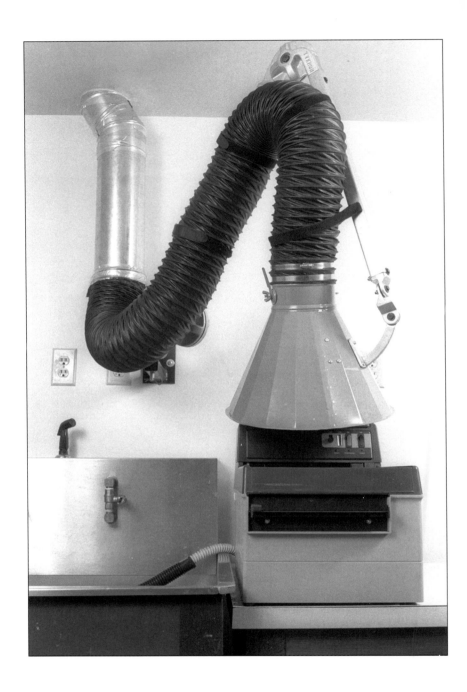

FIGURE 6-4
Vent hood. To satisfy OSHA requirements and to make the darkroom safer and more pleasant, this vent hood helps rid the darkroom of noxious fumes. (Courtesy of B.J. Graham.)

any tiny lights observed in the ceiling, and apply additional pieces of foam rubber to the door frame if any similar leaks are detected there.

Since proper light-proofing also restricts air flow, arrange for forced air ventilation in the darkroom.[1] Light-proof louvers and fans, sold through professional photographic suppliers, permit fresh air to replace contaminated air freely, while they simultaneously prevent light from entering the room. Since many processing solutions emit noxious odors and even toxic fumes, assisted ventilation is highly recommended for health and safety reasons and may be mandated by law in your state (Figure 6-4). To be certain that the air quality will be sufficient, considering the number of workers in the darkroom and the nature of the processes used, consult with an industrial hygienist or a ventilation engineer when planning any new facility.

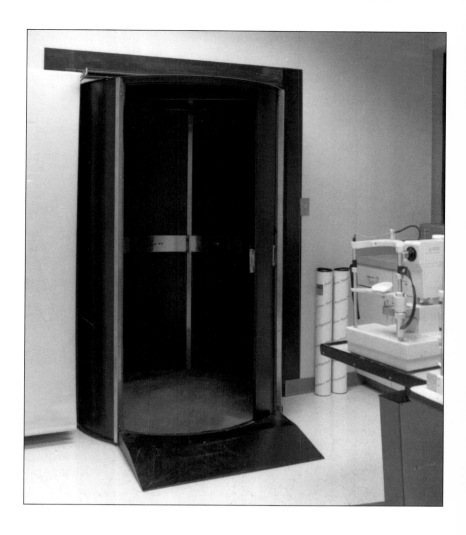

FIGURE 6-5
Drum door. These allow entry into the darkroom without permitting outside lighting to change the illumination chosen for work within the area.

Equip the darkroom with its own thermostat for heating and cooling. If the air temperature is kept at the same setting as the required temperature for processing (typically 68–72°F), then you can use stored chemical solutions immediately without requiring water baths to heat or cool them.

For most standard and advanced darkrooms, standard line voltage should be sufficient to operate timers, safelights, and enlargers. In North America, this means a 110-volt, 20-ampere circuit. Because the darkroom is a damp environment, use ground fault interrupter (GFI) outlets and three-wire grounding plugs to reduce the risk of electrical shocks. Make sure that outlets are placed behind the sink to provide current for processing timers, adjacent to the enlarger for its own power requirement, and proximal to the film or print dryer. The enlarger should be on a separate circuit to avoid voltage fluctuations. Safelights should have their own switch-controlled outlets. Many photographers arrange for a single master power switch next to the door, so all circuits may be shut off when processing and printing have been completed.

Exposed film is at its most vulnerable state when being transferred from its cassette to the processing reel and daylight tank. The film will be ruined if someone inadvertently opens the darkroom door at that moment. The most elegant way of avoiding such a catastrophe while providing easy access to the facility is the rotating drum door. These devices allow easy entry and exit without affecting existing darkroom lighting conditions (Figure 6-5). A less expensive alternative is to equip the door with a slid-

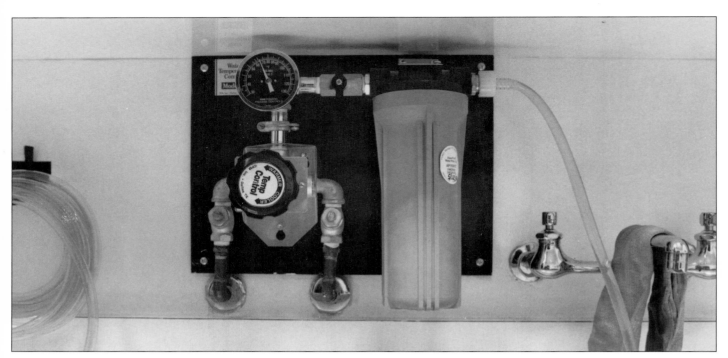

FIGURE 6-6
Thermostatic mixing valve. Photographic-quality valves allow the water temperature to be easily selected and maintained. This valve includes a water filter to ensure a clean water supply.

ing lock operable only from the inside, although some means of alternate entry from outside may be useful in an emergency. Illuminated "in use" signs may alert others to darkroom activities if they are mounted conspicuously outside the darkroom.

Although the design of the minimal darkroom does not absolutely require its own water supply (since you can use another room in the clinic to mix processing solutions and wash film), professional installations need both hot and cold running water. Depending on the cleanliness of the water supply, an inline water filter may prevent suspended grit or organic matter from adhering to the film. Typical black and white processing requires a flow rate of at least 3 gallons per minute and a temperature of 65–75°F; if your practice is in a warm climate, you may need to install a small refrigeration unit or "chiller" to cool the water in the summer. A photographic-quality thermostatic mixing valve is highly recommended (Figure 6-6) for convenient temperature control. These valves incorporate a gauge that allows the temperature of the water to be precisely set and easily maintained.

Standard and advanced darkrooms require a processing sink. These fixtures are designed to be set into a cabinetry base or may be supported by their own leg and shelf assembly and are used to provide a work surface to process film and printout media. The typical darkroom sink is about 4–6 inches deep. Determine its area by counting the number and size of processing trays to be used simultaneously, plus the area of the print washer. The ophthalmic darkroom should be able to process 8" × 10" material, since that is the minimum size for an angiographic contact print. Thus, a 2- × 4-foot sink is the minimum size for four 8" × 10" trays, though a larger sink will allow the trays to be manipulated with less congestion. On occasion, exhibition printing up to 11" × 14" may be called for. Rarely will the next larger size, 16" × 20", be requested.

Typical darkroom sinks are constructed of either fiberglass or stainless steel. Fiberglass sinks are lighter and less costly than steel but are also easier to scratch. They must be cleaned with special care using only nonabrasive cleaners. Stainless steel sinks are impervious to chemicals and last for many years with no sign of wear or breakdown of their surface. When either type of sink is installed, use shims under the sink or its legs to ensure that sufficient gradient is provided for proper water drainage. Without the slope, water will tend to pool in the sink instead of flowing out through the drain.

The last construction detail to consider is the finish for the walls, cabinetry, and floor. For a pleasant workplace that is easy to clean, paint the walls with washable high-gloss white enamel. White allows the room to be maximally bright under safelight illumination but will not contribute to fogging of sensitive materials.[2] Finish the walls directly behind or adjoining the enlarger with flat black paint to absorb stray reflected light when printing. Consider white plastic laminates for all work surfaces, table tops, and cabinet faces, since this material allows chemical spills to be easily cleaned. The floor must be waterproof, of course, and a central floor drain is good insurance against accidental water damage to adjacent offices if the sink leaks or a hose becomes disconnected. Either vinyl tile or sheet flooring material is a good choice. Install cushioned flooring material (i.e., Ace Koralite) on top of the standard floor to help prevent leg pain if darkroom workers must stand for prolonged periods.

Equipping the Darkroom

Because the array of hardware required for black and white processing is task-specific, the minimal darkroom requires only a few items. Standard and advanced darkrooms need a greater array of tools. These specialized materials are best found at professional photographic suppliers.

The following basic equipment is required for manual film processing:

1. *Thermometer.* An accurate thermometer is required because processing is a chemical reaction influenced by the temperature of the solutions. Fluid-filled glass thermometers are extremely accurate but quite fragile and difficult to read. Metal thermometers with dial faces are more durable and may be read even under safelight illumination. For the ultimate in accuracy, digital units are available. When first purchased, thermometers should be calibrated against a laboratory-quality instrument to verify their accuracy.

2. *Timer.* Timing the duration of the processing steps requires a timer that shows both minutes and seconds. Although one could use a standard clock with a sweep second hand, a far superior choice is a laboratory timer that counts down from the total required time to zero (Figure 6-7). Such timers typically have large luminous numbers and hands and also have an audible alarm buzzer that may be set to sound at the end of the time interval.

3. *Tanks and reels.* Film-processing reels and tanks are available in either plastic or stainless steel. The two materials have significant differences. To load steel reels requires greater manual dexterity, and thus practice is needed before loading can be confidently accomplished.[3] However, steel is impervious to chemical contamination and is an excellent thermal conductor (important when adjusting solution temperatures in a water bath). To load a steel reel, attach the end of the film to the center of the reel (with a spring clip, slot, or pair of prongs, depending on the model and brand) and then slowly turn the reel while the film is fed into it. Stainless steel reels may be loaded successfully when damp. However, if a steel

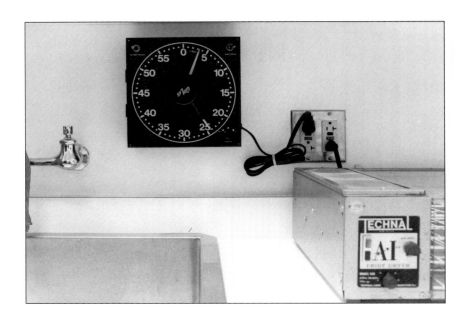

FIGURE 6-7
Laboratory timer. This unit features luminous hands that count down to zero, and a loud buzzer (that may be turned off) that announces the conclusion of each processing step. The timer is plugged into a ground fault interupter receptacle that provides an extra measure of electrical safety in this wet environment.

reel falls to the floor, it may be permanently bent (although this is less of a problem if high-quality, heavy-gauge reels are purchased).

Plastic reels employ a ratchet mechanism that semiautomatically pulls the film onto the spiral reel. Their construction style and material make thorough cleaning difficult. Even minimal moisture in the film track can prevent proper loading. The plastic tank is a poor thermal conductor, and thus its contents cannot be cooled or heated easily in a water bath. On the positive side, however, many novices find the semiautomatic loading feature much easier to master than loading a steel reel. If your darkroom uses an automatic film processing machine that uses plastic or stainless steel reels, then you have no choice in the type of reel to use.

Once loaded, the processing reels are placed in "daylight" tanks, containers that have a built-in light trap that allows the processing solutions to be poured in and emptied, rapidly, in bright room illumination (Figure 6-8). Tanks to accommodate one, two, four, and eight reels can be acquired. I have found it useful to equip my own darkroom with three tanks (one each of one-, two-, and four-reel sizes). With this selection, I can always process films efficiently.

4. *Solution storage tanks.* Mixed processing solutions must be stored in containers that limit evaporation and oxidation. Plastic or glass bottles with tight-fitting tops may be equally effective for small batches of solutions. However, if space permits, the use of storage containers with built-in spigots permits the easy transfer of solutions (Figure 6-9). These containers are available in 1-, 2-, and 5-gallon sizes and come with floating lids to limit oxidation caused by the large area of fluid surface in contact with the air. If the standard solutions are premixed to working strength and stored in these containers, then it is simple and quick to decant the required quantity.

Another alternative storage method is to use multiple small bottles to store chemistry. If 1 gallon of liquid is prepared, it may be stored in four quart-size bottles, each filled to the top, to limit oxidation.

Because many photographic processing solutions are colorless, be sure to label each storage container with its contents. Once the containers are labeled, you can avoid future contamination by only

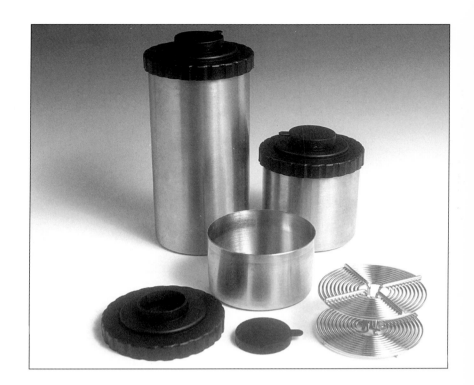

FIGURE 6-8
"Daylight" style tanks incorporate a two-part top that permits solutions to be poured in and drained without allowing the film to be exposed by light.

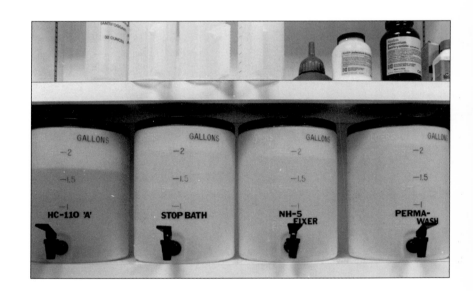

FIGURE 6-9
Two-gallon storage tanks with spigots. These allow solutions to be easily poured into measuring containers by simply opening the valve. The labels are created with self-stick black vinyl lettering. Be sure to follow OSHA labeling guidelines for hazardous substances.

refilling the container with its labeled contents. If you use a label-making machine to identify these containers, avoid red labeling tape, since it cannot be read under safelight illumination.

5. *Graduates, beakers, funnels.* Assorted measuring devices are required when processing film. Although photographic supply houses offer a variety of these items, try discount stores that sell them inexpensively as houseware items. Before use, verify their accuracy by comparing their marked volumes with a laboratory-grade graduate. Plastic is preferred over glass because of its durability and break-resistance. Translucent plastic allows the fluid level to be readily ascertained. (Although measuring utensils are also available in

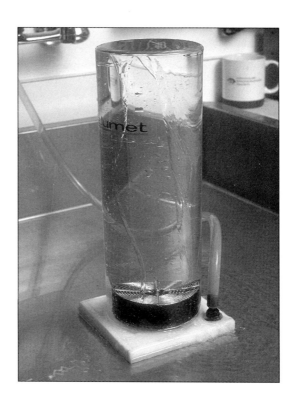

FIGURE 6-10
Film washer. This device allows flowing fresh water to cleanse the film of residual fixer and washing aid chemistry.

stainless steel, they are costly and are more difficult to read, since you cannot determine the exact location of the fluid meniscus for accurate measurements). A set of three each of 1-pint and 1-quart graduates, and a 1-gallon plastic bucket will be needed for solution mixing and film processing.

6. *Film washer*. After processing the film, it must be washed. You can wash film simply by setting the tank underneath a running faucet, but much more thorough washing can be accomplished (with less water!) by using a dedicated film washer. Such devices typically use a length of plastic tubing to connect to the faucet. The wash water is sent into the unit where residual processing chemistry is washed out of the film. Some washers introduce the water at the bottom of the unit, and it then exits by overflowing from the top (Figure 6-10). Others bring the water into the top and the waste water exits from the bottom. Still others use siphon action to completely fill and empty the washer in cycles. Each style of washer has its adherents, and each can be effective provided sufficient time is spent washing the film.

7. *Film dryer*. After washing has been completed, the film must be dried. For many years, film manufacturers recommended that the film be "hung to dry in a dust-free place." Although that suggestion is still applicable, film dryers speed the process and allow the angiogram to be safely examined in a fraction of the time air-drying requires. Film dryers incorporate a heater and a fan mounted in an enclosure, allowing the films to be suspended in a stream of warm air. Filters are used to ensure that the air is dust-free. The fastest dryers use a high-speed fan and allow the film to be dried on the processing reel; some will dry a single roll of film in as little as 2 minutes (Figure 6-11). If you use a machine that dries film while still on its reels, be sure to scrub the reels in hot soapy water

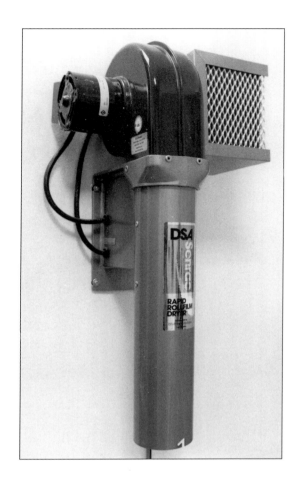

FIGURE 6-11
Forced-air film dryer. This unit is one of the fastest dryers available and is capable of drying a roll of film quickly while still wound on the processing reel.

thoroughly after removing the dried film. Otherwise, residues from the dried wetting agent will accumulate on the reels and contaminate the development process for subsequent rolls of film.

The items described in 1–7 allow standard processing of black and white camera film. The preferred method of angiographic analysis consists of directly viewing the processed negative. However, if positive copies are required (i.e., to send a copy of the study to the referring physician), a contact sheet may be produced. Either sheet film or paper may be used for this purpose, and either medium requires the following additional equipment for processing:

1. *Contact printer.* Contact prints are produced by placing the emulsion side of the negative onto the emulsion side of the paper or sheet film, pressing the two materials into firm contact, and then exposing the print medium to light through the negative. Specially designed contact printers may be used. These machines consist of a series of individually controlled lights, a fully adjustable timer, and a pneumatic pressure plate that maintains firm contact between the negative and the printout material (Figure 6-12). Such contact printers are perfect for ophthalmic use because you can customize their light pattern to produce multiple prints with precisely matched characteristics, but they are expensive.

   A low-tech, low-cost alternative consists of a standard photographic contact frame (Figure 6-13), comprised of a sponge rubber

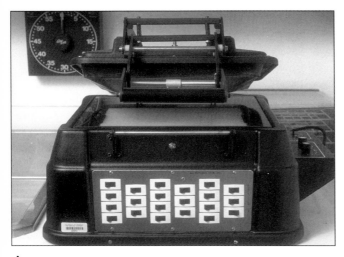

A

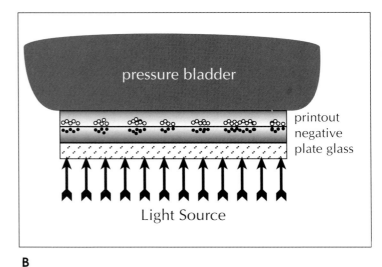

B

FIGURE 6-12
Professional contact printer. Ideal for producing high-quality single printouts or multiple matching prints (A). Its light source strikes the negative and printout from below (B).

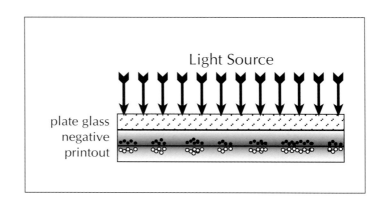

FIGURE 6-13
Photographic contact frame in cross-section. This simple device uses a controlled light source, such as an enlarger, to expose the printout.

or felt pad with a hinged plate-glass cover. With this device, the negative-printout sandwich is placed into the unit, the glass cover is closed, and the regulated light source is provided by either a low-wattage bulb suspended over the work or an enlarger with a timer to regulate exposure duration. For the ultimate in simplicity, some photographers use a single piece of plate glass and simply lay the glass on top of the negative-printout sandwich beneath the enlarger when contact printing. For either simple method, make sure that firm pressure is applied to the sandwich to counteract the natural curve of the film. If the negative and the printout medium are not in tight contact, the positive will not be sharp.

One problem associated with the use of high-contrast sheet film as the printout material is the inadvertent production of dust spots on the printout. These tiny white spots are caused by dust particles

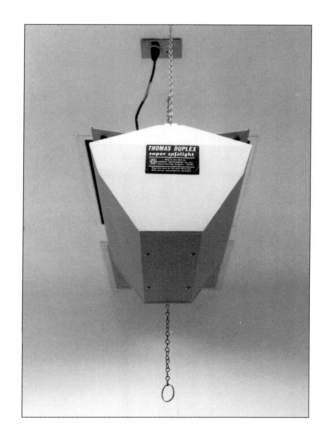

FIGURE 6-14
Sodium vapor safelight. This Thomas Duplex safelight produces enormous quantities of safe illumination from its sodium vapor bulb. Suspended from the ceiling, its light shines on the ceiling and walls, creating indirect illumination.

Testing Safelight Illumination

In spite of their name, safelights are not completely "safe." If the orthochromatic photo material remains under safelight illumination that is too bright or for too long, some fogging may occur. Under certain conditions, virtually all safelights may cause fogging.

To test your safe-light, in total darkness place a sheet of printout material you usually use (paper or sheet film) in the same location as the tray line would normally be and place several coins or other opaque objects on the sheet. Turn on the safelight and allow it to illuminate the sheet for two or three times the duration of the longest processing time. Next, turn off the safelight and, in total darkness, develop, stop, and fix the sheet. Turn on the room lights and inspect the printout. If you can see where the coins were placed, this indicates that the safelight fogged the adjacent areas. Either move the safelight farther away, replace its bulb with one of lower wattage, or shorten the exposure time for the next test until you have determined the maximum "safe" time and/or brightness.

that are caught in the beam of light and produce tiny unexposed shadows that appear white. Most of these artifacts can be prevented by changing the illumination from a point source to a broad, diffused one. This can be simply accomplished by fastening a thin sheet of frosted plastic (i.e., milky Plexiglass like that used on the front of x-ray viewboxes) or opal glass to the glass top of the printing frame. When the enlarger's illumination strikes this diffusion material, the frosted medium in turn becomes a broad, diffuse light source that virtually eliminates the spots without changing the sharpness of the contact sheet. The diffusion sheet must be homogeneous to produce suitable diffusion, so avoid rippled or textured materials.

2. *Safelight.* The film used in the camera for angiography is panchromatic (sensitive to the full spectrum of visible light). Before processing, this material must be handled in total darkness. Photographic paper and contact sheet film are usually orthochromatic (relatively insensitive to red or amber light). Safelights are designed to produce illumination that will usually not expose these orthochromatic materials (see the sidebar on testing safelight illumination).

Most safelights incorporate a low-wattage tungsten bulb in a fixture with a glass filter that limits the emitted wavelengths to either amber or red. The most efficient safelights use a sodium vapor lamp and adjustable louvers for maximal "safe" illumination (Figure 6-14). These lamps produce amazing quantities of light and thus enhance the working environment.

The color of the safelight illumination must be matched to the printout material. Many photographic papers require the use of an "OC" filter that produces a yellowish-orange illumination, while certain sheet films specify that a "1A" filter be used, producing a fairly dim red light. If your filter does not match the spectral requirements of the printout, fogging may result!

3. *Photo trays and tongs.* Following exposure, the printout material (sheet film or paper) must be processed. For manual laboratories, processing occurs in print trays. Sized for 5" × 7", 8" × 10", 11" × 14", and 16" × 20" print material, these are usually made of plastic. To minimize eye fatigue when working under safelight illumination, all-white trays are preferred to those made of red, black, or other colors. The bottoms of the best trays feature either raised ribs or buttons; these facilitate removal of the print when processing is completed. To prevent cross-contamination of chemistry, label each tray and tong (i.e., developer, stop-bath, and fixer).

Use a set of stainless steel or plastic tongs to transfer the paper from tray to tray. Some developing agents, such as metol, have the potential to cause an allergic skin reaction, so use tongs instead of bare fingers to decrease your chances of developing metol poisoning or contact dermatitis.

Of the tongs currently available, stainless steel ones are the most durable, although plastic tongs will work well if they are handled carefully. Avoid those made of bamboo with rubber tips, since they will retain chemistry and cannot be cleaned adequately to avoid future contamination of print materials.

4. *Paper safe.* A paper safe is a light-tight box with a hinged door that permits individual sheets of film or paper to be easily removed under safelight illumination. The safe uses baffles to prevent its contents from being accidentally exposed to white light. Even though the original packing container for paper or film may be used for its storage, the use of a paper safe streamlines printmaking.

5. *Print washer.* After processing the contact sheet, residual chemistry needs to be washed out of its emulsion. The simplest, least expensive washers permit you to use a standard processing tray to wash prints; these use a siphon that attaches to the tray to constantly circulate fresh water and drain contaminated water. More sophisticated units are made of Plexiglass and use water jets to continually bathe each print with clean water (Figure 6-15). Since fixer-laden water is heavier than clean water, one might assume that washers that drain from the bottom would be superior, although the turbulence caused by entering clean water keeps the fixer well circulated. Thus, either style of washer may be effective, provided that the prints are allowed to move around in the water stream and that sufficient time is permitted for maximal chemistry removal.

6. *Squeegees and print dryers.* After the wash has been completed, the print needs to be dried. If rapid turnaround times are not important, you may squeegee them to remove excess water and then clip the prints to a thin overhead wire or string (akin to a clothesline) and allow them to air dry (Figure 6-16). Some dryers use a heated forced air system to dry prints quickly, while others use an infrared drying element. Stationary units that direct the air flow onto the prints may be used for either paper or sheet film materials. Roller transport dryers that move the materials through the hot-air chamber can usually be used only for paper materials.

One of the best methods of drying fiber-based paper prints consists of placing the squeegeed prints onto clean fiberglass screens. This technique allows the prints to dry slowly in room air. Avoid the use of blotters or drum dryers for paper prints; both are prone to contamination and cannot be cleaned easily.

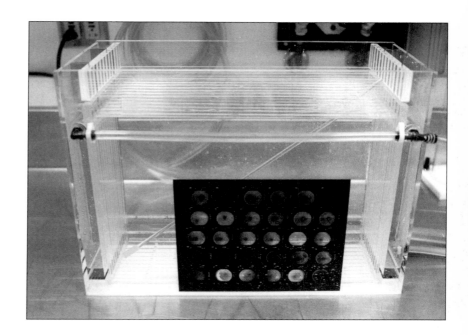

FIGURE 6-15
Plexiglass print washer. Properly designed print washers continually bathe both surfaces of prints with fresh water to remove processing chemistry.

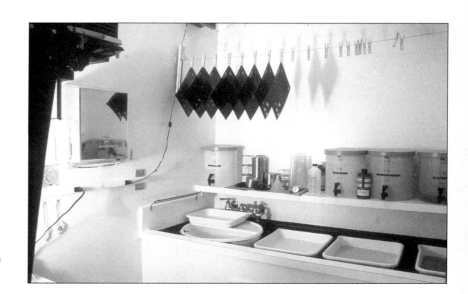

FIGURE 6-16
Printout drying. One of the simplest methods for drying sheet film or resin-coated paper prints is to hang them up to dry. This darkroom has been equipped with a sturdy metal wire line above the darkroom sink. Regular wooden spring clothespins are drilled and threaded onto the line and securely grasp each print for air drying. Note the tray line set up in the sink.

The Advanced Darkroom

The advanced ophthalmic darkroom has the capability of producing enlargements on paper. The following items are required for this assignment (see the sidebar on machine processing options for film and positive printouts).

1. *Enlarger.* The enlarger projects the image of the negative onto photographic paper to produce a positive print. Component parts of this device include a light source, negative carrier, lens board with an enlarging lens, support column, and baseboard. Condenser enlargers collimate the light and direct it evenly over the negative,

Machine Processing Options for Film and Positive Printouts

Within the last decade, automation has made steady advances in the ophthalmic darkroom. If your practice produces a high volume of angiograms, some degree of machine-processing technology may prove beneficial, since it may free the photographer from the darkroom and allow more time for patient contact. Of the various methods of processing automation, the two types most commonly used in ophthalmology are the rotary tube and the roller transport processors.

Both technologies automate the series of processing steps, and thus you only need to load the film and retrieve it from the machine when the steps have been completed. With manual processing, you must take care of each step yourself; machine processing permits you to leave the darkroom for the largest portion of the processing time.

In rotary tube processing, the film is threaded onto a processing reel, just as with manual "daylight tank" processing. The loaded reels are placed into the processing chamber. In some machines, this looks similar to the manual tanks, while others use a covered trough-like chamber. When the process begins, a motor starts rotating and sometimes oscillating the reels. Developer is automatically introduced into the processing container or trough. When the required development time has concluded, a valve opens automatically, permitting the used developer to exit the chamber. A brief water rinse typically ensues, followed by draining. Fixer is then admitted and the agitation cycle commences, followed by a water wash cycle. The film is manually removed from the machine for conventional drying.

In the health care field, roller transport machines were first used in radiology and dental departments. They consist of separate chambers that hold developer, fixer, and wash water. The rollers are made of rubber and consist of paired units that are motor-driven; they gently squeeze the film and pull it sequentially through the processing solutions. To begin processing, the film is removed from its cassette and taped to a leader card. This stiff piece of plastic sheet is then inserted into the first pair of rollers, and the angiographic film follows the card through the different chambers.[4] Several rolls of film can often be processed simultaneously, and once the film is inside the processor (or enclosed in a light-proof loading chamber), room lights may be turned on. Roller transport processors often incorporate a forced-air dryer, so the completely processed film emerges from the machine dry and ready to view. In addition to roll film, roller transport processors can also process sheet film and paper prints, often with the same processing chemistry.

Provided that regular and thorough maintenance is performed on the machines, films processed automatically are indistinguishable from those processed manually. In fact, the motorized agitation and the timer-regulated fluid transfer enable machine processing to potentially achieve a higher degree of uniformity and absolutely consistent results. These benefits are in addition to the fact that automatic processing frees valuable photographer time.

Although this technology is not inexpensive, a careful assessment of labor costs, personnel utilization, and patient volume may reveal a clear application for processing automation in your department.

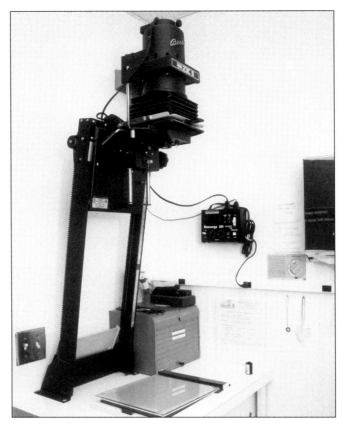

FIGURE 6-17
Photographic enlarger. Although 35-mm enlargers can produce acceptable work, those designed to accommodate larger negatives, such as this Beseler 23C enlarger, produce a wider field of even illumination

although after-market light sources are available to change the illumination quality.

Some ophthalmic photographers prefer point-source enlargers that produce extremely sharp prints but are prone to image dust, dirt, and scratches with equal precision. Others prefer "cold light" enlarging and use a fluorescent lamp light source. These enlargers minimize dust spots on the print and often reduce the need for burning and dodging. Like many other aspects of ophthalmic photography, the choice becomes one of personal preference, provided your enlarger produces the print quality you and your clients demand.

When properly adjusted, the enlarger's baseboard, lens board, and negative carrier are all perfectly parallel with each other and are held in rigid alignment. A well-designed enlarger column permits this to occur and allows the enlarger head to be raised off the baseboard for selected magnifications while maintaining structural rigidity.

For most applications, the best enlarger for any format is one capable of accommodating the next larger negative size. If 35-mm work is to be done, an enlarger capable of handling 6- × 6-cm negatives would therefore be chosen (Figure 6-17). This ensures that the negative is kept well centered within the illumination of the instrument and that no fall-off of density caused by diminished light intensity will appear at the edges of the resulting prints.

Most enlarger manufacturers offer negative carriers in a variety of sizes. Carriers are usually made of metal. Avoid those that incorporate glass windows that contact the negative, as the glass surfaces attract dirt. Many carriers have an aperture that is too small to permit the entire frame to be projected. If you cannot see clear film surrounding the entire image when it is projected onto the easel, you may wish to use a fine metal file to slightly enlarge the aperture. Following this operation, carefully apply flat black paint to the shiny metal edges.

2. *Enlarging lens*. The focal length of the enlarging lens is designed to provide a reasonable degree of enlargement at the baseboard and is different for each film size. A 50-mm enlarging lens is typically used to enlarge 35-mm camera negatives, although a longer lens (i.e., 80-mm) produces a slight improvement in the evenness of illumination. Unlike camera lenses, enlarging lenses are optically corrected for the limited range of magnifications typically needed to produce prints. Their maximum aperture is seldom faster than f2.8, and lenses with wide-open settings of f4 or f5.6 are common. Because print sharpness and resolution are a direct result of lens quality, it is logical to pay more for a high-quality optic, rather than to accept compromised quality for the sake of saving a few dollars.

If a condenser illuminating system is used, it must be adjusted to match the lens, not just the film size. Maximal sharpness and contrast can only be achieved with a precise match between the enlarging lens and the condenser.

3. *Enlarging timer*. When printing, minor differences in the duration of the enlarging exposure can show up as significant changes in print density. To do a proper job of enlarging, the enlarger must be controlled by a dedicated timer that turns its lamp on and off with precision. The simplest enlarging timer is the standard laboratory timer mentioned above; this unit allows the duration of each exposure to be set directly. More sophisticated timers incorporate an automatic reset feature that can be useful for local exposure control. The ultimate timer is a digital unit that incorporates a photocell in the lamphouse so the timer monitors the actual light output of the lamp in addition to the time (Figure 6-18); this feature may be crucial with cold light enlargers, since the light output from fluorescent tubes is known to vary considerably.

4. *Paper easels*. Enlarging paper must be held flat on the baseboard and must be positioned to include the selected portions of the negative. A paper easel is designed to accomplish both of these tasks. Most easels allow for a narrow (approximately ¼-inch) border to remain unexposed around the paper's perimeter. Adjustable units can accommodate paper of varying sizes and have either two or four blades that may be independently set for the desired image size. Those designed for fixed sizes of paper (Figure 6-19) permit speedy operation.

5. *Grain focusers*. The image must be critically focused when it is projected onto the easel. Because many modern films have fine grain, it is difficult to do this without optical assistance. A grain focuser is a low-powered microscope that uses a mirror to project the negative image to its eyepiece (Figure 6-20). While observing carefully through the focusing device, adjust the enlarger's focusing knob until a distinct grain pattern, representing the image itself, is observed clearly. Since grain focusers ensure critically sharp results,

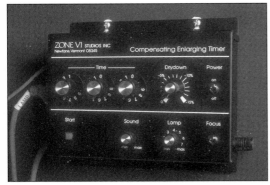

A

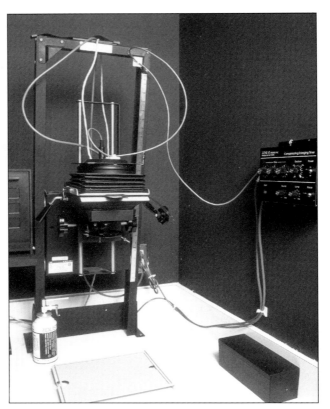

B

FIGURE 6-18
Enlarging timer. The Zone VI enlarging timer shown
here (A) uses a photocell that reads the actual light
intensity from its matching cold light enlarging head
(B), providing accurate exposure control for lengthy
printing sessions.

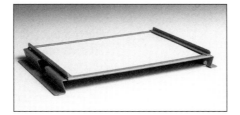

FIGURE 6-19
Paper easel. This simple paper easel is designed
exclusively for 5" × 7" paper and permits rapid production of paper enlargements.

choose a high-quality instrument. The best use precision glass
optics and a reticle eyepiece. Avoid those that project the image
onto a ground-glass surface, since the actual grain pattern cannot
be detected.

6. *Variable contrast filter set*. There are two basic types of photographic
paper. One style is "graded" paper and is available in fixed levels of
contrast. The levels may be assigned numbers or words; grade 1
("soft") has low contrast, while grade 5 ("ultra hard") has high contrast. The grade of paper is chosen based on the contrast of the negative; if the negative is "contrasty," a low-contrast paper would be
used. Obviously, to handle a variety of assignments, one needs to
maintain a supply of each contrast grade, which can be expensive.

The other type of paper is known as variable-contrast paper
(Polycontrast, Multicontrast, and Multigrade are trade names for

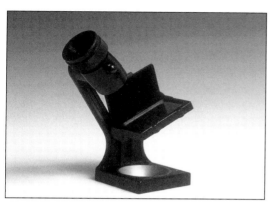

A

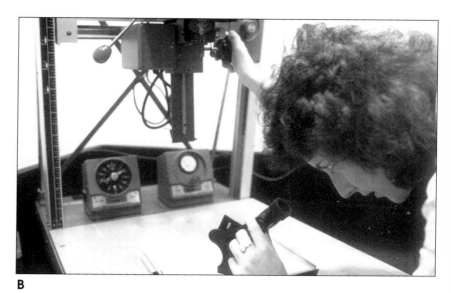

B

FIGURE 6-20
Grain focuser. To assist in obtaining optimal print sharpness, a grain focuser (A) is used to examine the projected image while the enlarger is being focused (B).

FIGURE 6-21
Below-lens variable-contrast filter holder. Variable-contrast papers require the use of filters to modify the projected light from the enlarger. Filters in plastic holders are designed to be placed under the enlarging lens.

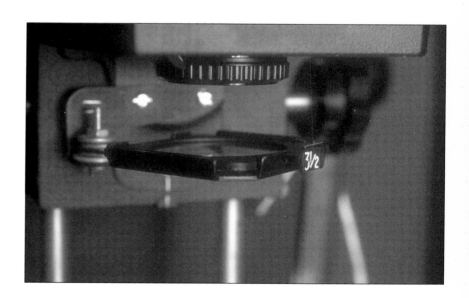

this type). Variable-contrast papers incorporate two emulsion layers of different contrasts, each designed to respond to light of different colors. The low-contrast emulsion is sensitive to yellow-green wavelengths exclusively, while the high-contrast layer responds to magenta light. A set of variable-contrast filters can thus be used to make the one paper act like four or five different contrast grades (as well as half grades between each full grade), depending on the relative amounts of each color of light the filter transmits. The most common set of filters are designed to be mounted below the lens (Figure 6-21), although some filters can be placed above the negative carrier. For the ultimate in sophistication (and cost), a dichroic color enlarger head, primarily designed for producing color prints, may be used to print on variable-contrast black and white paper by simply dialing in the amount and "flavor" of light required.

Processing the Negative

To process black and white materials, four separate basic steps are required: development, stop-bath, fixation, and washing. Each of these is responsible for another stage toward the completion of the final product: a permanent record of the pattern of fluorescent light that entered the camera from the patient's retina.

Film Processing: Concepts

Why is it important to understand the underlying concepts of film processing, when so many aspects of photography have become automated? If you are to be a professional, with the attendant self-esteem and respect from your peers and colleagues, then you should have a strong understanding of the reasons your photographic product looks the way it does. Professional photographers continually search for ways to improve their images, and this quest will help improve the quality of your diagnostic photographs. By understanding how each component of the various chemical baths influences the final image, you will be able to manipulate the process to solve difficult imaging problems, as well as to troubleshoot if something goes awry.

FILM

Of course, before decisions about development, the first choice to be made concerns the type of film to be used. In fluorescein angiography, the typical camera film is a black and white negative stock with a sensitivity rating of ISO 400. Black and white films are typically comprised of several layers including the base, antihalation backing, emulsion, and overcoat. The base provides a stable support for the film and is typically made of a transparent plastic material. The antihalation backing absorbs any light that passes through the emulsion from ricocheting off the back surface of the film and degrading the image. The overcoat is a transparent coating applied to the front surface of the film to make it more resistant to scratches.

The actual light-sensitive layer is the emulsion, which is made up of silver halide crystals suspended in a gelatin layer. The thickness of this layer and the physical shape of the silver halide crystals both play a large role in determining the characteristics of the final image. Historically, the emulsion layer was rather thick. At the instant of exposure, incoming light (image-forming rays) traveled through this layer, striking crystals haphazardly and spreading out as it traversed the emulsion. The resulting image was not critically sharp. Today's films incorporate thinner emulsion layers with flattened silver halide crystals that are more efficient at capturing the image-forming rays. Thus, the resulting image is significantly sharper.[5]

Another important aspect of film design is the manner in which the normally blue-sensitive silver halide crystals are made sensitive to a much wider visible light spectrum with sensitizing dyes. For fluorescein angiography, panchromatic (sensitive to the complete visible spectrum) film is used. In addition to broadening the color response, these dyes also increase the film's sensitivity, measured as ISO speed. The film's speed rating or sensitivity indicates that there is a specific quantity of light required to render it developable. If there is too little light, then the film remains unexposed and no image-forming density will be evident, even with prolonged development.

When the silver halide crystal is struck with light, a very subtle change occurs within the crystal. The light changes the makeup of the crystal at a point in its structure known as a *sensitivity speck*. This change primes the crystal to be developed.

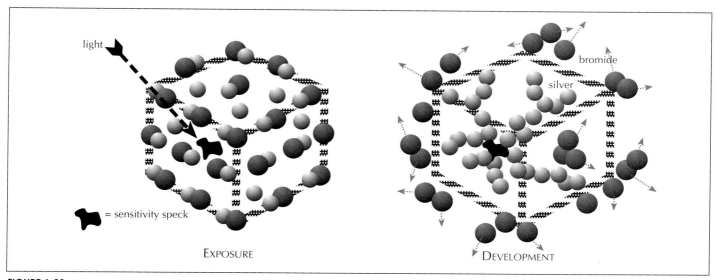

FIGURE 6-22
Photographic development. When film or paper is processed, developing agents convert the exposed silver halide crystal to metallic silver and then spin out filament-like strands of metallic silver to create a visible silver grain.

FILM DEVELOPMENT

During the process of development, the developing agent adds negatively charged particles (electrons) to those crystals that have been struck by light. The result of this reaction is the formation of a black, metallic silver image and the release of by-products into the developer (Figure 6-22). Chemists recognize this as an oxidation-reduction type of process, since silver is reduced to its metallic form while the developer is oxidized. Development is extraordinarily efficient at amplifying the effects of light on film. By making the sensitivity speck visible, development increases its size by well over a million times.

When developing film in daylight tanks, development requires periods of agitation followed by intervals where the tank is allowed to stand undisturbed. The agitation cycles introduce fresh quantities of processing solutions to the emulsion and remove waste products from it—the chemical action involves every part of the image during agitation. The quiet cycles allow the development of the highlights to slow down, since the relatively large areas of reduction liberate a commensurate quantity of waste products that prevent further highlight development from occurring. The regions of the film that have less exposure release fewer waste products and are thus permitted to continue development during the still interval.

As with any other chemical reaction, time and temperature play crucial roles. The reaction occurs more quickly at higher temperatures, and as the time increases, so do the number of silver halide crystals that are developed.

As development continues, contrast rises. Contrast denotes the separation between tones. The dark tones in a high-contrast image are extremely dark, the light tones are very bright, and the visual separation among the intermediate tones is likewise expanded. This fact is essential to the nature of black and white film materials; just as exposure creates density, development influences contrast. Excessive times or temperatures are harmful, however, since unexposed crystals may be converted to silver as well as those that were struck by light. This results in a "fogged" image of inferior quality. The physical size of the metallic silver grains also increases with prolonged development, and the resulting image appears "grainy"—almost sand-like in appearance.

Developers may be chosen depending on the type of negative desired. They are formulated with a variety of ingredients that work together to create an image with unique characteristics. Typically, these ingredients include developing agents, preservatives, restrainers, and activators. Angiographic negatives must be "readable"—that is, the information they record must be easy to ascertain through visual inspection. Areas of fluorescence, rendered as dark regions of the negative, must not be so dark that tonal variations cannot be differentiated. There should be only a few areas of maximum, deep black surrounded by regions of very dark gray, depending on the exact pathology recorded.

The developer's most important ingredient is the developing agent. Traditionally, two agents are combined: metol and hydroquinone. Developers such as Kodak's D-76, D-19, and D-11 feature these two chemicals in varying proportions. Ilford's Ilfotec, Kodak's HC-110, and other modern developers have used phenidone and other agents to replace the problematic metol, which can cause contact dermatitis. A preservative is added to prevent premature oxidation. Sodium sulfite is commonly used and allows the mixed solution to be stored for several weeks in a closed container without any deterioration.

The restrainer is used to help prevent fogging, or unintended development of unexposed silver halide crystals. Restrainers also are capable of increasing negative contrast. Potassium bromide is often used for this purpose.

The activator provides an alkaline environment that facilitates the action of the developing agents. Sodium carbonate and sodium hydroxide are two such activators. The latter is used in high-energy formulas, while sodium carbonate is a milder chemical that allows a slower rate of development.

Some developers are sold as liquid concentrates, while others are purchased as powders. Of the two choices, liquid allows fast mixing at temperatures at or near those used to process film. Thus, there need not be any delay between mixing the solution and using it. To mix powdered developers, a time-consuming regimen of alternately adding powder and stirring must be followed. Even after mixing, precipitates can form at the bottom of the storage container. If hot water is used to mix the powder, the solution must be cooled before use. Furthermore, mixing powdered chemistry liberates fine dust that may be harmful if inhaled. If you choose a powdered developer, be sure to use a mask and eyeshield when mixing.

Current practice in the United States for angiogram development sees a variety of developers in use. There are two families of developers used in angiographic processing: high-contrast and pictorial. High-contrast developers like Kodak D-11 and, to a lesser degree, D-19 are carryovers from the early days of fluorescein angiography, when wide-band filters were used and the resulting exposure allowed a significant amount of nonfluorescent light to strike the film. High-contrast development was required to expand the tonal values so a positive print could be made with adequate dye representation. These developers are chemically vigorous and disproportionately favor areas of hyperfluorescence. The darker areas of the angiogram are thus rendered too dark while the brighter areas may become excessively bright. Prints from 35-mm negatives processed in these solutions have moderately high granularity.

Developers like Kodak's D-76, HC-110, and T-Max developer, on the other hand, are designed primarily for pictorial photography in which an extended range of gray tones and fine grain are desired attributes. The gray tones associated with fluorescein angiography are at least as

important as specific areas of total hyperfluorescence or hypofluorescence. Angiograms processed in these pictorial developers exhibit a broad array of tones throughout the image.

Regardless of the particular developer chosen, it should be used only once and then discarded. Some developers offer a system of replenishment where the chemical activity is maintained by adding more components to the solution, but this can be complicated and time-consuming while offering little in actual cost-saving. Black and white processing solutions are quite inexpensive, and the only way to ensure consistency is to use fresh chemistry for each batch of film.

FILM AFTER-DEVELOPMENT PROCESSES

Once development has reached the desired level of completion, the chemical activity of the developing agents must be halted. The solution known as "stop-bath" accomplishes that goal. Since the developer is usually alkaline, a weak acid will effectively neutralize it. A solution of acetic acid is used, either with or without a chemical indicator that turns purple when the acidity drops below a certain point.

Some laboratories use a brief water wash after development instead of an acid stop-bath. Although water can slow the activity of the developer, it does not halt it completely. If any developer is carried over into the fixing bath, a subtle staining of the emulsion (dichroic fog) may result. To avoid this, and to obtain the most accurate timing (and thus consistency in processing), use an acidic stop-bath.[6]

After treatment in stop-bath, the film consists of a metallic silver image surrounded by areas of unexposed (and therefore nonreduced) silver halides. The developing solution has now been neutralized, but the silver halides remaining in the emulsion are still susceptible to darkening through exposure to light. To remove these crystals from the emulsion, you must use a fixing bath. Conventional photographic fixers mixed from powders use sodium thiosulfate as the active ingredient and typically require 5–10 minutes for adequate fixation to occur. When processing fluorescein angiograms, a rapid fixer is preferred to shorten the processing time. Fixing baths that are based on ammonium thiosulfate, available as liquid concentrates, typically require less than half the time of conventional fixation. Just as with development, fixation requires periodic agitation to allow fresh solutions to be brought to the emulsion surface.

At the end of the fixation process, the film is comprised of the metallic silver image surrounded by clear areas where the unexposed crystals have been removed. The entire emulsion layer is now impregnated with fixer. However, fixer acts as a bleach over time. Thus, the film must be washed free of this chemical contaminant so the image will remain stable throughout its required lifespan. Washing aids facilitate this procedure.

After fixation, rinse the film with water to remove the majority of fixer from the emulsion surface. Next, bathe the film for 1 minute in washing aid solution (sold by Kodak as Hypo Clearing Agent and by Heico as Perma Wash; other manufacturers have their own proprietary formulations). Without the washing aid treatment, at least 30 minutes in running water is needed to ensure an adequate wash. The washing aid converts the remaining fixer into readily soluble compounds and thus shortens the final washing step. Washing aids are recommended because they not only facilitate archival processing but also are ecologically sound—ethical darkroom work is "earth-friendly." Biodegradable compounds should be used and resources conserved whenever possible.

After the washing aid treatment, the final wash removes the remainder of chemicals from the emulsion. Washers should create some turbulence in the water flow to break bubbles free from the film surface and

Table 6-2. Manual Film Processing: Step by Step

Prepare	Set out film, reels, scissors, opener, tanks
	Fill graduates with correct quantity and
	    temperature of developer, stop-bath, fixer,
	    and washing aid
	Turn lights out

Load **Total darkness** ➔	Open film canister Cut film end Load film onto reel Place reel in tank with tightly fitting lid Turn lights on
Process	Set timer for development time Pour developer in rapidly, start timer, begin agitation Pour out developer, pour in stop-bath, restart timer Agitate Pour out stop-bath, pour in fixer, restart timer Agitate Pour out fixer, pour in wash aid, restart timer Agitate Pour out wash aid, wash with water Apply wetting agent Dry

allow fresh water to flow continuously through the processing reels. Fixer diffuses out of the emulsion layers, so at least five full changes of water or 5 minutes in a well-designed film washer are required.

When the wash cycle is completed, bathe the film in a wetting agent (such as Kodak's Photo Flo 200) to lower the surface tension of the water and promote even drying. Without such treatment, water spots are likely to form. These may be difficult to remove and can be seen in the final print.

Finally, the film must be dried. Air drying is effective but slow. Special care must be exercised to avoid a dirty or drafty place for air drying, since dirt and dust that come into contact with the wet emulsion are virtually impossible to remove, even with rewashing. To speed the diagnostic information to the physician, most ophthalmic darkrooms use a heated forced-air dryer.

Film Processing: In Practice

Manual processing of film in a small tank may seem daunting to a novice darkroom worker, but the task can be thought of as a series of simple steps: preparation, loading, processing, and finishing (Table 6-2).

If this is your first time doing film processing, do a practice run before attempting to process patient photographs. You might want to photograph some nonophthalmic subjects at home on a roll of black and white film, using a regular 35-mm camera, to provide the test roll for this first attempt. Alternatively, an evening class on basic black and white processing at a local college may provide you with enough experience to approach this task confidently.

PREPARE

To prepare for film processing, organize your work space and prepare your materials. Once the lights are turned off, it will be nearly impossible to locate any materials or supplies that are not first placed in a convenient location. Your sense of touch will be the only way to identify these items in total darkness.

Table 6-3. Angiographic Film Processing Parameters

Camera	Flash Setting	Film	Developer	Time	Temperature
Zeiss FF4	240ws	TMax 400	D-76 straight	12 mins	72°F
Zeiss FF4	240ws	Neopan 400	HC110 dil. A	6 mins	72°F
Zeiss FF4	240ws	TriX	D-19 (1:1)	6.5 mins	68°F
Zeiss FK30	300ws	TriX	HC110 dil. B	9 mins	70°F
Canon CF60UV	"angio"	TMax 400	D-11 (1:1)	7 mins	75°F
Canon 60S	"3"	TMax 400	D-11 straight	8 mins	70°F
Topcon 50VT	75ws	Tri-X	D-11 straight	5.5 mins	72°F
Kowa RCXv	"angio"	Neopan 400	HC110 dil. B	8 mins	70°F

Selecting a Film Developer and Its Proper Processing Parameters

Experienced ophthalmic photographers use developers and associated times and temperatures based on a long process of testing, analysis, and revision. Newcomers to the field must rely on previously published data to get started.

Manufacturers often include suggested exposure and development information in the film package. Unfortunately, that information is not applicable to the special requirements of angiographic imaging.

In 1995, several combinations of fundus cameras, films, and development parameters for fluorescein angiograms were in common use. Sample data are published in Table 6-3. Published data, no matter what the source, should always include a cautionary statement (i.e., "these data suggest starting points for individualized testing") because there are always local variables that will influence the results. While power supplies of fundus cameras are marked similarly, the output of the individual flash tubes may vary, and the light that actually reaches the film may have marked intensity differences between similar instruments. In spite of these differences, however, the data published above should provide usable negatives for direct viewing and interpretation.

When assessing the quality of an angiographic negative, you should make sure that the film leader and the angiographic timing data appear to be black on the negative and that the "clear" area surrounding the angiographic image is quite transparent and lacks obvious fog. For a more detailed account of the testing procedures for negative development, see Tyler's article on unusual film and developer combinations.[7]

Fill three beakers or other graduated containers with the proper quantity of developer, stop-bath, and fixer (see the sidebar on selecting a film developer and its proper processing parameters). (If you use stainless steel tanks and reels, use these amounts: 1 reel = 8 oz; 2 reels = 16 oz; and 4 reels = 32 oz.) All solutions should be at the same preselected temperature.

If your darkroom's air temperature is kept steady at the setting you select for processing, then it is a simple matter to pour the solutions from their storage containers and use them immediately. If the ambient storage temperature is too hot or cold, fill the sink with water at the correct temperature and then immerse the storage containers until their contents assume the temperature of the water (see the sidebar on Emergency Processing to Salvage a Study).

Next, lay the daylight tank, top, lid, and reels on the countertop. The reels should be oriented so that their loading slots all face the same direction. Place the film cassettes together on the counter and, next to these, a pair of scissors and a standard bottle opener. Remember precisely where these items are placed, because when the lights are extinguished, you will use them to complete the loading process.

LOADING

When all is ready, turn out the lights. (Caution: if your darkroom has fluorescent worklights, wait a minute or two before commencing, since fluorescent fixtures may have a residual "afterglow." Also make certain that any equipment indicator lights, or even telephone pushbuttons, are extinguished or covered before proceeding!) The darkroom must remain completely dark until the film has been loaded onto a reel, placed in the tank, and the tank covered.

Select a film cassette and hold it so the protruding end of the spool is facing downward. Use the bottle opener to remove the opposite, flat end cap of the cassette. Remove the spool and film and cut off the leader with the scissors—you will need to do these operations by touch; the leader is narrower than the rest of the film. Next, feed the end of the film into the processing reel emulsion side inward. If you use stainless steel reels, insert the end of the film under the spring clip located at the reel's center or into the central opening if there is no clip. Curl the film slightly by compressing it between the thumb and index finger while the other hand rotates the reel. The film is thus fed (emulsion facing inward) into the reel from the inside toward the outside of the spirals (Figure 6-23). Lightly touch the film to monitor the progress as the loading proceeds. It should smoothly fit into the spiral reels without bending. If the film starts to feel crooked, unwind it and begin again.

If you use a plastic reel, hold the film so it is parallel to the spirals of the reel. Slip the film end into the spiral groove at the outside edge of the reel; typically there are small plastic bumps adjacent to the loading spot to facilitate locating it in the dark. Then simply ratchet the film onto the

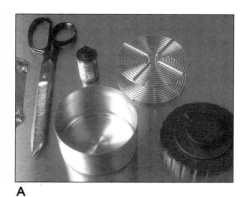

A

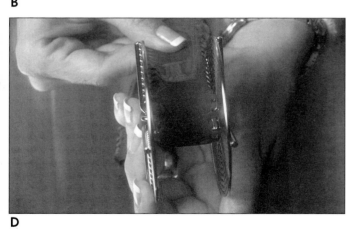

B

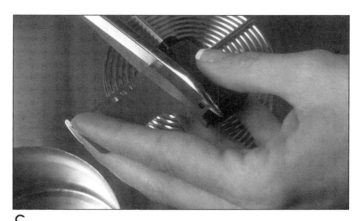

C

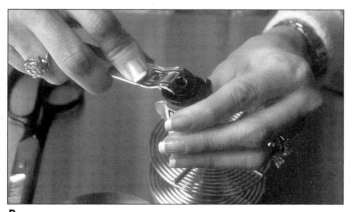

D

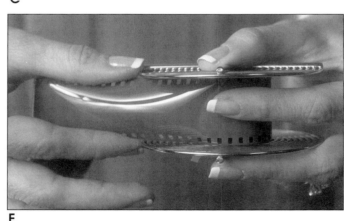

E

FIGURE 6-23
Film loading, using stainless steel reels. First, assemble the tank, film, reels, opener. and scissors on the countertop (A). Next, open the flat end of the cassette (B). Cut off the leader (C), and insert the cut end into the center of the reel (D). Gently squeeze the film's width into a convex curve as you roll the film onto the reel and be sure to lightly feel the film to ensure proper tracking (E). Finally, cut off the film spool, place the reel into the tank, and cover with the top.

spool by rotating the top and bottom flanges of the reel in alternate directions. The film will automatically feed into the reel.

To gain confidence and accuracy in loading film, repeatedly practice with a scrap roll of film until you can load the reel successfully (with your eyes closed!), allowing your fingers to provide you with all the information you need. Treat the film gently; avoid bending or crimping the film while loading it, since these acute pressures to the film's surface will result in small curved lines in the image itself, known as "cinch marks."

Emergency Processing to Salvage a Study

Even though the majority of angiograms are executed properly, on rare occasions technical difficulties arise during the photographic session. One such event that can create a terribly thin negative is the accidental extravisation of dye during the injection. In such an occurrence, only a small amount may be injected into the vein. The photographer may not visualize any fluorescence or a pronounced decrease in intensity through the eyepiece. To attempt to salvage useful information, you will need to overdevelop the film.[8]

Normally, processing times are selected to achieve a good balance between angiographic information and minimal granularity and fog. In an emergency, however, doubling the development time will increase the density of fluorescent areas and may allow even faintly fluorescein structures to become visible on the negative. The range of tones will be skewed, much detail in relatively hypofluorescent areas will be missing with such vigorous underexposure coupled with overdevelopment. The background will exhibit moderate chemical fog. However, such radical processing may provide sufficient diagnostic information so that a repeat injection at a later date will not be required.

Silver Recovery

Used fixer contains dissolved silver that is toxic to the environment and is not biodegradable. Many municipalities have strict laws that prohibit the discharge of heavy metals (including silver-laden fixer) into local sewer systems. Furthermore, silver is a nonrenewable resource that is essential to the photographic process. For these reasons, you should reclaim the silver from used fixer and make the solution safe for discharge into the sewer system.

Silver recovery machines are available in various sizes, and you should choose the model that is appropriate for the number of gallons of used fixer your facility produces. One of the least expensive units is the Silver Magnet. This device consists of a low-voltage power supply connected to a small, perforated plastic tray containing an anode and a cathode. This is placed in a storage container of used fixer, and the electric current slowly precipitates metallic silver out of solution and into the tray. When the tray is full, it may be sent to a smelter for reclamation. The smelter then sends a check to you for the current market value of the reclaimed silver. Once the silver has been removed, the remaining solution may be safely poured down the drain, since it no longer represents an environmental hazard.

If your laboratory is located within a hospital, an alternative to purchasing a silver recovery unit may be available. Some hospital-based radiology departments may allow you to add your used fixer to the x-ray machine's discharge for commercial silver reclamation. You may not receive any compensation for the reclaimed silver, but at least you will no longer be contaminating the local water supply.

When the entire roll is loaded, cut off the cassette spool and place the loaded reel into the tank. Press the top securely onto the tank, turn the room lights on, and complete the remaining processing steps in standard room lighting.

PROCESSING

Set the timer for the required development time. Start the timer and immediately pour the developer rapidly into the top of the tank. To speed this process, tilt the tank slightly to allow air to escape while filling the tank. During the pour, do not slow down or stop for any reason, since uniformity of development will be compromised. It is better to accidentally spill a few drops of developer while rapidly filling the tank! As soon as the tank is full, place the cap on it and bang the tank strongly on the sink or countertop. This dislodges air bubbles from the film that would otherwise cause undeveloped spots ("air bells") on the negative. After rapping the tank, begin agitation. Agitation techniques typically require a cycle of quickly inverting and righting the tank for a set period of time. This removes waste products from the film and allows fresh developer to act on the emulsion.

A typical agitation pattern consists of 5 seconds of agitation (one inversion per second) for each 30 seconds of development. Be sure to rap the tank on the counter after each agitation cycle. To promote uniform development across the entire surface of the film, a random movement should be used during agitation. To simply achieve this, rotate the tank about one-third of a turn when you complete each agitation cycle. Following each agitation period, the tank is allowed to sit undisturbed.

Developing is a highly individualized task. If several veteran photographers are asked to explain their technique, each may provide a different explanation. Like all other scientific disciplines, an extremely important aspect of photographic darkroom work is consistency. By working in a precise and repeatable fashion, you can more easily identify and remedy any problems that arise. Timing and agitation patterns are crucial to film development, so be sure to time the process and agitate the tank in exactly the same way for all standard angiographic film processing.

Fifteen seconds before the allotted time is up, begin emptying the tank. Time this so that the solution is completely drained as the timer reaches zero.

Quickly pour stop-bath into the tank. After a rap of the tank on a hard work surface, at least 30 seconds of continuous agitation in the stop-bath should provide for total cessation of development. This solution is then poured out. It may be saved for reuse.

Now reset the timer and pour the fixer into the tank. Three minutes is required for rapid fixer. Agitation cycles are required for fixation, just as with development, to ensure that the unprocessed silver halide is completely dissolved. As the timer nears zero, pour the used fixer into a temporary storage container. Rather than pouring used fixer down the drain, it should be saved for subsequent silver recovery (see the sidebar on silver recovery).

After fixation, the film is now processed and can be exposed to light without changing the image (see the sidebar on "Stat" film processing).

After fixation, wash the film. Fill the tank with water at the same temperature as the other solutions, agitate for about 1 minute, and then drain. This step removes much of the surface fixer. Next, fill the tank with a washing aid (i.e., Perma Wash) and set the timer for 1 minute. Agitate to ensure complete chemical conversion of the remaining fixing solution. When the timer reaches zero, drain the tank.

"Stat" Film Processing

Although most fluorescein angiograms can be processed efficiently in batches once or twice a day, occasionally the film will need to be processed while the patient waits. This may be due to medical necessity, as in the case of a patient with a choroidal neovascular membrane that threatens central vision and requires immediate laser photocoagulation. Rapid processing may also be requested for the sake of convenience. If the patient has traveled a great distance to the clinic, the physician may want to plan future visits or treatment strategies based on today's angiogram.

Using conventional film processing techniques, temperatures, washing aids, and efficient film dryers, it is possible to completely process a fluorescein angiogram in less than 30 minutes. The time allotted for each portion of the stat process is detailed below. Bear in mind, however, that the total elapsed time depends on the time required for each individual step (Table 6-4). The time in developer is crucial to image quality, and cannot be changed. Stop-bath acts quickly and can be effective in as little as 30 seconds. Rapid-fixing baths can achieve complete fixation in as short a time as 2 minutes. Washing aids can dramatically shorten the required final wash time. Some film dryers are much more efficient than others, although some clinicians will demand a "wet" reading and will want to examine the film as it is taken right from the washer. (Note: when wet, the film is extremely delicate and easily scratched. After the wet reading, return the film to the wash tank for wetting agent and proper drying!)

Even though rapid processing is possible, in the real world of clinical photography, ophthalmic photographers may not always be able to deliver the results with this kind of speed. You may have to exercise critical judgment, and hope for the clinician's understanding, to weigh the need for prompt results against the overall workload. At times, manual processing may be faster than automated film development, but doing the job by hand will obviously prevent you from taking care of other patients at the same time.

Table 6-4. "Stat" Film Processing Timeline*

Load film reels	30 seconds
Developer	8 minutes (adjust as required)
Stop-bath	30 seconds
Rapid fixer	3 minutes
Water rinse	1 minute
Washing aid	1 minute
Final wash	5 minutes
Dry	3 minutes
Scissor and insert	3 minutes

*The above data assume that all chemicals are already mixed and are at the correct processing temperature.

FINISHING

Remove the reels from the tank and place them in the film washer. Set the water flow to a moderate rate (2–4 changes per minute) and allow the film to wash for at least 5 minutes. If small bubbles seem to stick to the film, manually raise and lower the reels and tap the washer to liberate them and enable fresh water to cleanse the film. When the time is completed, turn off the water, assuming this will allow the water in the washer to remain in place.

Finally, according to its dilution directions, place some concentrated wetting agent into the water. Allow the film to rest in this solution for 1 minute, and then drain and dry in either a forced-air dryer or by evaporation. Although some photographers wipe the film with sponges, this practice may permanently mark or deform the film. When wet, the film's surface is very soft and fragile, so allowing it to dry in air provides the greatest margin of safety.

NEGATIVE STORAGE AND VIEWING

Once dry, the angiographic information is contained on a strip of plastic about 1 inch wide by 5 feet long. This format presents a rather unwieldy method of reviewing and filing clinical information. Furthermore, unprotected film is susceptible to physical damage. Dust, dirt, and fingerprints can each leave an indelible impression, and repeated exposure to such damage lessens the amount of information clearly visible at subsequent viewings.

The importance of caring properly for the angiographic negative cannot be overstated. In the representational aspect of scientific photography, the negative remains the only evidence of the transit of dye through the choroid and retina. The events recorded during angiography live on as delicate metallic silver tracings; for present and future review and analysis, the negative must remain in pristine condition.

Archiving requirements for medical images are based on legal requirements for record storage. In many cases, records must be retrievable for a minimum of 7 years following the patient's visit. Thus, photographic materials must be stored in inert materials that will not cause noticeable deterioration in image quality for at least a decade. Studies have shown that a variety of acids used frequently in modern paper-making are harmful to the photographic image. File folders, envelopes, and even glassine negative holders all incorporate materials that can attack and degrade processed photographs. However, by placing the angiogram in an archival-quality plastic holder, the image is protected from these antagonists.

Negative filing sheets of polyethylene, polypropylene, or mylar keep dirt and chemicals from harming the image and at the same time allow the entire angiogram to be viewed directly. These transparent plastic

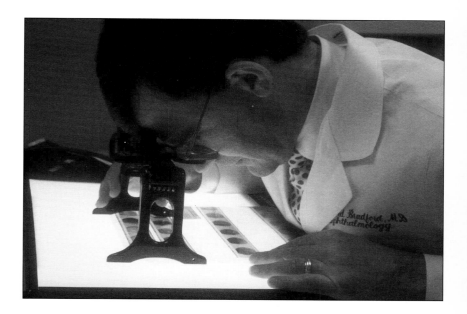

FIGURE 6-24
Viewing angiograms in stereo. When examining a fluorescein angiogram with a stereoviewer or loupe, the magnifying device is placed directly on the plastic negative sheet.

sheets typically incorporate a series of flat, narrow pockets with openings at either end. Cut the angiogram into five or six frame strips, taking care not to separate any stereo pairs, and then insert each strip into a pocket in the sheet. Once loaded, the sheet may be placed on a lightbox for viewing with a stereoviewer or loupe and then filed in the patient's chart or in the photographic records area.

An alternative method of storage requires that the negatives be individually cut, inserted into 35-mm slide mounts, and then placed into side-loading slide folio pages. This method is required by certain multicenter clinical studies.

To use a loupe or stereoviewer, rest the base of the device directly on the storage sheet or negative (Figure 6-24). These devices may be moved along at will, and detailed analysis of individual frames or stereo pairs may be made at any point during the inspection.

Viewers that are modified from microfiche or microfilm readers are an effective way of looking at angiographic negatives, since they can project an enlarged view of selected frames onto their self-contained viewing screen. However, those that incorporate a glass pressure plate require special care to make sure they do not scratch the negative if it is removed from its protective sleeve.

Negatives can also be reviewed on a video monitor. The Fotovix uses a small video camera and a transilluminated base to allow individual frames to be shown in this manner. Certain versions of this instrument come equipped with a polarity switch, so that the angiogram can be electronically converted from a negative image to a positive one. These devices also offer a zoom control so selected portions of the negative may be enlarged, as well as brightness and contrast controls.

The Positive Printout

Why Analysis of the Negative is Preferred

The vast majority of published fluorescein angiograms are produced as positives (dye depicted as white). While some resident training programs in ophthalmology use positive printouts to teach descriptive interpreta-

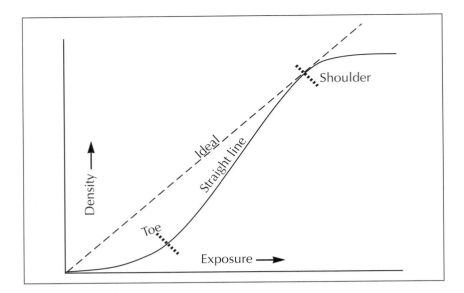

FIGURE 6-25
Characteristic curve. This line graphically shows how a film reacts to changes in exposure and development. Films cannot reproduce subject brightnesses with complete fidelity and have a tendency to compress information in the lightest and darkest parts of the image.

tion of these studies, the best way of reading and interpreting fluorescein angiograms is by direct analysis of the camera-original negatives. Issues of accuracy and timeliness support this statement.

No photographic medium reproduces the subject with complete accuracy. Every black and white film skews the reproduction of tonal values. To learn why this is true, a brief description of characteristic curves may be useful.[9]

The response of a given film and developer to changes in exposure can be graphically depicted as a characteristic curve (Figure 6-25). If a perfect film could be manufactured, it would have a constant, predictable response to changes in illumination. For every quantity of increased light exposure, the film would respond by creating density in exactly the same manner: one unit of light creates one unit of density. In reality, films do not respond well to either very low or very high levels of illumination. For low levels, seen as the "toe" portion of the curve, the film will receive a fair amount of exposure before it begins to respond by creating an image. This means that the very dim portions of the subject will be disproportionately dark. A similar situation exists in the "shoulder" of the curve, representing the effects of very bright illumination. As you can see by the flattening of the line, the film reaches a point where it no longer responds to increased light. The "straight line" portion of the curve represents the film's ability to respond straightforwardly to changes in illumination. In this area, every unit of light increase results in an equivalent increase in film density.

Film can only approximate the range of brightness values that is emitted by fluorescein. The darker areas of hypofluorescence are rendered somewhat darker than they really are; maximum areas of hyperfluorescence may be inaccurately portrayed with more brightness. When using printout materials to generate positive copies of the study, this second generation further warps the portrayal of densities.

The other reason for using negatives as the prime medium for communicating the results of angiography deals with speed. Simply stated, producing a positive printout can more than double the time required in the darkroom. With conventional hand processing, an angiographic negative can be fully developed, washed, dried, and delivered in less than 25 minutes. If one must cut it into strips, contact print it, process, and finally dry the printout, these subsequent steps may add at least anoth-

The Angiographic Zone System

As fine-art photography experienced a renaissance in the 1930s, Ansel Adams, Minor White, and others formulated a precise methodology for equating subject brightness with the values that result in the photographic print. The key to this scheme is the zone system. By assigning shades of gray to typical pictorial subjects, the photographer is better able to expose and process negatives so that the shades of gray that were previsualized at the instant of exposure are actually seen in the final print.

Adams' zone system is comprised of a series of nine shades ranging from pure black to pure white.[10] This represents a brightness range of 256:1 and is closely matched to the reproduction capabilities of photographic paper. Each zone is 100% brighter than the previous zone and is 50% darker than the next higher zone. The "twice or half" relationship is the same as that between one shutter speed and another and also between one f-stop and another. Thus, after metering a subject, the photographer can, at will, make an exposure that will produce the principal tone as an exact shade of gray.

The precision associated with the pictorial zone system is made possible by the fact that natural lighting can be measured easily with a reflected light meter. Various parts of the scene can be metered independently for maximal exposure control. After determining the intensity of the light and deciding on the required exposure settings, the photographer can exercise further creative controls in the darkroom through lengthening or shortening the development time.

In fluorescein angiography, the illumination is provided by electronic flash, and even though flash meters are used in conventional photography, none has been designed to measure small changes in retinal brightness during dye perfusion. The fact that exciter and barrier filtration is necessary for angiography further complicates accurate quantification of fluorescence.

However, in spite of problems with the previsualization of lighting effects, we know anecdotally that fluorescein dye behaves predictably based on the disease process being recorded. Thus, an angiographic zone system can be formulated (Table 6-5) that helps assign values to various areas of fluorescence.[11]

Adams further believed that the values recorded in the negative were similar to the score of a symphony; the print thus became a "performance." In fluorescein angiography, the maximum angiographic information resides in the negative; the positive printout's performance must be tailored to reproduce the negative's information as faithfully as possible.

er 30 minutes to the wait before the diagnostic information is presented to the physician and detracts from the efficient operation of the practice.

However, in spite of these objections to using printouts as the prime method of delivering angiographic results, there are several legitimate reasons for making positive copies of angiograms. These include referral of the patient to other clinicians when the original film must be retained in the medical record, the production of teaching materials for continuing medical education, the preparation of prints to illustrate manuscripts for publication, and the production of sample prints or slides for portfolios and professional certification.

Furthermore, having the capability of standard black and white printing will allow the photographic service to be more responsive, as public relations photographs, portraits, small object or surgical instrument photography, and other nonclinical assignments can be completed intramurally.

Positive printouts are produced in three basic formats: sheet film or paper contact sheets, paper print enlargements, or 35-mm positive slides. Even though there are significant differences between these media in terms of cost, ease of viewing, and brightness range, each must exhibit the proper distribution of tones (based on the characteristics of the original negative) to represent the original as faithfully as possible.

To communicate diagnostic information effectively, fluorescein angiography uses an array of blacks, whites, and shades of gray to represent the distribution of dye in the fundus. This assortment of tones can be organized into a scheme that takes into account dye concentration and the effect of overlying physical materials (such as tissue or hemorrhage). Using pictorial photography as a model, angiographic tonality can be organized into an angiographic "zone system" (see the sidebar on the angiographic zone system).

Sheet Film Contact Sheets

Sheet film contact sheets provide an expanded brightness range that allows the full range of angiographic detail to be observed. Two basic types of film are used for this printout technique: lithographic film and line film. The former is primarily designed to be processed in high-energy developers that produce black and white densities with virtually no intermediate steps. Dupont Cronar and Kodak Kodalith are trade names for such materials. However, processing these films in a continuous tone developer, such as diluted paper developer, can produce a range of gray tones that matches the requirements of fluorescein angiography.

In addition to accurately rendering black and white, line films can also reproduce a range of gray tones. Processing these materials (such as Kodak Fine Grain Positive film and Angiographics Photo Supply's Angiolith film) in diluted paper developer also produces positive prints with excellent gradation.

An annoying problem associated with the use of such high-contrast media is the appearance of small white spots on the printout (Figure 6-26). These are usually caused by dust specks that become trapped between the emulsion layers of the negative and the printout and thus cause a shadow to form during exposure. The shadow represents an area with no exposure and thus appears white (clear on the printout film). Because these white spots can mimic hyperfluorescence, on casual examination they could be misinterpreted as drusen bodies or microaneurysms. If your contact printer is not equipped with a frosted plastic diffusion layer, another strategy for avoiding these spots is to scrupulously clean the negatives and the contact printer before starting to print.

202 Ophthalmic Photography

Table 6-5. Angiographic Zone System

Zone	Tonal/Pictorial Representation	Angiographic Representation
I	Total black	Area adjoining angiographic image
II	First visible tone above black	Retroilluminated vessels in late phase
III	First texture in dark greys	Early choroidal fluorescence visualized through retinal pigment epithelium
IV	Normal grey value of skin in shadow	Vessels in recirculation phase
V	Middle grey (18% reflectance)	Later choroidal fluorescence
VI	Average caucasian skin (36% reflectance)	Diffuse dye from neovascular tissue
VII	Light grey	Near maximal dye in tissues or vessels
VIII	Lightest tone with texture	Drusen, microaneurysms, areas within neovascularization
IX	Paper base white (clear film)	Maximal dye concentration in filled vessels or in florid leakage sites (i.e., ICSC, NV)

FIGURE 6-26.
Dust spot artifacts. The tiny white spots that form on lithographic-type printout materials are caused by dust and dirt that is sandwiched between the negative and the printout medium. Besides their poor appearance, these may be mistaken for hyperfluorescent lesions. Notice that the dust spots are inside and outside the image area. (Courtesy of J. Balza.)

Continuous tone or line films are less likely to produce these spots than lithographic films.

Sheet film contact sheets provide an overview of the patient's angiographic status. By reproducing the angiographic series in total, contact sheets portray, in same-size positive format, every image originally captured on the negative.

To prepare for producing sheet film contact sheets, first set up the tray line. Assuming that four 8" × 10" trays will be used, fill the first tray with at least 1 liter of diluted paper developer. Many photographers use Kodak Dektol developer, diluted 1:1 with water. Fill the second tray with 1 liter of indicator stop-bath, and the third tray with with at least 1 liter of fixer. Finally, set up the last tray as the wash tray, or set up and fill the print washer if available. Turn on the safelight and extinguish the room lights.

Your enlarger is a fine light source for contact printing. To use it in this manner, first turn on the lamp and adjust the height of the enlarger so that its light shines onto the baseboard in a large enough area to cover the size of the contact frame. Roughly focus the lens to produce a sharp edge of the negative carrier. You may want to mark the projected area on the baseboard with black tape to aid in positioning the contact printing frame when you are ready to expose. Once this has been checked, turn the enlarger lamp off temporarily.

If you use a simple contact frame, place a sheet of printout film (emulsion side up) onto the frame. Next, carefully position the angiographic

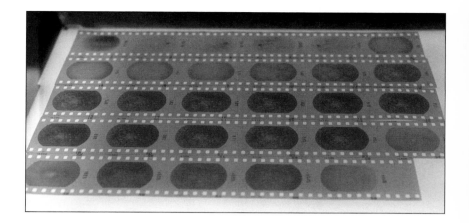

FIGURE 6-27.
Placing negatives in a printer. When arranging the negatives, spend a few seconds to make sure the edges of each strip touch, and align vertically the circular angiographic images to produce a truly professional product.

negatives (emulsion side down) onto the film, keeping them in correct order (Figure 6-27).

To produce a contact sheet, the negatives must be clean and already cut into strips of five or six frames (ideally, they will already be stored in negative filing sheets in this configuration). For maximal image quality, the negatives must be removed from their plastic storage sheet to be contact printed, since contact print sharpness requires intimate contact between the negative's image layer and the printout sheet's emulsion.

Lower the glass top plate onto the materials and latch if required. When assembled correctly, this "sandwich" will feature the film emulsion (right below the top glass plate) in direct contact with the sheet film's emulsion. The light from the enlarger will pass through the film first and then strike the printout material.

Make a test print to fine-tune the exposure time. Even though this print will be discarded later, it will still help you determine valuable exposure and processing information. To create the test print, use an 8" × 10" piece of cardboard. Set the timer to 3 seconds and cover the contact frame with the cardboard, leaving about 2 inches uncovered at one side. Start the timer; the enlarging lamp will expose only the uncovered strip for 3 seconds before turning off. Next, slide the cardboard laterally so that an additional 2 inches are uncovered. Repeat the exposure of 3 seconds. Repeat again and again, until the entire contact sheet has been sequentially exposed.

Next, open the frame, remove the negatives, and carry the exposed sheet of printout film to the tray line. Set the timer for 2 minutes. As you start the timer, quickly slide the print, emulsion side up, into the developer. Immediately begin agitation by lifting one corner of the tray about half an inch and then setting it down again. Repeating this cycle rhythmically will move the solution briskly in the tray, but don't do this so vigorously that the solution spills out! Every 5–10 seconds, use the tongs to lift the film out and replace it turned over. The aim of the agitation and manipulation is to ensure that the action of the developer is uniform across the entire surface of the film. Resist the temptation to short-circuit the process because the print looks too dark; this is a typical mistake when viewing prints under safelight illumination. The printouts must all be developed for the same length of time (use 2 minutes as your initial standard).

When the timer is down to the final 15 seconds, carefully lift the film with the developer tongs by one corner and allow excess developer to drain into the tray. As the timer reaches zero, place the film immediately into the stop-bath without permitting the tongs to touch any of this solution. Make sure it is completely submerged, and agitate for at least 30 seconds in this tray.

Next, pick up the film again by a corner with the stop-bath tongs, allow excess stop-bath to drain back into the tray, and transfer the printout to the fixing bath. Set the timer for 2 minutes and again begin the agitation cycle used previously. You may turn on the room lights after 30 seconds—the remaining steps are performed in room lighting.

Drain the printout of excess fixer, and as the timer reaches zero, place it into the wash. Set the timer for 4 minutes. The print should move around in the wash water. You may want to manually move, invert, and agitate it while this process continues (you may use your bare hands for this step). When the timer reaches zero, drain excess water, squeegee it if desired, and hang it up to dry or place it in the print dryer.

Carefully inspect the test printout on a lightbox to determine the proper exposure time. Exposure primarily affects density. Examine the highlights, or areas of hyperfluorescence. The brightest regions of fluorescence should *just* be clear, barely lighter than very pale gray. Ideally, the strip of exposure that produced the proper highlights should be neither the first nor the last strip but instead should be located toward the middle of the strip series. Based on the exposure time for each strip, calculate the time it took to produce the correct exposure (Figure 6-28).

Next, produce another test, but this time, apply the newly determined correct exposure time to the entire contact sheet. Develop again for precisely 2 minutes, stop, fix, wash, and dry. Look critically at this sheet, and this time examine the darkest areas. Maximum black tones should surround the angiographic image, and there should be clearly differentiated gray tones throughout each frame. If the sheet film looks flat (without much contrast), extend the time in the developer for your next effort by another 30 seconds. If the film has too much contrast, you may wish to reduce the developing time by 30 seconds. By continually refining the processing times and exposure times, you will approach just the right combination to consistently produce good prints (Table 6-6).

Throughout this process, you should remember two fundamental concepts that influence your results:

1. *Exposure creates density.* The effects of exposure changes are seen primarily in the highlight areas.
2. *Development creates contrast.* Changes in development are chiefly noted in the darkest areas of the print.

Although these factors are not mutually exclusive, their effects are quite selective. Without sufficient exposure, you cannot develop to obtain a strong black. And development by itself is not sufficient to create density in the highlights—only proper exposure will create that level of tone in hyperfluorescent regions of the printout.

Of the two factors, exposure is more straightforward. By creating and analyzing test strips, correct exposure can always be determined. Correct contrast is more difficult to determine directly. If development is prolonged, you run the risk of fogging the image. If you extend the time to 4 minutes and a strong black and good tonal separation have not been achieved, you may want to use a less-diluted developer. Similarly, if the print has too much contrast (i.e., an image that seems to be made up of just black and white tones with a poor intermediate gray scale), dilute the developer further.

Another simple method for adjusting contrast is to adjust the relationships between exposure and development. To increase contrast, slightly underexpose the printout and then overdevelop. To decrease printout contrast, slightly overexpose the sheet and then underdevelop. Agitation is extremely important when underdeveloping, since positive printouts subjected to short developing times may appear mottled with patches of uneven maximum density.

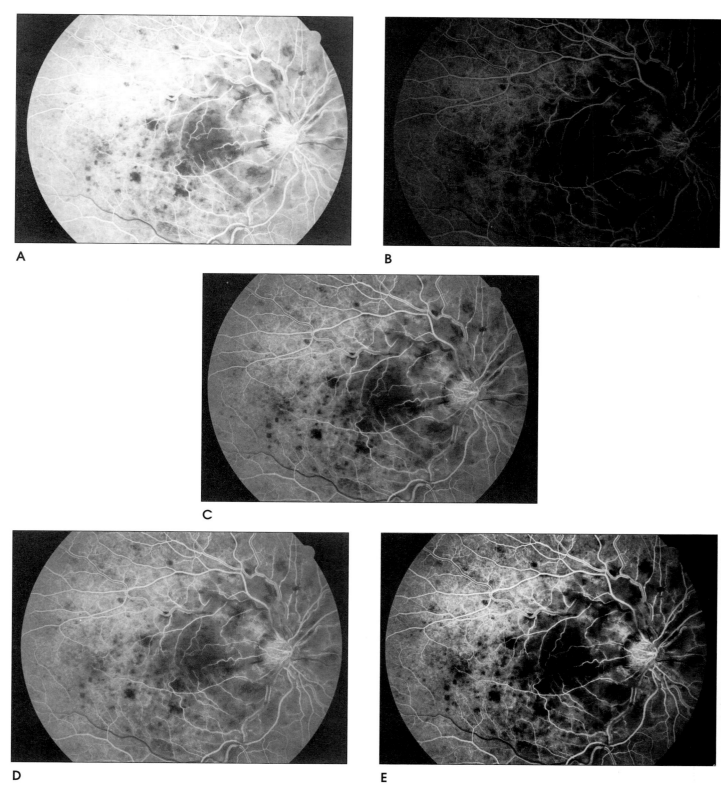

FIGURE 6-28
Exposure and development testing. (For clarity, full-size images are reproduced here, rather than test strips.) Changes in exposure are shown in A, B, and C. A. An underexposed print; the hyperfluorescent areas are too light. B. An overexposed print; all detail is too dark. C. A properly exposed print, in which tonal information is seen in the highlight areas. A, B, and C are all exposed to the same contrast (grade 3). The development or contrast test, will not appreciably alter the highlight tones but rather will dramatically change the darkest areas of the print, as seen in C, D, and E. D. A print made on a grade 1 paper. The detail created by the exposure found during exposure testing provides for good tonal reproduction of the highlights, but the dark values are flat and do not produce any crispness. E. A print produced on a grade 5 paper, resulting in good highlight detail but dark areas that are so black that no detail can be differentiated. C, produced on grade 3, again represents the best combination of exposure (for highlight detail) and contrast (for dark tones).

Table 6.6 Exposure and Contrast Testing

I. Make test strip for exposure. Analyze for highlight detail and select best exposure time
II. Expose full sheet for selected time.
   A. Analyze for shadow detail.
      1. If there is adequate separation of the dark areas, adopt developer time and temperature in step I as your standard.
      2. If shadows are so black that no detail is visible:
         a. Shorten development time or
         b. Use a more dilute developer, or
         c. Use lower-contrast paper
      3. If shadows have no blacks and are just dark grays:
         a. Increase the time in the developer or
         b. Use higher-contrast paper
III. Repeat step II using new development parameters to confirm the choice.

Paper Contact Sheets

Paper contact sheets are the least expensive printout medium. They are relatively easy to produce and, like sheet film contact sheets, only require a printing frame and a controlled light source (i.e., an enlarger—or even a bare light bulb—connected to a timer). Although room light is sufficient to view them, paper contact sheets have some significant liabilities in terms of their ability to convey information. First, the small size of the individual frame makes magnified viewing a necessity. More seriously, the brightness range of any paper print is considerably less than transparent media (a maximum range of 50:1, compared to film's 1,000:1). However, paper prints can be used as a simple record to give an overview of the patient's angiographic status.

Most photographic papers used in routine angiographic printing are resin-coated (RC). This material is comprised of a layer of paper, sensitized on one side, sandwiched between two thin layers of a plastic material. Some RC papers also incorporate a developing agent within the emulsion and lend themselves well to automated processing.

When first introduced, RC papers were considered to be inferior in quality to conventional papers, but today's RC papers are excellent for routine work. The only important processing technique to remember is the importance of accurate timing of the various processing steps. Prolonged times in fixer or in the wash may have deleterious effects on the image, since moisture can penetrate along the paper's edges and residual chemistry will be much more difficult to remove. Most RC papers require 2 minutes in fixer and a maximum of 4 minutes in the wash.

To achieve the proper exposure and development when using paper, follow the same process of test strip production and analysis described previously for sheet film contact sheets. Because photographic paper is available in a variety of contrast grades, contrast can be controlled easily by changing from one grade to another without the need to adjust developer dilution. As a starting point to determine optimal contrast, use a grade 3 paper for your printout tests.

Exposure regulation to establish proper highlight density will be the same as for sheet film printouts. Remember, unless sufficient exposure is given to the printout, no amount of development will bring tone to the highlight areas.

On occasion, to maintain proper tonality within the image, the overall print contrast may need to be reduced slightly. This will cause the edges of the negatives and the film's sprocket holes to be barely visible, rather than being processed to maximum black. However, the most important aspect of the printout is the angiographic information within, rather than outside, the retinal image itself.

35-mm Positive Slides

Sheet film or paper contact sheets provide a single viewer with the means of viewing the entire angiogram. However, contact sheets cannot easily be used to communicate diagnostic information to a large group. The projection of individual 35-mm positive slides solves this problem. Although single frames can be cut from a sheet film contact sheet and secured into slide mounts, you must print more frames than you will use, since some frames will be discarded. Furthermore, you cannot tailor exposure and development to yield optimal quality on selected frames, since the entire contact sheet must necessarily be exposed and developed uniformly.

The alternative, producing individual frames, relies on the use of any of several styles of slide duplicators. With these, selected frames from the angiographic negative can be rephotographed onto line-type black and white negative film, processed, and placed into slide mounts. The resulting slides exhibit high sharpness and a gray scale that reproduces the tonal range of the negative. To produce these slides, use a 35-mm single lens reflex camera equipped with a slide duplicator attachment. Typically, the duplicator attaches to a macro lens capable of a 1:1 reproduction ratio, either via an extended helical focusing mount or by way of a bellows unit. This permits the original negative frame to be reproduced as an identically sized positive. This simple duplicator requires a separate light source.

Professional duplicating cameras incorporate a transilluminating base with tungsten and/or electronic flash lighting, and a sturdy camera column with bellows unit onto which a 35-mm single lens reflex camera is mounted. Both duplicating systems require placing the negative into the duplicator, focusing the camera lens onto the image precisely, transilluminating the negative with tungsten or electronic flash, and finally making the exposure.

Use 35-mm line film (Kodak's Technical Pan Film is recommended for this application). If the camera's internal meter is used to regulate the exposure, an exposure index of EI 100 may provide a basis for further testing and refinement. The film may be processed along with angiograms if high-activity developers are being used, or in Kodak Dektol, undiluted, for 4 minutes at 72°F with regular agitation. Just as with other development data in this chapter, use this reference as an approximate starting point for additional testing. This is particularly important when testing relatively high-contrast materials, since these have much less latitude for errors in exposure and development than continuous-tone photographic media.

An especially useful modification to either a simple duplicator or a full-featured professional unit is to add the special strip film carrier from an enlarger (such as a Beseler Negatrans) that facilitates moving from frame to frame for selected duplication.

Unlike contact sheets in which all frames received the same exposure, 35-mm positives from a slide duplicator permit the exposure to be individually tailored for each frame. With this technique, multiple slides of a single frame can be generated. This can be particularly important for teaching programs, since each resident may be given selected slides to begin their own collection of instructional materials.

Paper Enlargements

Though the brightness range of a photographic enlargement is identical to that of a paper contact print, the enlarged size allows fine angiographic detail to be more easily seen. Enlarging is a photographic skill that is useful in many clinical, research, and general photographic assignments. Good printing is an art, and mastery requires time and effort.

An important need for paper prints arises when submitting a manuscript to a medical journal. Printing for publication is challenging; high-quality work is required, and otherwise excellent manuscripts have been rejected solely because of deficient photographs. Typically, matched sets of 5" × 7" enlargements are required.

The first step in making an enlarged angiographic print is to select the image. Inspect the negative carefully with a high-quality loupe. Depending on the precise focus and the patient's tear film, there will probably be certain frames that are sharper than others within the same angiographic phase. Carefully examining the negative will help identify the best candidate for enlargement. Be sure to alert client-physicians to this fact before printing, in case a substitution is not acceptable!

To begin printing, set up the tray line with trays of paper developer (diluted 1:1 with water), stop-bath, fixer, and running water wash. Turn on the darkroom safelight, and if you use a cold light enlarging head, turn on its heater unit.

Clean the selected negative thoroughly before printing to minimize the need to correct dust spots on the final print. Examine the negative under strong lighting and use film-cleaning solution (either a commercial preparation or 95% ethanol) to remove any fingerprints. Next, place the negative in the negative carrier. Inspect the negative again and use a soft brush or compressed air to remove any last specks of dust just before setting the carrier into the enlarger.

Open the enlarging lens to its widest setting, turn on the enlarger's lamp, and adjust the height of the enlarger so the projected image is approximately the size of the required print. Place the print easel on the baseboard, roughly focus the negative onto the easel, and adjust the orientation of the negative carrier, easel, and enlarger height until the easel shows the required image projected onto its surface. Carefully inspect the edges of the easel; make sure that the projected image extends just slightly past the edges of the easel mask. Use tape to secure the easel to the baseboard, thus preventing accidental movement during the printing session. Also, lock the enlarger head height adjustment to prevent it from moving while the negative is focused. If you use variable-contrast paper, now is the time to install the filter into its holder. Begin your tests by using a grade 3 filter for an angiographic negative.

To critically focus the negative, set the grain magnifier onto a scrap piece of photographic paper placed on the easel. The paper must be of the same thickness as the material you will use to make the final print. Look through the magnifier's eyepiece as you adjust the enlarger's focusing knob. When the image is sharp, you will see the negative's grain pattern sharply through the magnifier. Don't be surprised if you cannot recognize the image; many magnifiers use high-powered optics, so pictorial elements in the negative may not be appreciated.

Once these preliminary steps have been accomplished, turn the enlarger's light off and set a sheet of enlarging paper in the easel. Use the same process for making test strip exposures as when printing contact sheets. Incrementally expose the paper, sliding a cardboard mask across its surface so about 1–2 inches of paper is exposed for each step. Develop the print the same way you did for a paper contact print, for 2 minutes, then agitate it in stop bath for 30 seconds. Place in the fixing tray and agitate for 2 minutes, then wash for 4 minutes. Since papers typically darken slightly when dry, assess contrast and density after the test print is dry.

Remember the all-important rule of printing: Exposure creates density, and development influences contrast. Make certain that the enlarger exposure is sufficient to render areas of hyperfluorescence that are not too bright; most vessels can be printed so they have a just perceptible hint of tone darker than the pure white of the paper base. After the highlights have been suitably printed, look at the darkest areas of the print. If they approach true black, then the contrast is probably correct. If the area surrounding the angiographic image is only gray, try switching to a higher contrast paper or develop the grade 3 paper longer to increase the contrast. A cycle of printing, processing, assessing, and reprinting is almost always required by even the best printers.

At times, local exposure control may be required to permit the print to more closely approximate the range of values seen in the negative. "Burning in" describes the process in which a selected portion of the print is exposed longer than other areas. "Dodging" denotes lessening the exposure selectively for specific parts of the image. Both are performed manually, using either your hands or specially made tools (Figure 6-29). Both tasks require a sensitive touch; when properly done, the edges of areas that have been dodged or burned-in should not be noticeable in the final print. The secret is to keep the light modifier (hands or tool) constantly moving; it must also be suspended some distance from the paper surface to cast a very soft edge to its effect.

Local exposure control has ethical implications. Photography has long been assumed to have an intrinsic honesty and objectivity—the main reason that science has adopted photography as a relatively impartial medium for recording and disseminating data. In that spirit, local exposure control should be used only to correct technical deficiencies (i.e., to overcome limitations in matching the printout medium to the negative) and not to artificially create or suppress the distribution of fluorescence.

Advanced Printmaking Techniques

Even though exhibition printing usually plays a small role in ophthalmic photography, at times it may be advantageous to produce a print that reflects the highest levels of photographic quality. When producing an exhibition-quality print, the same techniques are used to determine contrast, exposure, and processing factors as discussed above. However, special photographic paper stock, exposure techniques, and processing chemistries are used to produce a print that has enhanced aesthetic qualities.

The first difference in exhibition printing concerns the choice of paper stock. Even though RC papers could be used, many experienced printers choose fiber-based paper. This stock is not coated with plastic. Instead, the image is directly incorporated in the emulsion layer bonded to the paper support material and thus appears almost tangibly closer to the viewer. The subtle texture of the paper substrate is detected within the image itself. The image will appear slightly sharper, brighter, and of higher contrast than it would in an RC print. Fiber-based papers are available in either graded or variable-contrast. Most fine printers choose the "F," or glossy surface; when air-dried, this surface takes on a most pleasing luster.

A special exposure technique using the unique characteristics of variable-contrast papers will also enhance the quality of your exhibition prints. This technique is called *split filter printing* and is equally applicable to RC media.

Selecting a single filter to print on variable-contrast paper always represents a compromise, as the filter works only for the average contrast value of the negative. In this case, highlight tones (i.e., hyperfluorescent areas of the angiogram) often require burning in, while dark areas may require dodging. Cold light heads help bring the extreme values into a

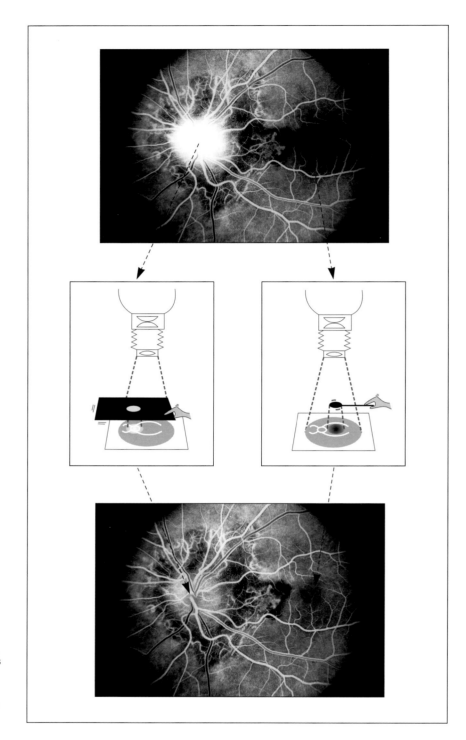

FIGURE 6-29
Presumed ocular histoplasmosis syndrome with choroidal neovascular membrane. Depending on the distribution of dye and the negative's processing, at times a straight print will show an optic nerve that is too bright and a macular region that is too dark. This can be corrected by applying extra exposure (burning) to the nerve head, while a portion of the base exposure is subtracted from the macular area (dodging) to bring the photo into better tonal balance.

closer alignment with the abilities of the paper to depict them[12] but do not solve this problem completely.

Split filter printing employs two filters: a high-contrast (magenta) filter (i.e., grade 5) and a low-contrast (yellow) filter (e.g., a grade 0 or a –1). The low-contrast filter has its greatest effect on the highlights, and the high-contrast filter influences the contrast in the darkest values.

For split filter printing, first place the lower contrast filter in the enlarger. Make a test print (by sequentially exposing strips across the print), develop, fix, wash, and dry. Examine only the lightest tones; choose the final exposure to give proper density in the highlights. The low values will appear flat in this print, however. Next, make another test print giving the selected grade 0 exposure to the entire sheet and then exchange the grade 0 for the grade 5 filter and give the same sheet (already exposed to grade 0) sequential test exposures to the high-contrast filter. Process and examine the results. You will find that the grade 5 filter has little effect on the highlights, but the dark values will show much improvement. Select the grade 5 exposure strip that shows the desired contrast in these areas. To make the final print, expose first to the grade 0 filter for its proper time and then to the grade 5 filter with its distinct time requirement. Obviously, the enlarger must be locked securely and the easel taped down to prevent any movement between the two exposures. The final print will show excellent detail in the highlights, pleasing gradation throughout the middle tones, and just the right contrast in the darkest areas.

When you print on a single-contrast grade paper, you select the proper grade based on the negative's middle values. Customarily, the highlights may require burning and the shadows need dodging. With split filter printing, the highlights and shadows are each exposed through precisely matched contrast filters, and the middle values take care of themselves.[13]

Kodak Dektol or similar paper developer is used to develop fiber-based paper. A worthwhile enhancement to the developer comes from adding benzotriazole to the solution. One ounce per liter can slightly increase print contrast as well as slightly cool the print color.[14] Also, for the finest print quality, the fixer should not include hardener solution since it prevents uniform toning effects and also lengthens the required duration of the wash cycle.

Most photographic papers have a distinctive print color. Even though they are called "black and white," most papers appear to have a slightly olive-green tint once they have been processed. Many find this color to be unappealing. It can be shifted to a slightly cooler, more purplish color using a toner. After the stop-bath, fix the print for 2 minutes. Then place the print into a bath that consists of 1 liter of Hypo Clearing Agent or Perma Wash, to which has been added 1 oz of rapid selenium toner. *Caution: selenium is toxic.* Use tongs or rubber gloves when processing prints in this material! Constantly agitate the print while observing its overall color carefully (an untreated print next to the tray will provide a useful comparison). After several minutes, you will be able to detect a subtle shift in color towards a cool purplish brown.[12] When the desired color has been reached, remove the print and place it in the print washer. If the print stays too long in the toning bath, it will eventually turn noticeably brown. The intended goal of this bath should be a subtle color shift; at a glance, the finished print should still appear to be black and white.

Fiber-based papers naturally absorb more chemistry than RC materials. They must be washed much longer to ensure long-term stability. At least 1 hour in an efficient print washer is required to achieve a chemical-free condition. RC papers typically dry flat. Fiber-based papers, on the other hand, have a tendency to curl as they dry. For best results, they should be allowed to dry on fiberglass drying screens—these look like screen windows and permit air to dry both the front and the back of the print simultaneously. The emulsion surface of a wet fiber-based print is quite delicate; it is best to place these prints face-up on the screen to avoid any chance of imprinting the screen's texture on the print. Avoid the use of photographic blotters or drum dryers, as these cannot be kept perfectly clean. Drying may take anywhere from several hours to overnight, depending on the relative humidity of the environment. When completely dry, these prints may be flattened under a weight (i.e., a stack of books) for several hours.

Carefully inspect the final dried print for white specks. If they are present, they should be spotted as a last step in finishing the print. In this process, tiny white spots in the print caused by dust, scratches, or other defects on the negative can be retouched by carefully painting them with dyes. These dyes are formulated to match common print colors and are usually sold in sets of three. Use an extremely fine sable watercolor brush (i.e., size 00) to pick up a minute quantity of the selected dye. The brush must be nearly dry to avoid placing an uncontrolled drop of dye liquid onto the print surface, where it could spread and darken surrounding tones. Under strong illumination (and with the use of a magnifier if you have presbyopia), fill in the white spots by repeatedly touching the tip of the brush to the offending speck of white, periodically charging the brush with more dye as required. A light, delicate touch is needed for this work. As the pigment from the brush penetrates the paper, the spot will slowly merge into the surrounding tone. Work slowly, and periodically rotate the print's orientation to help see new spots that need correction. If the white speck is linear, it is best to first break it up into short segments and then to fill in each segment, rather than trying to paint out the line in one or two strokes. Every few seconds, sit back from the print to measure your work's progress.

Acknowledgment

This work was supported in part by a grant from Research to Prevent Blindness, Inc., New York.

References

1. Shaw SD, Rossol M. Overexposure: Health Hazards in Photography. New York: Allworth Press, 1991.
2. Spencer DA (ed). LP Clerc's Photography Theory and Practice. Vol. 4: Monochrome Processing. Bath, England: Focal Press, 1971.
3. Thall L. Survival of the stainless steel developing reel. Photo Electronic Imaging 1994;37:50.
4. Frohlichstein A. Automatic processing of fluorescein angiographic film with a modified MohrPro 8 print processor. J Ophthal Photography 1991;13:77.
5. Merin LM, Lewis RA. New film alternatives for high resolution fluorescein angiography. J Ophthal Photography 1988;10:36.
6. Scott ML. Understanding the Photographic Process. In JP Vetter (ed), Biomedical Photography. Stoneham, MA: Butterworth-Heinemann, 1992;14.
7. Tyler ME. Total tonal information in fluorescein angiography. J Ophthal Photography 1979;2:62.
8. Merin LM. A pragmatic approach to "technical difficulties" in ophthalmic photography. J Biological Photography 1994;62:113.
9. Hurtgen TP. Understanding photographic parameters—guides to film selection and use. In Biomedical Photography, a Kodak Seminar in Print. Rochester, NY: Eastman Kodak Company, 1976.
10. White M. Zone System Manual. Hastings-on-Hudson, NY: Morgan & Morgan, 1968;7.
11. Merin LM. Aesthetics in angiographic imagery. J Ophthal Photography 1981;4:22.
12. Picker F. Zone VI Workshop. Garden City, NJ: American Photographic Book Publishing, 1974;51–52.
13. Vestal D. The Craft of Photography. New York: Harper & Row, 1972;251.
14. Adams A. The Print. Boston: Little, Brown, 1983.

Suggested Readings

Blaker AA. *Handbook for Scientific Photography*. San Francisco: WH Freeman, 1977.
CBE Scientific Illustration Committee. *Illustrating Science: Standards for Publication*. Bethesda, MD: Council of Biology Editors, 1988.
Graves C. *The Zone System for 35mm Photographers*. Stoneham, MA: Focal Press, 1982.
Kelly J (ed). *Darkroom 2*. New York: Lustrum Press, 1978.
Lewis E (ed). *Darkroom*. New York: Lustrum Press, 1977.

Chapter 7

Electronic Imaging of the Fundus: Principles and Technique

Marshall E. Tyler

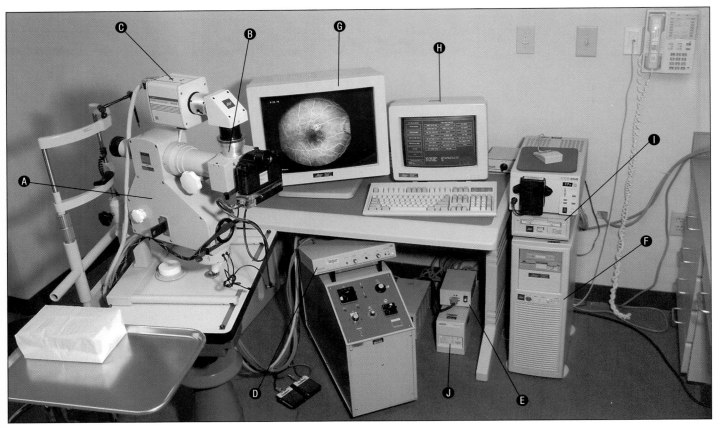

FIGURE 7-1
Digital fluorescein angiography system. A. Fundus camera. B. Optical port for digital camera. C. Digital camera head. D. Digital camera control unit (CCU). E. Synchronizing "black box." F. Computer with image grabber board. G. Image monitor. H. Text menu monitor. I. Archival mass image storage device (optical laser drive). J. Uninterruptable power supply (UPS). Some systems use one monitor for both the image display and the software menu. (Note: This image and Figures 7-9 and 7-15 were photographed with a Kodak DCS-460 digital camera.)

Introduction

Digital imaging provides faster results and diagnostic capabilities that were heretofore not possible with conventional photographic techniques. With the rapid advances in economical personal computing power and high-resolution imaging technologies, there has been a move to incorporate these technologies from research facilities into the academic and clinical ophthalmic photography setting (Figure 7-1).

We present the topic of electronic fundus imaging in its own chapter because we believe it has its own subject matter and vocabulary unique and separate from those of fundus photography and fluorescein angiography, the mainstays of ophthalmic photography. Angiographic studies, which are quickly made available for diagnostic interpretation, account for the majority of this chapter.

Why Electronic Imaging?

There are several forces driving the acceptance of electronic imaging into the practice of ophthalmic photography. Electronic imaging permits the physician to receive diagnostic information—chiefly from fluorescein angiography—in a timely manner. Additional computer imaging tools increase the level of diagnostic information. Computer manipulation and analysis have advantages over more conventional photographic processes, including image enhancement and imaging tools such as

Terminology Note: Photography

The term *photography* is used rather than electronic imaging or diagnostic imaging because we continue to be concerned with the properties of light and how to represent it. We would rather not dwell on the recording medium (film or silicone). It is the light that must be controlled to achieve the required images. The recording and display media in electronic imaging must be understood to be part of the total "photo-graphic" process.

image overlays. Indocyanine green (ICG) angiography, which was technically very difficult to perform with infrared (IR) photographic film, received little clinical attention until IR-sensitive electronic cameras became available. Finally, the competitive marketplace demands that a patient be offered treatment in the same visit. This is particularly true if patients have traveled for hours to see the retinal specialist.

Environmental concerns continue to affect the chemical darkroom as well. While the production of computer chips and other electronic components is not without its environmental concerns, electronic imaging does not produce an ongoing stream of waste products from the computer itself. Concern still exists about by-products from the printing systems.

Computers and electronic imaging cameras are tools that assist in creating images (see the terminology note sidebar). The light sources and optics of electronic imaging systems are similar to those of their film counterparts, but their "photosensitive" material is very different. These systems now include video and digital cameras for fluorescein angiography and ICG angiography.

Following is a section on scanning laser ophthalmoscopes (SLOs) used for angiography, both fluorescein and ICG angiography, nerve fiber layer (NFL) studies, and systems for optic nerve analysis and retinal topography. This chapter also describes the various technologies used to create and analyze posterior pole images. The components of the systems, how they work, and how they differ from each other as well as from comparable conventional photographic systems are discussed. Cost considerations in purchasing and using the new technology are included. After a historical review, there is a discussion of the differences between video and digital imaging, followed by a technical comparison of film and electronic imaging. Each section starts with a technical description of the instrumentation, followed by a description of how to use it, and then by a discussion of equipment selection.

History of Video and Digital Technology

Video Fluorescein Angiography

Throughout the history of video fluorescein angiography, many manufacturers and system integrators have made amazing progress in providing ophthalmic photographers with new tools. As early as 1951, Ridley[1] reported television applications in ophthalmology. In 1970, Dallow[2] wrote a treatise entitled *Television Ophthalmoscopy*, in which he briefly discussed Image Orthicon cameras but chiefly reported on Vidicon cameras (Figure 7-2). His concepts of ophthalmic image analysis stand today as testimony to his ophthalmic and technical insight. Of particular historic interest was his advanced work on monochromatic imaging.

During the 1970s, van Heuven and Schafer used black and white video (TV) cameras to record fluorescein angiograms on videotape.[3–6] The first video cameras received images using specialized photo-multiplier tubes coated with phosphors. Image intensifiers allowed fluorescein angiographic images to be recorded since conventional video camera tubes did not have adequate sensitivity. The videotaping process degraded the resolution and added even more noise to the image. The limitations of the video camera and recorder resolution and the expense kept video fluorescein angiograms from gaining wider acceptance.

van Heuven and Mehu used a high-intensity Vidicon camera tube coupled to a three-stage image intensifier, which replaced the eyepiece on a Zeiss fundus camera. A sliding mirror was substituted for the illu-

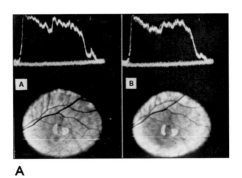

A

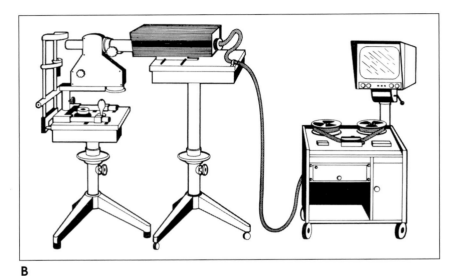

B

FIGURE 7-2
Early video fluorescein angiography system. A. Television monitor image of selected lines in monochrome illumination. B. Perspective drawing of a television ophthalmoscope. (From RL Dallow. *Television Ophthalmoscopy: Instrumentation and Medical Applications.* Springfield, IL: Charles C Thomas, 1970.)

minating beam splitter. This increased the intensity of the viewing lamp at the patient's eye. They stated: "The positive public-relations aspects of this fast service are not without reward," and mentioned that recording a fluorescein angiogram as a kinetic event was of potential importance.[7]

I have always marveled at the feeling I get when seeing the true dynamic nature of a fluorescein angiogram on a continuous medium such as videotape. Even when you take a film fluorescein angiogram, there is usually a mirror that blanks out the view of the fluorescein image each time you expose an image. A technological change to include continuous imaging would provide for analysis of the choroidal and early arterial angiographic phases.

In the 1980s, Vidicon video camera tube(s) were replaced with silicone chips. The imaging chip technology used is a charged coupled device (CCD).

Video Camera with Computer Digitizer

As computers became less expensive, smaller, and more powerful, the next generation of imaging systems began with the introduction of video frame grabbers. A personal computer–based video frame grabber permits an analog video signal to be digitized.

In 1980, at the University of Pittsburgh, Paul Rehkopf and Joseph Warnicki, with Stuart Brown, M.D. (Chairman of the Department of Ophthalmology), began developing an ophthalmic video digitizing system. In late 1982, they worked with James Cambier at PAR Microsystems to develop the first marketable electronic ophthalmic imaging system. This system was a Unix-based computer running a Motorola 68000 processor on a S-100 data bus. Red, green, and blue (RGB) or National Television Standards Committee (NTSC) video images were digitized to a 512×512 resolution with rectangular pixels using seven imaging boards. There was a capture and a memory board for each color (red, green, and blue), as well as a controller card. The color images were used for stereo glaucoma studies. The system sported an 80-megabyte (MB) hard drive and an optical drive for direct recording of images. The computer did not have enough hard disk space for the temporary storage of images, so all images were recorded to the optical disk. Final proof sheets could be built without any "bad" images, but they still wasted space on the nonerasable optical disk. It took approximately 1 second to record just a single memory plane for a black and white video image. The initial system was wired for the electronic interface and flash synchronization circuits of the Topcon fundus camera, although shortly after that, supplementary interfaces were made for the Zeiss fundus camera and slit-lamp.

The program screens were in monochrome but had "windowed" control areas, and a mouse was used as a pointing device for image selection and contrast manipulation. Quite a few of the image manipulation routines seen in current systems were implemented in this system, although processing speeds were much slower. Image sharpening took 2–3 minutes and image registration took well over 5 minutes. Remember, this was a 512-resolution system. In a personal memorandum, Mr. Warnicki stated, "There were 24 ribbon cables with more than twelve hundred connections for just the video capture and memory boards. These connections were very touchy. We regularly had to clean them to keep the system running."

This imaging system was marketed in 1983 by PAR Microsystems as the IS-2000. The cost of the basic system was $150,000. This included a S-100 based 68000 computer with Unix operating system, two monochrome vt-100 computer terminals, two color monitors, and a 12-inch optical disk recorder, which could store 1 gigabyte of data. The disks cost about $400 each. The basic system was rack mounted in a cabinet about 30×30 inches wide and 6 feet high.

Ophthalmic Imaging Systems, Inc. (OIS), founded by Dennis J. Makes and Steven Verdooner, shipped its first FA-512 system in 1986. It consisted of an Ikegami video camera on a Topcon TRC-50VT fundus camera and an IBM-compatible computer using an Intel 80286 processor. Their first FA-1024 system (1989) used a Dage 1-inch Vidicon tube type video camera, and the analog video signal was converted to a digital file in a PC.

In 1987, Topcon America purchased the system marketed by PAR Microsystems and released the product under the IMAGEnet name. Three models were available: fluorescein, color fundus, and stereo.

In 1988, Olendorf Research, now owned by Tomey, Inc., introduced its Zeiss-adapted digital camera using a Kodak camera. This digital camera back was mounted on a Nikon F-3 35-mm camera and used a Macintosh computer and National Institutes of Health (NIH)–based imaging software (NIH Image). Later models used the Kodak DCS-100 and DCS-200 camera backs. These digital backs use the Kodak M2 and M3 chip technology, which digitizes the image at the chip level.

In 1989, OIS and Topcon introduced 1024 models using the Kodak Videk camera to create the first commercially available high-resolution system with analog-to-digital conversion within the camera control unit (CCU). This was used for fluorescein angiography. The Intel-based computers (80386) were slow at acquiring images. To speed up the process, one manufacturer skipped the recording of every other line of the image and later extrapolated it to synthesize a 1024×1024 image. When computers became faster, they offered a full-resolution system. The other system was slower but maintained full-image resolution.

In 1991, both OIS and Topcon moved to the Kodak Megaplus (model 1.4) camera. This was a high-resolution video camera based on Kodak's M1 chip technology. Like the Videk, it contained an internal digitizing board, but the image was not digitized near the chip.

In 1994 and 1995, OIS and Topcon America brought Microsoft Windows-based software to ophthalmic photography. This advance assisted in getting the images onto computer networks and facilitated the sending of images out of the camera room. Systems with a single monitor showing both the menu text and the images were brought to the marketplace in the mid 1990s as a space- and cost-saving measure.

Cameras and Instrumentation

Electronic Fundus Imaging and Angiography

When film is replaced with its electronic counterpart, the digital camera, there are additional technical challenges for the photographer. The technical differences between video and digital imaging discussed here form the basis for all the discussions that follow: how the components are integrated and how to use this new technology for fluorescein and ICG angiography, monochromatic imaging, and color fundus photography. There are many basic components to be discussed: fundus camera, optical interface, electronic image camera (digital camera), computer (with image digitizing board, image display board, archiving system, and network connection), software, and printer.

This section describes how the components function; the next section describes how to apply an electronic system to ophthalmic photography.

A complete explanation of the electronics of the digital camera, the computer interface, and the mathematics of image enhancement is outside the scope of this book. The information presented here about the functioning of this equipment is sufficient to allow the photographer to understand the capabilities as well as the limitations of digital imaging. You may want to skim the technology section and then review it again as your needs arise. First, however, see the sidebar on video and digital terminology.

Angiography System Components

Integrators of electronic fundus camera systems have attached a digital camera, computer, and software onto a film-type fundus camera to create a comprehensive ophthalmic instrument. This is not a simple task. When making a photograph, you are asking the system to do the following: clear the previous image from the computer's image capture board, clear the previous image in the digital camera, and then synchronize the fundus camera's solenoid eyepiece head, electronic flash, and digital camera image capture with the computer's image capture board. Systems from all vendors use similar components to accomplish digital imaging (see Figure 7-1).

SYSTEM SYNCHRONIZATION

A synchronizing device coordinates the flash, digital camera, image capture, and computer to receive the image. Each system manufacturer has its own name for this synchronizing "black box," which is one of the most important proprietary components of the system. Without the synchronizer, the image capture sequence cannot be coordinated.

(the number of capacitors selected is a precise number), or "0s" and "1s" in a computer.

If the signal is turned into an analog signal in the camera, then, by definition, the camera is an analog video camera. If the camera maintains the digital information all of the way from (next to) the CCD to the recording medium, then the camera and system are digital. Some cameras have a high-resolution (greater than NTSC) analog signal going to the camera control unit (CCU) where it is digitized. An example of this technology is the Kodak Megaplus, model 1.4, which uses what Kodak calls M1 chip technology.[9] The model 1.4i has no separate CCU and has computer-adjusted controls.

The brightness of the video image is represented by a voltage level (Figure 7-4), which is changed in the computer on the digitizing board (frame grabber) into a digital signal for each relative position on the video signal (Figure 7-5). The advantages of this transformation of the video signal to a digital signal are twofold. First, the image saved in the computer is of a higher quality than the same signal recorded and played back on videotape, because the process of recording and replaying an analog videotape degrades image quality. Replication (attempts of duplication) further degrades image quality. Computers that can record continuous video signals are expensive. Duplication of a computer (digital) image is not degraded when copied, whereas in photographic or video replication the image is modified when one attempts to duplicate it.

Second, the digitally recorded video frame may later be manipulated in the computer. Overall contrast expansion and control of brightness is similar to changing paper grade and/or exposure when printing in the darkroom. These brightness and contrast expansions allow the viewer to see the desired image.

A video camera can be a cost-effective input device for low-end electronic imaging systems. Do not forget that not only is the image of lower resolution but it is not a true "digital imaging" system since the image was once an analog signal. Thus, it should be referred to as a *digitized* video imaging system.

Resolution of digital camera is limited only by the levels of present technology and cost. Digital cameras with image resolutions of 2k × 3k are now available.

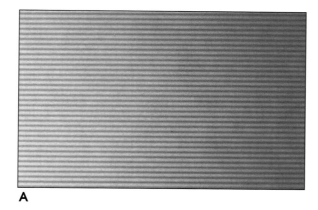

A

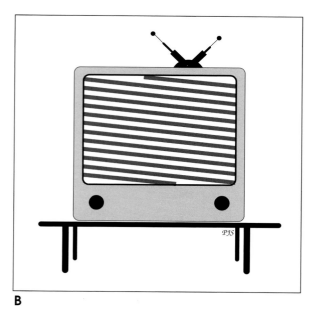

B

FIGURE 7-3
Scan lines on an NTSC television screen. A. Close-up of scan lines. B. Scan lines, even and odd.

DIGITAL CAMERAS

Photographic film responds to light by creating image density that relates to the intensity of the light that exposed it. The resultant density is a very accurate (although not linear) representation of the degree of illumination or subject reflectance. An almost infinite number of shades of gray, with a dynamic range of 160:1, are created in the photographic negative. In a digital camera, electronic approximations are created to represent the illumination on the camera chip face (Figure 7-6). The following section describes how this is accomplished.

The digital camera receives the image of the fundus after the fundus camera illuminates the eye with its electronic flash. A digital camera's CCD sensor contains a grid of many thousands of discrete locations, each of which is uniquely identified. These locations on the sensor are called *pixels*, short for *pic*ture *el*ements. The smaller the pixel the finer the resolution, given the same size of active chip area.

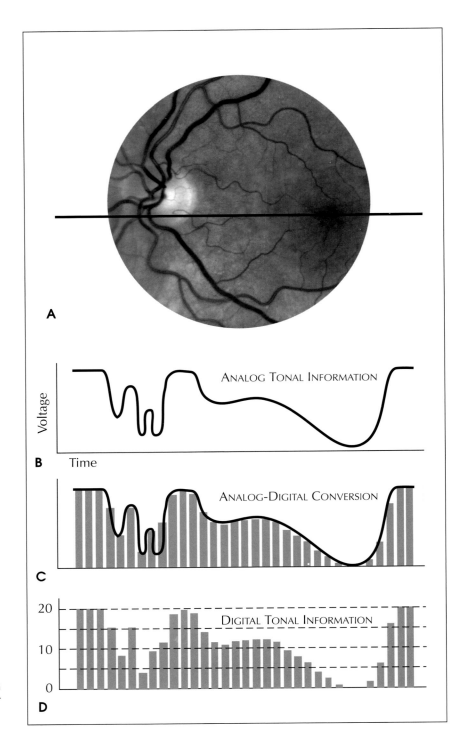

FIGURE 7-4
The fundus photograph (A) has a single scan line drawn through the image. Relative brightness (expressed as voltage) at approximate positions on the video screen (B) and its transition and conversion from analog to digital signal (C) are precisely recorded brightness at exact locations on the digitized image (D).

The camera then translates the analog world into numbers, which can be sent directly to a computer for storage. Making a photographic slide from a digital original creates an analog image from a digital image. Compared to video images, the digital camera typically has higher image resolution and a lower signal-to-noise ratio. In image duplication, the digital image does not induce image distortions (tonal shifts) or increase image noise as does replication of videotapes (attempts at duplication).

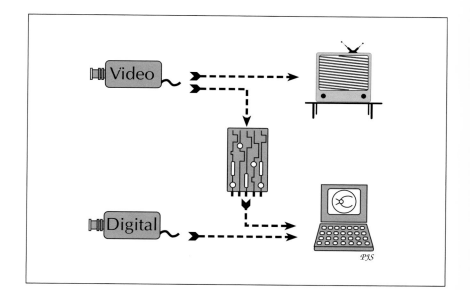

FIGURE 7-5
Integrating video or digital images. Electronic angiography systems use either a video or a digital camera. A video camera produces an analog signal, which can be recorded in analog on videotape or translated into 0s and 1s by a digitizing board in a computer. A digital camera provides a digital image directly to the computer.

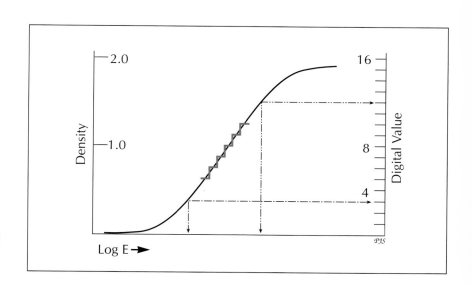

FIGURE 7-6
Analog film density versus digital camera output. The digital camera creates discrete values for each level of illumination and produces values that represent the linear nature of the imaging devices.

IMAGE DEPTH

A digital camera receives light onto its CCD, where the light on each pixel generates a number that represents the brightness of the light. Eight-bit cameras generate a number between 0 and 255 ($2^8 = 256$) and 12-bit cameras, 0 to 4095 (2^{12}). This number approximates the amount of light that falls on that specific pixel. Some cameras use a 10- or 12-bit dynamic range for image capture but save the image as an 8-bit image. There are also 16-bit cameras, and these store 65,536 gray-level values (2^{16}).

Pixels may be numbered starting in the upper left-hand corner of the image sensor. This location is 0,0 for the row-column location. The next pixel in the first row would be number 0,1. Since the pixels are read off in order, there is little reason to note the actual location of the pixel once the total array dimension (in pixels) of the CCD is known. Just the brightness (luminance) values are noted as discrete values—for example, 0, 127, 255. These values represent black, medium gray, and white.

Table 7-1. CCD Pixel Defect Ratings (Simplified)

C0	No point defects*
C1	Five or fewer total point defects with two or less within the central 35% of the image and none in an adjacent row or column.
C2	Ten or fewer point defects (total) with five or less within the central 35%.
C3	Twenty or fewer point defects (total) with 10 or less within the central 35%.

*Point defect: A pixel that deviates by more than 6% from neighboring pixels when illuminated to 70% saturation.

PIXEL DEFECTS

Most cameras have some defective pixels. A typical bad pixel will return a value of 0 (black) no matter how much light falls on it. (Note also Kodak's definition of a "point defect" at the bottom of Table 7-1.) Camera grading is based on the quality of all of the pixels and their placement. The higher the pixel defect grade, the less distracting the bad pixels will be. There is a significant cost premium for perfect and near-perfect cameras. Cameras with a few bad pixels are considered the standard grade, and cameras with multiple central defects are sold at a discount (Table 7-1). In Kodak terminology, a class C3 camera would be the lowest quality. A class C2 or C3 camera would have a reasonable price-quality balance for clinical applications. When buying a camera, be sure you are getting what you are paying for. Software can change the value of a bad pixel and give it a value similar to adjacent pixels, which visually masks the defective pixels.

SENSOR SIZES AND ASPECT RATIOS

Imaging chip measurements are based on standards developed in the video industry. The first TV camera tubes, image orthicons, were referred to as "2-inch tubes." This was the measure of the diagonal of the rectangular scan area of the image on a round tube face. Video camera chip sizes are also referenced by the diagonal measure of the active chip area. Typical diagonal measurements are ⅓-inch, ½-inch, and ⅔-inch.

Digital cameras are often referred to by the number of active pixels on the CCD or by the physical size of the active area of the chip—for example, 1035 × 1370 pixels or 8.98 mm × 7.04 mm (camera that was used on the OIS and IMAGEnet 1024 systems in the early 1990s). The pixel count reflects the resolution of the system, and the image area is used to calculate the magnification of the images (Table 7-2). An early series of cameras had pixel counts of 1012 × 1524 and an active image area of 14 mm × 9.3 mm. Later units had more pixels, 2024 × 3072, and a larger image area, 18.4 mm × 27.6 mm.

The height-to-width ratio is different for different imaging technologies: 35-mm, 2:3; video, 3:4; and round fundus images, 1:1. When these media are mixed, there will either be some black area added or some cropping of the images (Figure 7-7).

COMPONENTS OF VIDEO AND DIGITAL CAMERAS

In addition to the camera head, there may be a camera control unit (CCU) (see Figure 7-1C, D). The CCU separates some of the electronics so that some of the weight and size of the unit may be located away from the camera-lens assembly. This separation also permits electronic adjustments to be made remotely. Cable connections to the computer are also easier to establish, since the CCU can be located conveniently. Some newer cameras are designed to be controlled from the computer and are not equipped with a separate CCU.

Table 7-2. Imaging Devices Tube and Chip Sizes

Format	Diagonal (mm)	Height × Width (mm)	Pixels	Image Size (MB)	% of 35 mm
⅓" video	8.5	5.1 × 6.8			4
Megaplus 1.4	11.4	7 × 9	1035 × 1370	1.4	7.3
½" video	12.7	7.6 × 10.2			9
Digital (DCS-100)	16.8	9.3 × 14	1012 × 1524	1.5	15
⅔" video	17.0	10.1 × 13.5			15.8
1" video	25.4	15.2 × 20.3			35.7
Digital (DCS-460)	33.2	18.4 × 27.6	2024 × 3072	6.1	58.8
35-mm film	43.3	24 × 36			100
2" video	50.8	30.5 × 40.6			117

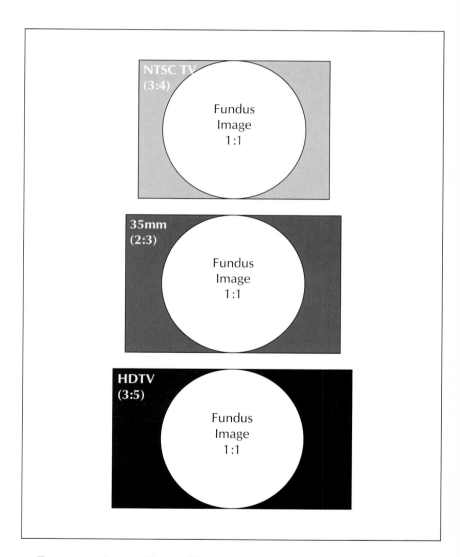

FIGURE 7-7
The aspect ratios of NTSC-TV, 35-mm film, and HD-video.

For comparison, a 35-mm film image size is 24 mm × 36 mm. Typically, digital chips are smaller (see Table 7-2). This means that an optical adapter is required to make the image the correct size for the physically smaller electronic imaging sensors.

Optical devices (photo adapters)[8] that relay the image to the video or digital camera often are referred to by the diagonal size (diagonal measure) of the video image they support—for example, ½-inch. Calculations must be made to show the magnification of the image and therefore how the image will be displayed by a particular chip size. When selecting an imaging system, ensure that the image is filling the full area of the chip.

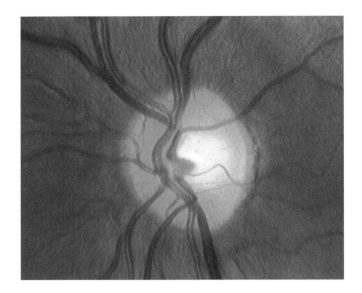

FIGURE 7-8
Color video fundus image. The video image is reproduced to show the anticipated detail that would be seen on a 5 × 7 print. Evaluate the image sharpness on an actual print from any system you are evaluating—does it meet your needs?

Using as much of the chip's active area as possible helps create the highest resolution image. Check this by increasing the brightness control on the monitor to reveal the edges of the chip's active scan area.

COLOR FUNDUS ELECTRONIC IMAGING
Video CCD cameras may continue to be integrated into electronic ophthalmic imaging devices to reduce expense. The rest of this chapter includes this technology as well as true digital imaging. Keep in mind that the resolution of video systems is only about one-third that of even the most basic digital cameras (Figure 7-8).

Video imaging systems sometimes use color cameras that give the system color fundus recording capabilities. The quality of these images is comparable to those produced on instant film materials and perhaps, therefore, are not of adequate quality as the only documentation of the color fundus. However, these images may be used as a convenience to remind the clinician of the previously examined fundus. Video will not replace the need for high-quality images. There are now digital video cameras that are used in high-end television broadcast applications—high-definition television (HDTV). These cameras maintain a digital signal all the way to a video recorder and editing equipment. Digital satellite distribution systems now bring digital quality into the home, and analog signals may soon be a thing of the past. Fortunately, digital cameras with the resolution for both high-quality color and black and white imaging are now available.

The greatest advantage achieved by replacing video with digital signals is the freeing of the resolution of the image from the NTSC standards. The first digital cameras that were affordable to clinical ophthalmology had resolutions of 1024 × 1280 pixels. Cameras that will image more than three times (total area) that resolution, 2048 × 2048 and 2036 × 3060, are entering the imaging market. Time will drop the cost of these cameras as well as the computers that manipulate the images.

In a true digital camera, the digital signal is maintained from the sensor, the camera head, and the CCU, all the way to the image grabber card in the computer. This card receives a digital signal directly from the digital camera. Whenever there is an analog-to-digital (A/D) converter, some information is lost, whereas no information is lost with reproduction using the digital signal (Table 7-3). The picture is then moved from the image grabbing card to the computer memory or, in some systems, directly to a fast hard drive.

Comparison of Film and Electronic Imaging

Most of the components of digital fundus cameras are similar to those of photographic film cameras, but the former have additional components (computer parts) that replace the film and the processes that film usually undergoes. Film is first processed (developed, stopped, fixed, washed, wetting agents, dried, printed, and stored) and then the images are reviewed. The digital camera replaces these "film steps" with electronic substitutes (amplified, digitized, enhanced, archived, and displayed). Since black and white cameras made the first inroads into ophthalmic digital imaging, I will discuss that technology first. Color digital cameras have the same types of imaging components, but the concept of digital imaging will be easier to understand if we first think only of black and white images.

Let us first look at the flow of the electronic image through the electronic system and compare it to film (Table 7-4). Exposure latitude and technical considerations of dynamic range are discussed later in the sidebar on exposing the image.

After the digital camera's CCD is exposed to the image-forming light, the digital signal is created in the camera head. There the picture is made into a formatted digital image, which is then sent to a special electronic circuit board (imaging board) in the computer. This board acts as an interpolator of the electronic image and the computer memory. With the use of software, the computer controls where and how the image is stored in the temporary computer memory, called the the random access memory (RAM). After images are stored in the RAM, the software permits the user to delete any of the unwanted images and then save the desired images onto the hard drive.

The image stored in RAM is like the latent silver image on the film. It is volatile (nonpermanent) and, just like exposed but unprocessed film, the image stored in RAM can be destroyed. If the computer loses its power (including any backup power supply), the images in the camera, on the image capture circuit board RAM, or in the computer RAM will be lost. Just as a film image is stable once the film is processed (developed and fixed), light will not damage the silver image; once the digital image is copied onto the hard drive, it will be preserved even if the computer power is turned off. These stored images can then be enhanced, printed, reviewed, and finally archived.

For film images to be usable in the future, the film must be dried, labeled, and stored in a filing system. Likewise the digital image needs to be copied onto a mass storage device, typically an optical disk or a CD-ROM.

Table 7-3. Analog and Video Equipment: Which Equipment Uses What Technology?

Camera Type	Still (Single Image)	Motion (Continuous Imaging)
Analog	Still video	TV cameras, camcorders
Digital	Megaplus, DCS	Broadcast: Digital-TV

Table 7-4. Comparison of Film Imaging and Digital Imaging

Film Term	Digital Term
Developed	Digitized
Fixed	Archived
Printed	Displayed

Note that while the Kodak Megaplus 1.4 has been generally known as one of the first "digital cameras" used in ophthalmic photography, it uses Kodak's M1 chip technology, which is a high-resolution analog chip that digitizes the images in the CCU, not next to the chip.[8]

Color digital cameras generate a red, or green, or blue value for each pixel location. Color chips are usually 28–30% less sensitive to light, due to the red, green, and blue filters that have been placed in front of the pixels. When used in a monochromatic imaging situation (e.g., fluorescein angiography), color cameras will have less resolution (because of the extra pixels required to capture the color information for the same size chip) than their monochrome counterparts.

As the technology matures, digital color cameras will become just as useful for color fundus photography as monochromatic digital cameras are for angiography (see the sidebar on the comparison of film and electronic imaging). Complementary metal oxide semiconductors (CMOS)–active pixel sensor imaging technology may provide reduced sensor costs while providing electrical power and size advantages. In addition, there may be improved reliability through a reduced overall system component count.

Image Capture

The computer controls all the image acquisition steps as well as the mechanism by which the image is manipulated, printed, and stored. Let us first look at acquisition.

After patient data are entered and the camera is prepared for patient photography, you are ready to begin a dye study. To start the timer on a fluorescein angiography series, most computer-controlled systems use the same device as a film-based fluorescein system. This is typically either a button located on the camera positioning joystick of the fundus camera or a foot pedal. Pressing the joystick button signals the solenoid eyepiece to move the viewing mirror to send the image to the imaging chip (Figure 7-9).

A signal from the mirror is sent to the computer and, in combination with the control box, a signal is sent to the digital camera's CCU. The signal then travels to the computer's central processing unit (CPU) with its image capture board, and finally to the fundus camera's flash tube trigger circuit to initiate the firing of the flash. If a digital camera is mounted on the video port on the fundus camera, the fundus camera synchronizes the image going to the video port and the triggering of the digital camera. When a digital camera back is used, as

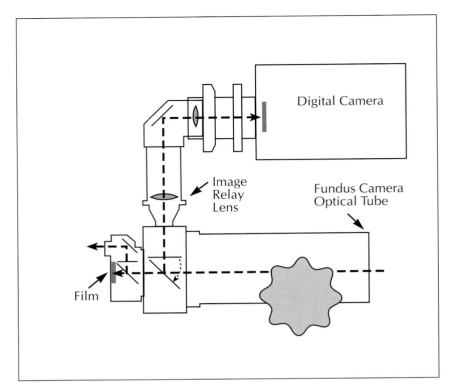

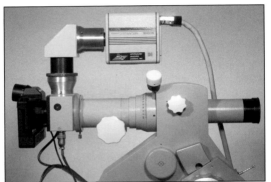

FIGURE 7-9
Digital camera eyepiece head and optical schematic. Note the position of the additional mirror and the relay lens. In this system, the viewing mirror moves into place to shift the image upward to the digital camera.

opposed to a digital camera mounted on a video port, then coordination of these signals is taken care of by the digital camera back, the same as with film.

Each of these components must be ready to record the image. Upon receiving instructions from the computer's CPU, the camera's CCU tells the imaging chip in the digital camera to get ready to receive an image. The chip is set up to receive a new image by clearing any image that may have been stored on it. The frame grabber is told to go through the same process: It is cleared and put into a ready state. After the imaging chip and the frame grabber are prepared, the fundus camera is signaled to fire the flash, which illuminates the fundus. The image is received by the digital camera and sent via its CCU to the frame grabber board in the computer and displayed on a monitor. The image is off-loaded into the computer's random access memory (RAM) to free the capture board so that it can acquire another image.

HOW MUCH RAM IS NEEDED? HOW MANY IMAGES DO YOU WANT?

After a series of fluorescein angiographic images are acquired, they must be moved from the RAM to make room for more images. Images are typically a minimum of 1 MB in size. The amount of RAM is usually the limiting factor on how many images can be recorded quickly before some must be saved. Some systems may use fast hard drives to save each image just after it is acquired. No matter which system is used, check the minimum time for continuous image acquisition to make sure it meets your needs. Shorter is better.

The computer's operating system and the image acquisition program will use 1–4 MB. If a system is configured with only 16 or 20 MB of RAM, then that RAM only permits 12–16 images to be acquired before they must be transferred to the hard drive to make room for more images. If a system has 32 MB of RAM, then 26–30 images may be stored in the RAM at one time. Some systems may keep one or two images on the frame grabber board and then transfer them to the hard drive. As computer processors and hard drives become faster, it may be possible to write unlimited numbers of images directly to the hard drive.

Monitors

Monitors are the prime viewing devices for viewing images and for reading the menus from the computer software. Some systems have a separate monitor for the images, and some share one monitor screen between the images and the software menu. The advantages of using dual monitors are twofold. First is that the angiography monitor can be black and white. Not only does this reduce the cost of the larger monitor, it also increases the sharpness of the black and white image. However, if the image monitor is in color, it can be used for color fundus images, and other imaging work is more convenient with a larger monitor. Second, having a separate image monitor keeps the software menus away from the images. Disadvantages of a two-monitor system include greater cost and the need for greater space.

While monitors are typically of a resolution similar to that of the images that are to be displayed, the resolution of the image is not limited by monitor resolution. The stored image should be kept on the computer at the fullest resolution that the camera and optical system are capable of producing. The image can be displayed on computer monitors by using a software package that permits "zooming" the image to reveal the full resolution of the image.

Image Processing and Enhancements

Before printing, you may choose to modify the images through enhancement techniques, imaging tools, or both. The imaging software and your computer are the workhorses of this phase. How you use these tools is discussed later in the section entitled "Digital Angiography: Using the System."

Printing

Several printing technologies have been used in electronic ophthalmic imaging. Printers range in price from less than $1,000 to more than $20,000. Obviously there are some differences in these printers. When you are ready to print, the software will permit you to select the number of images to be included on a single sheet of paper. Typical formats are for 1, 4, 9, or 16 images to be printed on 8½" × 11" paper or transparency. Image resolution and image size should be appropriately balanced for cost and quality. Note the decrease in sharpness as more images are put onto a single screen or print (see Figure 7-26).

VIDEO PRINTERS

Video prints are much smaller than their digital imaging counterparts, because video resolution is so low that a large print would look very poor. In the 1-up mode on a 5" × 7" video printer, the images may reveal the image resolution limitations of video (see Figure 7-8). With the decreasing cost of digital printers, low-end digital printers are sometimes used for video images. Large video images will not be sharp despite the larger size printers.

OFFICE LASER PRINTERS

Laser printers (office type) provide an economical as well as a high-contrast and low-resolution solution to producing a chart copy of the digital image (Figure 7-10A, B). A laser printer can be driven via the normal printer ports or with a special cable and a card, which, when placed inside the laser printer, can increase the printing resolution and speed. The images that can be achieved from the systems in which the laser is driven directly from the computer have resolutions of 1200 dots per inch (dpi). However, there are limitations as the laser cannot create true tonal information, but rather produces the appearance of tones via a screening process. Screening creates black dots of different sizes, which, when placed close together (and seen at the proper viewing distance), create the illusion of an image with continuous tones. Computer-generated halftones include some additional methods such as frequency modulated screening (or stochastic screening). These methods randomize the dot patterns that were used in the older screening processes and hide the method of screening from the viewer. The effect is to produce higher-resolution halftone representation of grayscale images with lower-cost printers. The results with these printers are very good considering both the initial cost and low per-print cost. Although the image is not of sufficient quality to diagnose or treat a disorder, it is sufficient for noting the diagnostic information that was read from the computer screen.[10]

DYE SUBLIMATION PRINTERS

Dye sublimation printers can print true tonal information. The process takes a digital image comprising shades of black from 0 to 255 and places a dot of the corresponding darkness on the paper. The paper (substrate) is not a light-sensitive material. These printers use a ribbon whose pigment is moved via a transfer roller to the paper or transparency. The transferred image is then heated in the "finisher" to stabilize the image onto the substrate. Black and white prints can be ready in less than 3 minutes.

Dye sublimation printers at 200 dpi have greater apparent sharpness than office laser printers at 600 dpi, because they can reproduce dots of appropriate density and they do not use any of their resolution for screening the image (see Figure 7-10C).

Dye sublimation printers can also use a color ribbon that has three separate color transfer strips that are sequentially transferred onto the paper (Figure 7-11A). The ribbon passes across a 200-dpi linear laser printhead; the printhead heats the ribbon, causing the ribbon dyes to change directly from a solid to a gas. Sublimation is the scientific term for this phase change, which skips the usual liquid stage. The gas is then condensed and diffused onto the paper's surface. The paper, which is attached to a transfer roller, sequentially receives each of the colors. An additional clear ribbon may be used to overcoat the image to protect it from chemical contamination, chiefly formaldehyde, and the resultant fading of the image.

Although dye sublimation prints are very stable under a variety of test conditions, if they are left in contact with polyvinyl choroid (nonarchival) slide pages or acidic paper (patient chart folders), there can be a dramatic shift in their print densities as well as a color shift toward a reddish brown. These effects can be seen within weeks of a polyvinyl choroid slide page being placed in a file folder. Newer printers reduce this problem by overcoating the print with plastic. However, two recommendations have merit: First and foremost, sleeve your dye sublimation prints in Mylar jackets, and second, use archival quality pages to hold your 2 × 2 transparencies.

The heat and noise from older dye sublimation printers can be more than most camera room personnel (patients, physicians, and photographers) will tolerate. Unless it is a cool and quiet model, the printer should

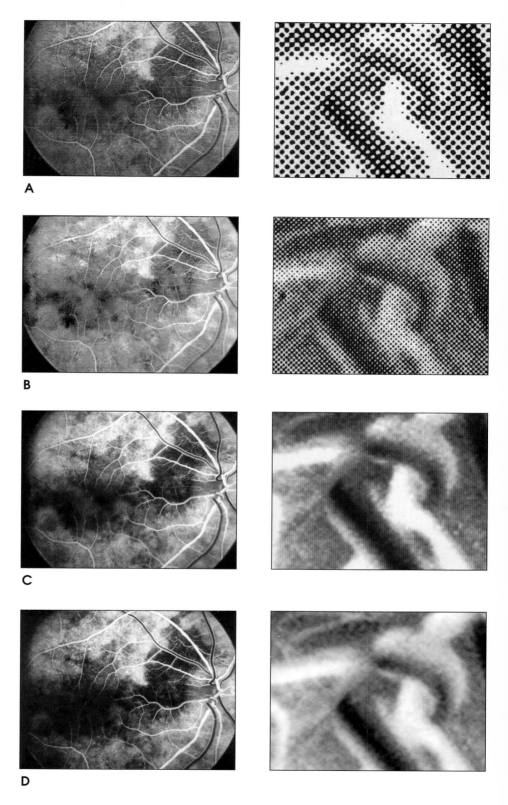

FIGURE 7-10
Magnified views of sample prints from different printing technologies. A. Laser print 300-dpi Hewlett-Packard LaserJet III. B. Laser print with photo-realistic software on 600-dpi Hewlett-Packard LaserJet 5 printer. C. Dye sublimation print, Kodak XL-7700, black and white media ribbon. E. Photo-graphic quality laser, Fuji Pictographic 3000 laser printer.

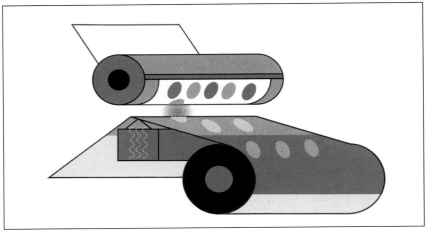

A

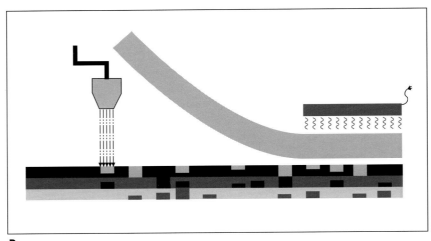

B

FIGURE 7-11
Color digital printing processes. A. Dye sublimation
process showing the image being transferred *onto*
the paper. B. Fuji Pictographic 3000 system using
Pictographic process, roller transport. Pictographic
one-pass dye transfer *into* the receiving paper.
Evaluate the image quality for sharpness, color
accuracy, and image evenness (lack of image
banding).

not be in the same room as the fundus camera. There are technical limitations on how long the printer cable may be, so be sure to examine those.
Placing the image acquisition station and the printer on a network can
overcome these limitations as well as make the printer available for other
applications.

DIGITAL-PHOTOGRAPHIC PRINTERS
Higher-resolution digital printers can use a true photographic process
with a laser imaging engine. The output medium is color photographic
paper, which is processed with conventional color photographic chemistry. The image quality is not that of "digital imaging," but if the image
file resolution is adequate, these printers achieve marvelous near–photographic quality images. These printers accept digital computer files or
can directly scan a slide into the printer.

The *pictography* (Fuji) silver halide printing technology creates images
without photographic chemistry (see Figure 7-10D). A light-sensitive
(silver halide) material, called the donor, is exposed simultaneously by
three laser diodes for each pixel value in the digital image file. The
donor is then moistened with distilled water. This is the only wet part
of the process. A receiver sheet is bonded to the damp donor with pressure, and heat is then applied to activate the thermal development

process. The self-developing dyes from the donor migrate into the receiver paper. The donor is stripped away, revealing the photographic-quality image (Figure 7-11B). Prints made with this technology are sharper than prints made with dye sublimation, since not only are all of the pixels transferred in a single pass but also the image is transferred *into* the receiver instead of *onto* it from the dye sublimation ribbon. At 400 dpi, the potential image sharpness is four times greater than that of a 200-dpi dye-sublimation printer.

Databases

The computer database tracks images and patient information. Important information to be entered includes the patient's last name, first name, middle name, hospital number, Social Security number, physician, referring physician, photographer, procedure, and camera. The software should also enter the date of the procedure, the location of the patient's images (disk and path), the time each image was taken, and, in the case of a fluorescein angiogram, a method of recording or calculating the lapsed time after the start of the angiographic injection.

The ability to export the database to a network database will become more important as more ophthalmology practices use networks for patient information and patient records. Once new patient data are entered at the acquisition station, the ability to query the network for patient demographics not only saves time but also reduces data entry errors. Databases are discussed further in the section on equipment purchasing.

Image Storage and Archiving

Digital images, in uncompressed form, are a minimum of 1 MB per image. At 20 images per angiographic study, it does not take long to fill up even a large hard drive. The images that are on the hard drive must then be moved to make room for images of new patients. Hardware options include high-speed optical drives and slower, but less expensive, recordable CD-ROMs.

Digital Angiography: Using the System

There are a number of differences between digital imaging systems and film-based systems. Some of these differences are obvious, but some may not be at first. On all of the systems, the greatest benefit to you, as the photographer, is the instant feedback you receive when your images appear on the monitor. This assists you in understanding how the session is progressing. Focus, exposure, the dynamics of the dye flow, and patient cooperation are all easily monitored, so that you can clearly see and analyze diagnostic information.

Although each imaging program and computer platform has its own way of doing things, all the same steps need to be included. In the same way, different photographers may do things in a different order or in a different style of working (Table 7-5), but they must accomplish the same tasks.

The imaging software will give you functions (choices of things you can do). The main categories are image acquisition, saving images, enhancement and printing, archiving images, and utilities.

Getting Ready for the Patient

All the preliminary photographic tasks, as well as the setting up of the medical supplies for the fluorescein angiography, should be completed

Table 7-5. Digital Angiography Steps

Getting ready for the patient
   Power up equipment—internal computer system diagnostic checks
   Monitor setup and adjustment—black level and contrast
   Enter patient information into a database
   Ready medical supplies for the angiographic injection
With the patient
   Review the procedure with the patient
   Take color slides on photographic film, or color electronic images
   Take monochrome and preinjection digital images
   Have the IV puncture made ready for the injection
   Set the timer to start
   Call for the injection and start the timer
   Acquire the early angiographic images
   Delete blank images and duplicates (extras)
   Save images to the hard drive
   Acquire additional images
Patient may leave
   Review images: enhance, combine, and print
   Send images to laser suite or other physician-reviewing area
   Archive images

before the patient enters the room. The system must first be turned on. This is done, just as for a fundus camera, with an electrical power switch. Since there are many components to the digital system, there may be a master power strip with a single power on-off switch. This could also be the on-off switch on an uninterruptable power supply.

Once turned on, the computer will go through its internal diagnostics and then load the computer operating system (OS) from the hard drive. After it loads its OS, it will present an opening prompt or menu. If this is a dedicated digital system, this menu may be that of the digital imaging system. If not, you must enter the program name to start the imaging program. The imaging program will be loaded into RAM and the imaging software menu will appear on the monitor.

MONITOR SET-UP

Quality control is paramount in achieving an optimal quality fluorescein angiogram, whether digital or film. In a digital system, the first step is to adjust the image monitor with a standard image. This should be done under the same viewing conditions you will have when you actually acquire the images. This includes room light level, the amount the door is open, and so forth. You will be making decisions that require you to make a judgment call about image quality, including brightness and contrast. For example, if the image monitor is adjusted to give too dark an image, then you might select totally black images for deletion, when, in fact, they may be high-quality images of the early choroidal phases of the angiogram. The system integrator/manufacturer should provide a "Shirley" (the trade nickname for a standard image), which includes a full tonal range image, a stepped grayscale tablet, as well as a continuous grayscale (0–100% illuminance). This image should be presented before every fluorescein angiographic study, not just the first time the system is turned on for the day. The standard image should be readily available at all times so that you can recheck the monitor (Figure 7-12).

To adjust the monitor, after setting the room illumination, I suggest the following order: First set the monitor black level using the brightness control so that the "black" background of the image is slightly above the true black of the non-image area around the test image. Then, using the

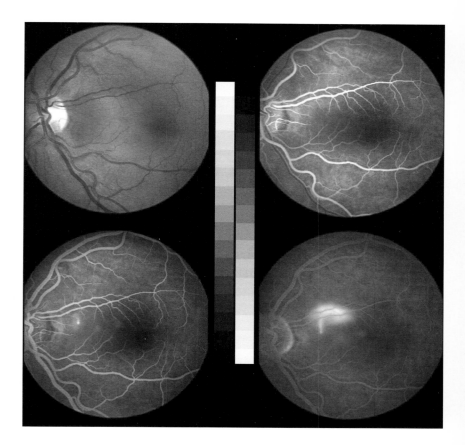

FIGURE 7-12
A standard image is used to adjust your monitor. It should reflect the uses to which the monitor must be adjusted. In addition to a grayscale. The "Shirley" should contain all the pictorial elements for which you might be using the monitor. For fluorescein angiography, a monochromatic green and a few key dye phases are the minimum. A color scale and additional color images can be useful if the system is also used for color image acqusition.

monitor's contrast adjustment, change the highlights of the standard image so that they are just below the brightness level where these areas bloom—that is, blend together into a white mass. This will maximize the brightness dynamics of your monitor when it is used in that particular level of room illumination. If the printer look-up table (LUT) is properly calibrated, the print will closely approximate the image on your monitor. Keep in mind, however, that while there is a greater dynamic range (contrast) on the monitor than on a print or transparency, all of the tones should be maintained on the print.

PATIENT INFORMATION DATABASE

Enter the patient information into the imaging database. If the database is kept on a local area network (LAN), then you may only need to enter the patient hospital number, since all of the other information is already on the LAN.

Working with the Patient and the Digital Imaging System

Review the procedure with the patient. This provides time for the patient to get additional information and to ensure that the patient understands the procedure. It is important to establish good rapport to achieve the optimal clinical information. The conventional color slides and/or color electronic images are exposed first.

Some systems build a "contact sheet" of images to let you monitor the procedures. Some systems permit you to view full screen images, allowing you to check focus and alignment. A system that allows you to choose between the large-picture mode and the contact sheet mode is the best-of-both-worlds since a hybrid system could show the most recent image

Exposing the Image: Digital Camera Sensitivity and Dynamic Range

Current digital cameras do not have the dynamic range of exposure that film cameras possess, the dynamic range (or exposure latitude) being the range of exposures from which the camera will produce information that represents the original subject.[14] The size of the pixel affects the dynamic range of the camera. A camera with a 6.8-micron square pixel (Kodak Megaplus, Model 1.4, M1 technology) will not be able to accept as many electrons as a camera with a 16-micron square pixel, (DCS-100, M3 technology). This ability to hold electrons is called the *well capacity*. The Megaplus 1.4 has a well capacity of 45,000 electrons while a DCS-100 has a well capacity of 250,000 electrons. This gives the Megaplus 1.4 a dynamic range of 60 db and the DCS-100 a greater dynamic range—70 db. Kodak has some digital cameras with even better light-gathering capabilities that use more advanced (Kodak DCS-420 using M5 and the DCS-460 using M6 technology, etc.), and therefore more expensive, technology. Time will bring the cost of these and other new technologies into the everyday practice of ophthalmology.

What are the implications of this potential limited exposure latitude? While Tri-X will give a high-quality fluorescein angiogram without changing the relative exposure to the film, an M1 technology camera may not accept the large dynamic range of illumination that is required to image a fluorescein angiogram. To compensate for this limitation, you will need to adjust the flash output on the fundus camera's power supply and/or adjust the electrical gain (like film ISO) on the digital camera. If the flash is properly set, then there can be an adequate exposure range for a high-quality individual image during the fluorescein angiographic sequence. There are additional problems if the power supply does not allow the output to be adjusted in smaller than full f-stop increments. Images are either over- or underexposed (Figure 7-13). This situation occurs with older Zeiss fundus camera power supplies. A "workaround" is to use a half f-stop (0.15 log units) neutral-density filter in the flash light path. This is accomplished by placing a filter in the slider filter holder (Figure 7-14). Finer gain adjustments (e.g., 3 db) on the digital camera would also be helpful. It would be ideal if the changes in the amount of illumination on the fundus were documented with each individual exposure.

If exposures are too great and the flash setting cannot be adequately reduced, then the gain control of the digital camera can be used to reduce the camera sensitivity. This is not usually needed during fluorescein angiography but may be needed during monochromatic photography. If this maneuver does not reduce the light level sufficiently, such as you might need for monochromatic red images, you may need to turn off the electronic flash and use only the viewing light. However, you might then need to add camera sensitivity by turning up the gain on the digital camera (+6 db to +12 db) and adjusting the viewing light to get a good exposure.

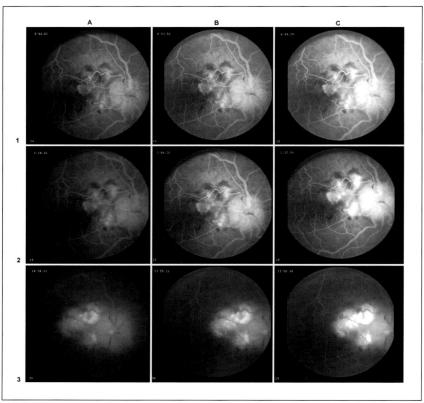

FIGURE 7-13
The exposure latitude of some digital cameras is limited. Three different fluorescein dye phases are shown on lines 1, 2, and 3. Each column represents a different exposure. The middle column (B) is properly exposed. The first column (A) is underexposed by ½ f-stop and shows a lack of shadow detail. The last column (C) is overexposed by only ½ f-stop and shows "blocking" in the highlights.

as a large image with the previous four images being displayed as "proof sheet–sized" images. With the press of a button (function key or mouse click), you can toggle between the two.

MONOCHROMATIC IMAGING

Photographing nerve fiber layer images with blue light and choroidal images with red light may provide additional clinical information.[11, 12] Digital systems lend themselves to imaging the fundus with monochromatic light. As with film systems, insert a filter into the optical path of the illuminating light of the fundus camera. Spectral sensitivity of the digital camera must be analyzed using the same considerations as for film, to ensure compatibility with the selected color of the monochromatic filter. Make sure that the digital camera is sensitive to the color that you want to record by checking the spectral sensitivity curve of the camera. Also find out if the optics in the fundus camera, including any filters, will pass the desired color of light. Later you may use image enhancement techniques to—pardon the redundancy—enhance the ability to read these images.

After you acquire the images, you should be able to select bad or redundant images for deletion (see the sidebar on exposing the image). The best systems have a method of editing images at each natural break in the procedure. A full-screen image displays image detail that is very helpful when choosing images to delete. You may use the proof sheet

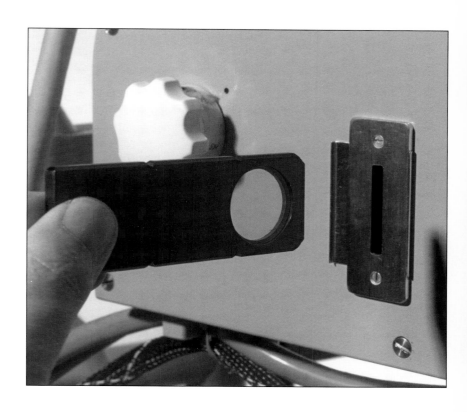

FIGURE 7-14
Filter slider for use in the Zeiss fundus camera with a
0.15 log neutral density filter, which provides a ½
f-stop exposure difference.

mode to see if there are redundant frames and the full-screen mode to see
which frames are the sharpest. Most systems also use a keyboard key
(delete or backspace) to delete the last image. It is important to see, on
the image monitor, the result of pressing this key—that is, continuously
revealing the next image that you are about to delete. An "undo" function or an "image trash can" function is also useful.

Fluorescein Angiography

Continue by making the patient ready in the same manner as for a film
angiogram. There is the customary timer to record the lapsed time after
the start of the injection of fluorescein sodium. The exciter and barrier filters are selected for insertion into the light path.

It is important to know how many images may be saved into the
image buffer RAM before you must stop acquiring images and save the
images to the hard drive. Unlike your routine with a 36-exposure roll of
film, if you can only acquire 16 images, you must plan how to handle the
early-image acquisition sequence. If you have a patient who has delayed
filling and you are at frame 14 when you first see the dye, you may miss
many of the arteriovenous images. One solution is to upgrade the imaging system to allow more images to be acquired. Each 1024×1024 image
will take 1 MB. In addition to the RAM, which you need for images, you
may need 1–4 MBs to be used by the computer OS. With appropriate software and high-speed hard drives, unlimited images can be written continuously and directly to the hard drive. The number of images is then
limited only by the amount of available space on the hard drive.

If a system upgrade is not possible in your practice, there are a few
other ways to manage this limitation. The simplest way is to wait to
take images until you see the dye. This results in nice arteriovenous
phase images but denies the physician the important choroidal and

early arterial frames that may be crucial in demarcating the edges of a subretinal choroidal neovascular complex. Another strategy is to try to shoot for the early phases, and if the dye does not come when you expect, delete these pre-choroidal flush "blank" images. Some photographers bounce back and forth—taking a frame, quickly looking to see if any dye shows on the monitor, and then deleting the single frame if needed. If the dye shows, they continue to shoot. With this last method, there may be lost early frames when the dye is not quickly appreciated on the monitor. The best solution is using an imaging system with enough RAM to acquire these important early frames.

After the early frames are acquired, they can be examined, and the redundant or poor-quality images can be deleted from the RAM. This is a time-saving step, since only needed images are copied to the hard drive. If time permits, you should then write the images to the hard drive. This usually can be done 2–5 minutes after the dye injection. It may take a minute or so to store 16–20 images. Writing images to the hard drive frees room for more images to be stored in the RAM as well as moving the previously acquired images to a safer place. After all the additional images are acquired, the process of selecting for saving or deleting is repeated, and the completed study is saved to the hard drive. Again, some systems use fast hard drives to overcome limitations in the RAM.

A discussion of image compression, either the technical aspects or the medical implications, could fill entire books. Please see the discussion on image compression later in this chapter.

CONCURRENT ANGIOGRAPHIC PROCEDURES

If a second patient requires an angiogram and images of the first patient are desired beyond 10 or 15 minutes, most systems permit you to start the second angiographic study. There is a second timer so that you can use the software to alternate between patients. The times must be linked to the patients' database records. It is usually a requirement of the system that you save your images to the hard drive before switching between patients, so that you avoid having two patients in the RAM at the same time. This capability has limited use in a high-quality photographic service but might be used to keep a timer running to document late images in a patient with suspected cystoid macular edema (CME). Dual timers are also useful for combined fluorescein angiography and ICG angiography procedures to keep track of both injection start times. Make sure that your software will permit a single patient to have two timers running concurrently, and that the two studies can be added to separate contact sheets.

Retrieving Images

After the angiogram has been completed and the images have been saved from RAM onto the hard drive, it is time to review your work. There are several ways to view digital fluorescein angiograms. The computer monitor is the best way. Other output devices include paper prints from office-quality laser printers, full-tone high-end printers (dye-sublimation can print onto paper or transparency material), and photographic-quality digital printers or slide-imaging equipment. The digital images also can be sent to other computers via removable media (e.g., optical disk) or a local area network (LAN), and to distant locations on commercial networks using modems and telephone lines or high-speed data lines.

There are several steps involved in getting the image to the person who will be reviewing the angiogram (Table 7-6). The order of the steps may be different with each vendor's system.

Image Enhancement: An Educational Responsibility

The process of photography has always required the photographer to work with the light that falls onto the film, with the tonal information that is produced on the negative, and with the densities that are produced on the final print. These basic steps comprise a multitude of small processing steps, requiring decisions about how the image will be represented and being subject to the variabilities of the photographic processes.[16]

Technical limitations of the printing processes that are used in textbooks and journals have always required compromises in the tonal information that is reproduced. To maximize the limited tonal range, photographers will work with their images to provide the maximal information to the viewer as presented on the final printed page.

The photographer who uses film has always had a variety of tools that can be used to modify the image. With the digital image, these tools are easier to access (Table 7-7).

It is important for you, and for anyone who is reading diagnostic information, to be completely cognizant of the extent to which an image has been enhanced and the type and magnitude of that enhancement. In addition to having the responsibility of maintaining image integrity, you have an "educational responsibility" when giving the physician an enhanced image.

We recommend that a complete imaging system record and display the type and magnitude of the enhancements that the original image has undergone. There are many types of image enhancement, so each system integrator or software manufacturer may have slight variations in its naming system for the enhancement tools. Nonetheless, some naming conventions and standards should be used. If an image is enhanced before publication, it could become common practice to include an explanatory statement on the type and/or extent of enhancement. That said, it is also the responsibility of the viewer to understand normal and accepted darkroom practices, which may now, via the computer, be used in printing the image.

Some image enhancement systems perform their functions quickly by letting you work on a low-resolution version of a larger image. The desired manipulation, when completed, performs those functions on the high-resolution image. This type of software produces a small script file that records the desired enhancement functions. This approach allows the original file to be maintained and the enhanced image to be recreated at any time.

The following statement should be obvious, but it must be made. *Image enhancement and manipulation have always been within the working tools of the photographer.* The ability to mislead has always been within the capabilities of the photographer and the photographic technology. These new (computer) tools make it easier to create misleading images. The responsibility and integrity remain the same: Has an image been modified to clarify it for the viewer or has it been changed to misrepresent reality (Figure 7-15)? An image, like other academic work, is the responsibility of the individual who represents the work as truthful.

Table 7-6. Steps in Printing an Image

Select patient and visit date
Show proofsheet(s)
Select image
Enhance image (contrast, brightness, dodge and burn tools, etc.)
Save enhanced image
Use imaging tools (measurement, overlays, etc.)
Group images for printing
Print images or send images to a review station or network

PATIENT DATABASE

First, the patient and visit must be selected. The patient database is your inroad to recalling (finding) the images you need. A good patient database will show your most recently recorded patients even without your having their names or ID numbers. Look for databases that display the informational fields you would find most helpful. Would you rather look at a patient number (without the name being displayed), the date of the procedure, and the disk where it can be found, or would you rather look at the patient's name, diagnosis, date, and disk number?

After a patient and visit date are selected (the patient may have been photographed on more than one visit date), the software will display small (thumbnail) images. These are small versions of the images that were acquired during the photo session. Some manufacturers call the display of these small images a proof or contact sheet, after the photographic counterpart. The number of thumbnail images the manufacturer chooses to display at one time is a function of the type and size of that manufacturer's monitor and software. These images may start in the top left or top right corner. Images should be sorted to permit stereo imaging on the monitor.

Selecting the file should display the thumbnail images of the procedure. Selecting an image will pull up a full-screen image on the monitor. In addition to viewing a single image, you may wish to group images using the appropriate choices from the software menus. These images may be enhanced and then printed.

Image Enhancement Software

Computers can change an image to reveal information in a photograph that could be difficult to see without the enhancements (see the sidebar on image enhancement). Some of these are similar to the enhancements we routinely perform in the darkroom, while others would be difficult or impossible to do in the darkroom. Small local-area contrast enhancements are more complex if performed in the darkroom, and the image overlay functions are almost impossible to replicate in the darkroom.

After the images are safely stored on the hard drive, a copy of the image(s) can be loaded back into the computer RAM for manipulation. Once you select an image from the proof sheet, a full screen-sized image is displayed. You could, at this point, simply select one or more images and send them to a printer. Don't forget that if you were simply to adjust the controls on the monitor (brightness and contrast), the print of the image would not reflect the changes you made to the monitor. Adjust your monitor (see the earlier section on monitor set-up) before modifying or printing an image.

CONTRAST STRETCH

Some of the easiest manipulations are of the contrast and brightness ranges. This is equivalent to selecting different contrast grades of paper

Table 7-7. Photographic Tools for Image Modification

Darkroom	Computer
Using the correct contrast paper	Contrast stretch
Burning and dodging	Area darken/lighten ("contrast enhancement")
Modified tone-line process	Sharpen
Photo montage	Cut, paste, blend edges, FundusMap

and different enlarger exposure times, or to adjusting the brightness and contrast settings on a TV. The results of your image manipulations are seen on the image monitor.

The variations of illuminance (brightness) levels that the monitor displays are much greater than either reflective or transmission print materials can record and display. This is the same type of limitation that occurs between the information that is on a photographic film negative and the information that can be displayed on a print. When the brightness range is compressed for producing a photographic print, the printed image may look flat (inadequate contrast) unless some photographic compensations are made.

Contrast expansion, or contrast stretch, is a helpful tool to allow rapid expansion of the available tonal information. The viewing of this image on the computer monitor may be adequate, since the dynamic process of expanding the contrast window allows you or the physician to expand a particular part of the "tonal window." If the computer equivalent of high-contrast paper is used to accentuate detail in one part of the image, then other parts of the image will suffer. This is an unacceptable method of manipulating an image for printing, since shadow and/or highlight detail will be compressed, with the resultant loss of information. While this contrast and density-shifting technique may be adequate for dynamic viewing of the information on the monitor, the result is unacceptable for a print. Local-area contrast expansion (see the next section) is helpful (Figure 7-16).

LOCAL-AREA CONTRAST EXPANSION
Burning and dodging in the photographic darkroom allows the tonal information in a local area to be expanded for easier viewing (Figure 7-17). In a fluorescein angiogram, the relatively dark area of the fovea is difficult to print while maintaining the detail of a hyperfluorescent disk or a neovascular complex. In the darkroom, when the negative is printed, there may be some burning and dodging of the appropriate light and dark areas to maintain tonal information in all areas of the print. Fortunately, good imaging software will allow you to perform the same type of manipulation that you would do in the darkroom. The computer's ability to take predefined mathematical algorithms and apply them to the image is very powerful.

Local-area contrast enhancements help to overcome the limitations of the dynamic range of the monitor and the printing media. Some of the parameters used are image resolution and magnification, the size of the dodging tool, the duration of dodging, and the range of contrast needed for the image. This computer technique is essentially an electronic burning and dodging tool kit.

Local-area contrast expansion tools increase the tonal contrast throughout the image or in a selected rectangular area. There may only be one contrast enhancement tool to choose from, and all or most of the values are preset. It is important to understand how your image is being manipulated and the limitations of having predefined tools.

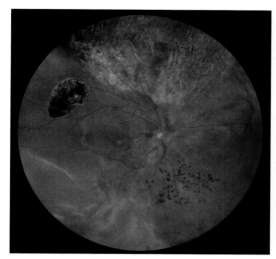

FIGURE 7-15
Computer-manipulated composite illustration from multiple fundi was created from photographs of multiple patients with multiple conditions. While this combination image may be a useful teaching tool, it is not an accurate representation of a single patient's condition. (FundusMap by Richard E. Hackel.)

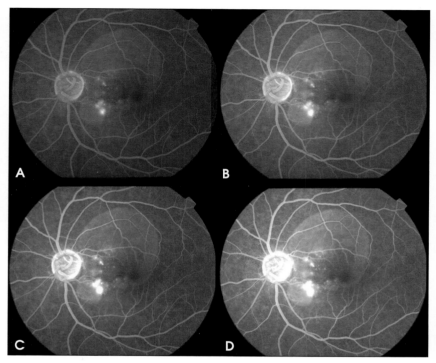

FIGURE 7-16
Printing limitations and controls in fluorescein angiography. A. Image printed "straight" to retain all tonal information. The print does not use the full tonal range of the print material (flat print) B. Image printed with the maximal contrast stretch without clipping either the shadows or the highlights. C. Image printed with a computer to simulate a higher-contrast paper and adjusted to expand highlight detail (shadows lost). D. Image printed with a computer to simulate a higher-contrast paper and adjusted to expand shadow detail (highlights lost).

Some systems may have several predefined tools for use on different image magnifications.

There are multiple mathematical algorithms for determining this "average" value.[13] Some mathematical models use pixels within a horizontal and vertical distance of the base location or use a neighborhood pattern (Figure 7-18). Better models use values that attempt to approximate a radius distance, which reduces the squaring off of the image as it is enhanced (Figure 7-19).

Three basic values in the model can be changed: the area of neighborhood, the weighting of the values, and the amount of change. This strategy is called the *neighborhood area of influence*. The fall off of the average value can also be changed. How the average brightness is calculated (center weighted, even distribution, etc.) is similar to the changes that are made in the relative distance between the enlarger lens and the photographic print paper. Finally, there is the amount of change or, in darkroom terms, how long did the dodging tool block the light?

The first choice is how far (what distance) from the pixel you wish the influence of the enhancement to extend. If there is a 1024 × 1024 pixel image, you could choose to influence an area 20–50 pixels to provide a pleasing smoothness of the tonal levels. If you were to apply this same algorithm to a page of 20 thumbnail images, the result would be reduced tonal shifts. The selection of this value is akin to the selection of a particular size of dodging tool and its distance from the paper used while printing a photographic print (Figure 7-20).

The software examines the average brightness at each point in the image. The brightness of pixels within 16 pixels of the pixel at the top left-

FIGURE 7-17
Localized tonal enhancement. Burning and dodging in the computer can enhance the presentation of the image, providing additional information to the clinician. A. Original. B. The same image with burning and dodging in the computer (e.g., Adobe Photoshop). Then the image is adjusted to expand the image's tonal range to take full advantage of the printing medium (contrast stretch).

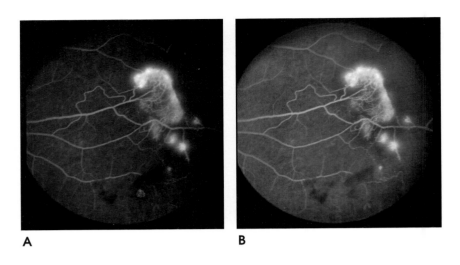

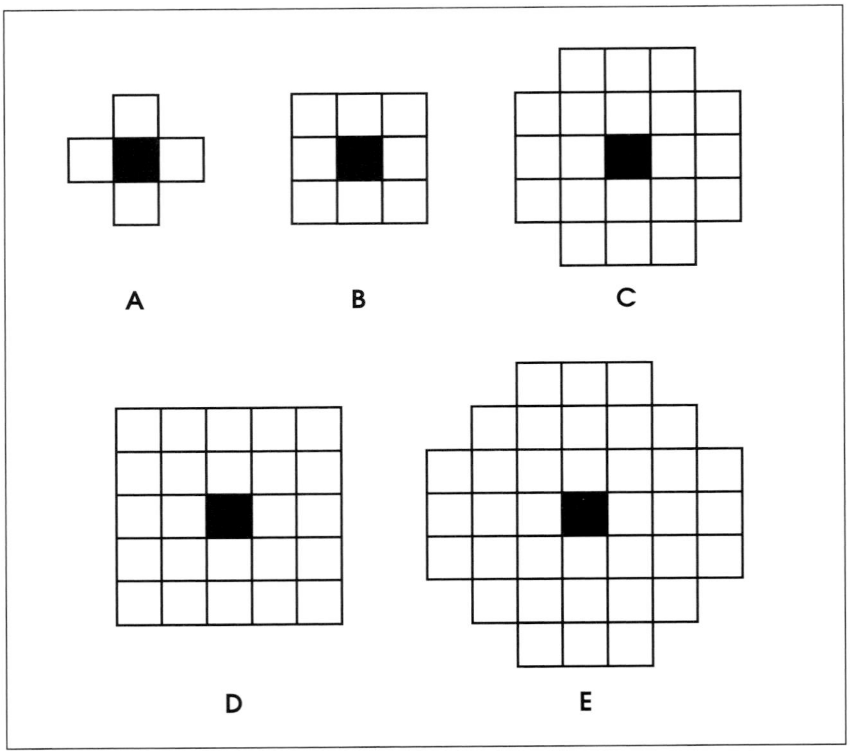

A   B

FIGURE 7-18
Neighborhood patterns are used for local contrast calculations. A. Nearest-neighbor cross. B. 3 × 3 square containing nine pixels. C. 5 × 5 octagonal region containing 21 pixels. D. 5 × 5 square region containing 25 pixels. E. 7 × 7 octagonal region containing 37 pixels.

A   B   C

D   E

hand corner (pixel 0,0) is logged, averaged, and tabulated. The next pixel (0,1) is examined. The average brightness of pixels in the neighborhood of this pixel is also recorded. This is repeated for every pixel in the image.

Finally, the table of average values may be adjusted for the amount of increase or decrease in contrast that is desired. This will adjust the local contrast of the final image and is a measure of how severely the mask is applied. With these tools, an image's tonal information can be enhanced to show you information that may not have been obvious previously.

SHARPENING
Increasing edge definition is a feature that would seem valuable, especially when trying to sharpen a blurry image. Sharpening routines define

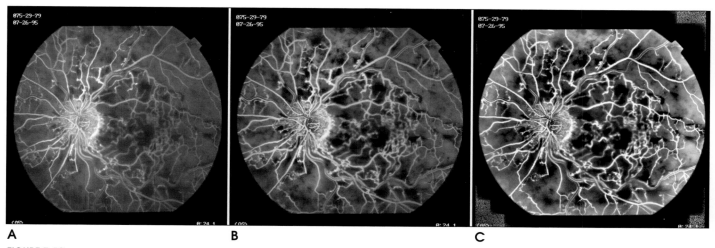

FIGURE 7-19
Enhanced images with neighborhood pixel level adjustments. A. Original image. B. Image enhanced with a radius-based algorithm. C. Image enhanced with contrast enhancement software, which uses a neighborhood square algorithm for increasing local area contrast. Notice also that the black "background" is reflected into the image area with this algorithm (C).

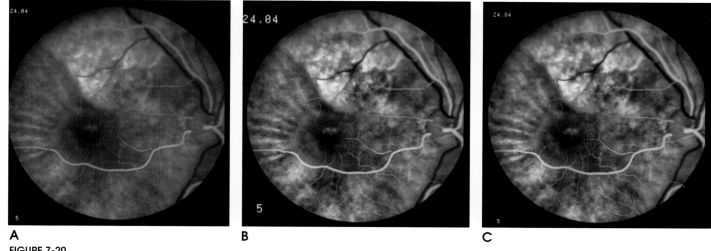

FIGURE 7-20
Burning and dodging different sizes of images. A. Original image. B. Image enhancement performed on a contact sheet–size image. Note the darker central foveal zone and the lighter choroidal flush visible in the branch of the supratemporal vein. The same enhancement routine was performed on the full-screen image (C) and shows less extreme changes in density in small areas.

an edge by increasing the contrast where there is a small rapid shift in density. This edge is defined by a mathematical model. The computer then makes this transition from one tone to another in a fewer number of pixels. The resulting apparent sharpness of the image is increased. Sharpening actually reduces the information in the image but may make the image more visually pleasing.[13] Sharpening should be used in moderation and with great caution, as it can be a destructive tool (Figure 7-21). Sharpening may be even more destructive on an original image without fine detail (Figure 7-21, column C). This tool should be used last (just before viewing or printing) to prevent interfering with other enhancement tools. Check your system to see if the order of enhancing and sharpening makes a difference. Zoom in to check. It may be safest to use the sharpening function last since sharpening creates the most

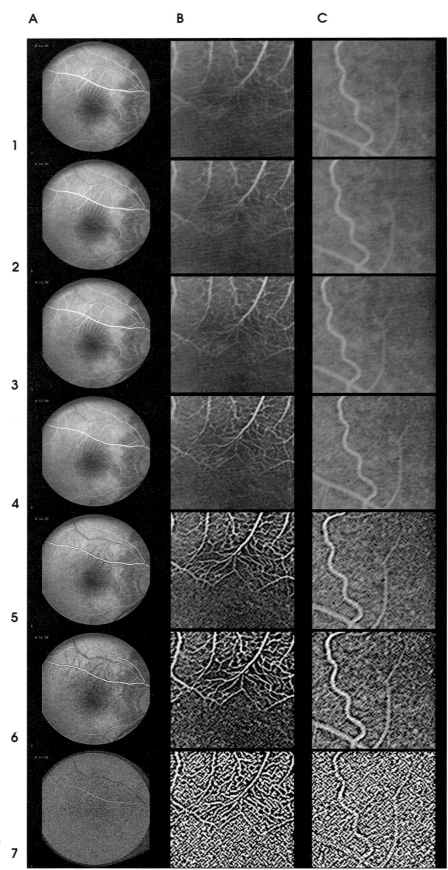

FIGURE 7-21
The sharpening tool is used with increasing degrees. The original image is on the left. Three columns of images—full image and two sections of the image at ×8 magnification. The first column (A) shows the original with levels of sharpening (rows 2–6) and finally sharpening level 5 repeated two times (row 7). The second column of images (B) shows image sharpening on part of the image with fine detail. As sharpening is increased, it reaches a level where the image becomes degraded. Imaging degradation appears earlier in an image that does not contain fine detail to be sharpened (column C). The image appears to be degraded at a lower level of sharpening.

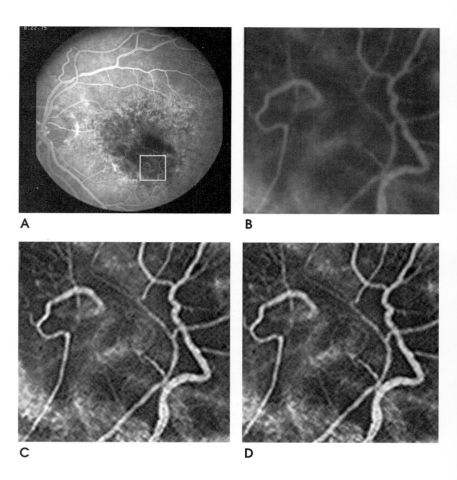

FIGURE 7-22
Sharpening versus enhancement order. A. Original.
B. Enlargement of original. C. Image enhanced, then
sharpened. Note the accentuated highlights on the
larger vessels and a decrease in shadow detail.
D. Image sharpened, then enhanced. Note the
increased shadow detail.

change to the detail of the image (Figure 7-22). Finally, never sharpen a destructively compressed image (see the discussion of compression later in this chapter).

Other Imaging Software Tools

ZOOMING
Image enlargement by zooming the image on the monitor provides visualization of important details that might otherwise be difficult to see. A larger image will not provide more information (unless your monitor shows you less resolution and detail than your image contains), but the image is easier to see. This may be particularly helpful in the laser treatment area where the monitor may be placed more than a few feet from the physician. You should be able to position a zoomed image on the monitor so that the area of interest is centered. Printing the zoomed image is particularly useful if you print with a lower-resolution laser printer.

IMAGE OVERLAYS
Computers can do things that are impossible (or, for practical reasons, nearly impossible) in the darkroom. These programs allow a lesion to be outlined on one image and the outline to be overlayed from that image onto another image can provide feedback to the physician about the relative position and size of the lesion and the treatment (Figure 7-23). To make sure that the overlayed information is placed correctly on the image, there must be a mechanism to ensure that the fundus on the two images

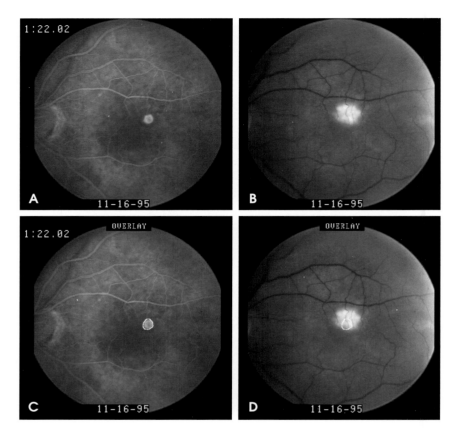

FIGURE 7-23
Overlay function. A. A fluorescein angiographic image taken at 1 minute, 22 seconds showing a subretinal net. B. After laser photocoagulation, a monochromatic green photograph shows the extent of treatment. After registering the two images with the overlay software, the neovascular complex is traced (C). Then the the defined net is placed onto the monochromatic green photograph of the laser-treated eye (D). Note that the entire area of juxtafoveal subretinal neovascularization had not yet been treated. (Courtesy of Richard E. Hackel.)

is in identical registration. Accurate placement of the outline of a lesion, as seen in a fluorescein angiogram, onto another image, such as a monochromatic green post–laser treatment photograph, is accomplished with sophisticated image alignment software. With this tool you can manually trace the borders of a laser treatment area onto the fluorescein angiographic image of a neovascular complex. To create the overlays you must first get the two images into perfect registration—that is, one image on top of the other. This can be done manually or with semiautomated computer routines.

With the manual method, the two images are usually presented next to each other on a single screen. You then alternately select similar points on each image to act as tie-points (which will serve to tie the images together). If you are placing tie-points by eye, make sure that you have enough magnification on the images so that you can place the points with certainty and precision. After a reasonable number of pairs of tie-points is selected, the computer then warps (stretches) and/or rotates one image to make a "best fit" on top of the other image. You then select the lesion outline that you wish to be presented onto the other image.

Some computer programs even assist in accurate placement of these points. In a semiautomated system, you assist the computer in finding similar tie-points on each image. The program then identifies the geometry of the points. These points are used for the overlay.

Selection of these tie-points is important. Vessel crossings and bifurcations are usually the easiest structures for both a person and the computer to see. Structures that are easy to see in both images are a prerequisite. The best starting points are those located near the area of interest. Additional points should be selected throughout the image to

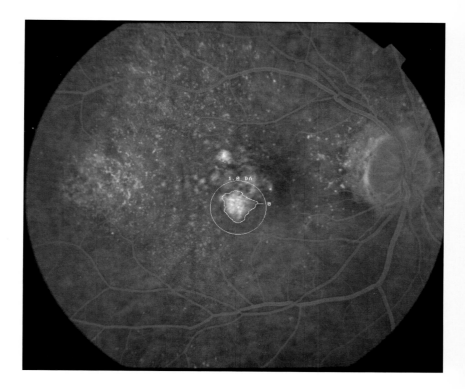

FIGURE 7-24
Macular photocoagulation study (MPS) rings. A disk diameter ring overlying a subretinal neovascular complex (SRNV) assists the physician in assessing the size of an SRNV. Sizes can be adjusted: 1 disc diameter (1-DD), 1.5 DD, 2.0 DD, etc.

give as much area to the tie-points as possible, in order to enhance the accuracy of the warp and rotation.

If you are using automatic alignment software, it should be reliable enough to register with consistency even images of marginal quality. The software should have an option to display the number and location of tie-points that are matched on the two images. This information should be transferred to the print so that any future viewers of the image are informed of the quality of the overlay match. Running the local contrast enhancement tool on both images before starting the overlay function may increase the quality of the overlay "best fit."

An area of interest is then traced with a pointing device onto one image. This trace also appears on the other image. Overlaying the area to be treated onto a post-treatment image permits analysis of the laser treatment. This type of image overlay also enables the physician to treat only the necessary retina and thus avoid over-treatment. Since the entire overlay process takes quite a bit of time, the ability to save the overlayed images is important.

MACULAR PHOTOCOAGULATION STUDY RINGS
Software that meets the Macular Photocoagulation Study (MPS) protocol assists the clinician in judging the size of a lesion relative to the size standard of disk diameters.[15] This software permits circles of multiple disk diameter sizes to be placed over an area of subretinal neovascularization (Figure 7-24).

OTHER IMAGE ENHANCEMENT TOOLS
Imaging systems can provide additional tools (Figure 7-25). Their inclusion here should not be taken as an endorsement of their usefulness.

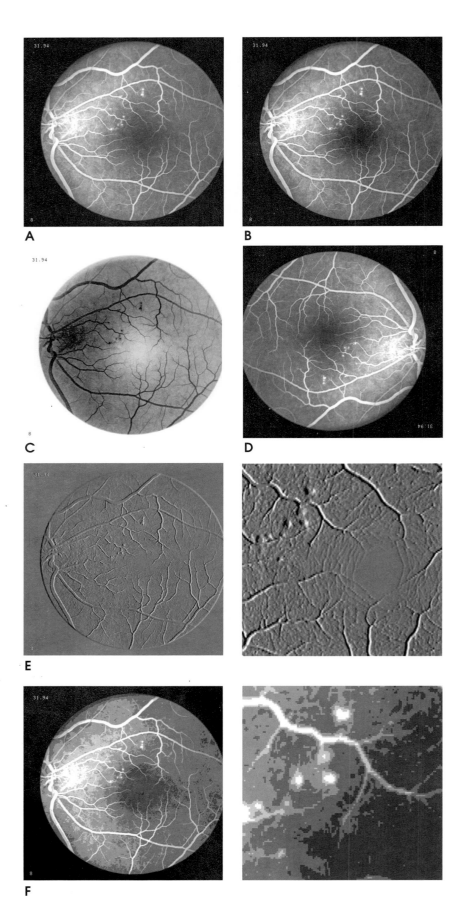

FIGURE 7-25
Other imaging tools. A. Normal/original. B. Contrast
stretched. C. Negative. D. Rotated (indirect ophthalmoscope view). E. Grayscale contour map
(tone-line process with lateral shift) with enlargement of contour map. F. Posterization (reduced
number of tones of gray) and enlargement of
posterization.

1. Expanding the contrast (B) to the full tonal range of the monitor or print.
2. The ability to present an image as a negative (C) (black-white tone value reversal) may permit viewers to look at an image in a familiar manner.
3. Inverting the image (D) so that it will be oriented to match the view seen through an indirect ophthalmoscope may be helpful in some situations.
4. A relief-mapped (E) image displays a rapid left-to-right tonal threshold increases as black lines and decreases as white lines. The image does not show a true shadow but a pseudo-shadow.
5. Posterizing (F) changes an image so that there are fewer tonal values of gray, or in color posterization, fewer values of gray are represented with different colors. This may be interesting for illustrative purposes.

Saving Enhanced Images

Once you have done considerable work to enhance an image, you may want to produce additional copies at a later date. The ability to save this new image with the patient record is important. The type and amount of enhancement the original image has undergone, or at a minimum, an indicator that the image is not an original but a modified image should be saved with the image file.

SCRIPT FILES

A shorter way to save modified images is to record the program commands that are used to create the desired enhanced image. This file can be stored with the proof sheet (thumbnail) image of the enhanced image. Advantages are threefold:

1. The script file is much smaller than a full image file and therefore transmits much faster over a network.
2. The original file is (and must be) kept unmodified.
3. Script files may be modified to change the outcome of the image appearance.

Disadvantages are twofold:

1. Imaging software is needed to recreate the modified image from the script file.
2. The recreation of the image takes more time to recreate than the time it would take to display a saved image.

Printing

The job of printing is to make visual the digital information contained in a computer file available for interpretation without computer hardware. Printing lets you put the digital computer images onto paper or transparencies to be used for chart copies. These copies can be used to indicate diagnostic notes or to accompany interpretation of the fluorescein angiography. The original image is the digital file and the print is only a representative copy. Because the tonal range of the monitor is greater than the print, local-area contrast expansion tools (discussed above) are important to assist in creating a printed image of the best quality.

While prints are convenient, quality interpretation and/or treatment of the patient should be performed only from the computer monitor image. Since the monitor is a light source unto itself, the available dynamic range is greater than that of a (reflective) print. The informa-

Table 7-8. Print Image Size (Active Image Area 8" × 8" on 8½" × 11") Paper

Number of Images	Image Diameter (inches)	Image Area (square inches)	Pixels per Image Full Resolution (K)	Pixels per Image Screen Resolution (K)	Screen Relative Size (%)
1	8.0	50	1024	1024	100
4	4.0	12.5	256	256	25
9	2.7	5.6	455	114	11
16	2.0	3.14	256	64	6.3

tion contained in even a high-quality print conveys less tonal information than a computer monitor. This is analogous to directly reading the film negatives on a fluorescein angiography study or reading the positives: The negatives always contain more information. Also, the ability to enhance and zoom an image permits the highest quality of diagnostic information to be shown. As we say in the film world, "read the negatives," and now in the digital world, "read the screen (and not the print)."

Prints from office-type laser printers may be an extremely cost-effective "chart copy" of the photograph. However, it is paramount that these lower-quality images not be used for diagnosis or treatment; they must be used for reference only. For responsible treatment, a computer for image review must always be accessible in the laser suite.

Although stacks of full image prints are impressive, sometimes the ability to put multiple images onto one sheet of paper may be not only more convenient but also more economical (Figure 7-26). The choice of the number of images to be printed on the paper is interrelated with the final image size and the image resolution (Table 7-8). Additional selection factors include the cost of the print material, storage costs, ease of handling (if there are fewer sheets of paper), and, most important, size and resolution of the final image. Considering that there is a 56% increase in image area from the 16-up to the 9-up image, the 9-up printing format is very useful. Nine images are adequate to represent many studies. Also useful are 4-up images, which give greater magnification, but obviously they use twice the paper as a single 9-up image. Some software even permits an "enlarged version" by magnifying the image while trimming the edges of the circular fundus image.

The image area is typically less than the full size of the paper, so that patient data can be printed on the paper as well. In addition to the desired images, database information, such as patient name, number, visit date, physician name, and photographer's name may make the print more useful. Examine how your clinic functions when determining which database fields are to be included on the print.

Manufacturers should permit you to print the information the way you want. Some information is taken from data that is the same for all prints—for example, the name of the institution. Other information is taken from the database and is unique to that patient—for example, the patient name. Some databases permit the fields to be changed for each patient visit or photo session—for example, the diagnosis for different sessions can change from macular degeneration to subretinal neovascularization to status post-laser treatment with an overlayed image. Be cautious when a manufacturer tells you that the physician's name can be put on the print if what you really need is for the physician's name *for that patient visit* to be on the print. Having the correct physician name on the prints will make it easy to sort and deliver the prints, and recording the diagnosis for each session will permit accurate photographic records.

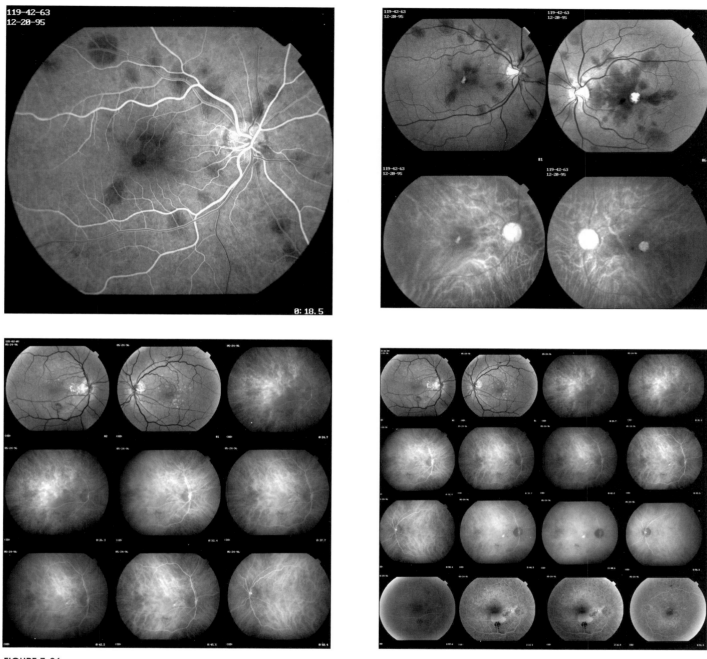

FIGURE 7-26
Printing layouts: 1-up, 4-up, 9-up, and 16-up. These show the relations of image size and the final resolution of the image.

Image and Printing Resolution

Maintaining image quality is important in maximizing diagnostic information. If an image is reduced in tonal information or resolution, then there may be a decrease in the quality of the diagnostic interpretation. Ensuring that the full resolution of the captured image is maintained throughout the image storage, retrieval, and printing functions is sometimes difficult but nonetheless paramount in preserving image quality.

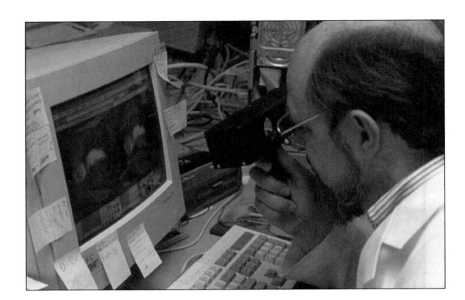

FIGURE 7-27
Four-mirror stereo viewer permits viewing of side-by-side stereo images. A lever adjusts one mirror to view different sizes of stereo images. (Courtesy of Ophthalmic Imaging Systems, Inc.)

If four 1-MB images are printed on a single 8½ × 11 page with a high-end printer, it is important to have the full resolution (information) in the images reproduced on the print. Taking a 1-MB screen image "screen dump" and sending it to the printer will produce results different from those produced by taking four separate 1-MB images and sending them, with their full resolution, individually to the printer. Printing four 1-MB images as a 1-MB file will produce four prints that are only ¼ MB in size. This is less than the resolution of the original image and of the printer; the software is not giving you the image that you have worked so hard to produce. The manufacturer should be able to tell you if you are getting a "dump" from a 1-MB monitor image file or actually going back to the original image files and printing them as four separate 1-MB files.

Stereo Image Viewing

The ability to view stereo fundus and fluorescein angiographic images has always been an important diagnostic tool. (See Chapter 3 for information on the viewing of stereo images.) Electronic stereo images can be viewed in the same way as conventionally produced images, as well as using several additional techniques.

Sixteen or 20 image contact sheets, when displayed on a 20-inch image monitor, produce images that may be too large for easy free viewing. Base-out prisms combined with a +4 diopter lens will help most viewers view the stereo images on the monitor. Viewers with mirrors make the viewing of 4-up images easy (Figure 7-27). Capabilities to display zoomed stereo images would reduce limitations of screen resolution.

The software must be capable of rearranging the position of the images on the monitor and onto the print. Check the software you are thinking of purchasing and try to rearrange the images on both the screen and for printing. Software capable of marking the images as a stereo pair permits easy identification.

Of particular note are systems that can use the color image monitor to align stereo images one on top of the other, and to display them simultaneously, one in red and the other in blue—an anaglyph. The images are viewed with red-blue glasses without requiring convergence or divergence from the viewer (see Figure 3-34). This technology can also be used to overlay hyperfluorescent lesions over a monochromatic green image. It is important to know how much time it takes to prepare two stereo images for viewing. If a procedure is too lengthy, it may not be convenient to view a stereo image. If it takes a while to create the stereo image, it is important that the image can also be saved and/or printed.

Image Storage and Archiving

A photographer would never consider keeping only prints and throwing out the original negatives. Likewise, the digital angiographer needs to store the original digital (computer) image files and keep the images on a long-term storage medium. Images will quickly fill up the hard drive. In order to keep using your imaging system, you will need to move and then delete images from the hard drive to make room for additional fluorescein studies. Later you may make archival copies of the image files. Remember that at 1 MB per image and 20 images per patient, even a gigabyte hard drive would fill up with less than 50 patients.

First the images are recorded onto the computer's hard drive. This storage is fine for the day's work. For easily accessible storage of images taken during the preceding weeks, some form of rapid, online, mass storage is usually needed. Finally, some form of less-expensive storage medium is needed for archiving the images.

Since the ability to retrieve images quickly is important in ophthalmology, the current medium of choice is the optical disk. Removable disks, which run at the speed of hard drives, can store over 5 gigabytes, enough room for several hundred angiograms. Multiple drives may be combined to form a drive array if more studies need to be available. The cartridges cost less than $1 per angiogram.

For less frequently needed images or images to be sent to a referring physician, the images may be moved onto less expensive (and usually slower) storage media. The CD-ROM is usually considered for this task. The first CD-ROMs held 650 MB of data. Obviously data storage systems will continue to provide greater amounts of data online with decreasing costs.

IMAGE STORAGE

Storage of your images should be completed after printing, so that any extra images (combinations, overlays, etc.) may be saved with the original images. You need a smooth way to move images from the hard drive onto the storage media. You may use one of several types of media, but the way that you interact with them is similar. Here I use the generic term *laser disk* to refer to either an erasable optical disk or a CD-ROM disk.

Storing images is a two-part process: copying and then deleting the original. First the images are copied onto the laser disk and the database is updated to document the new location of the copied files. If the files are left on the hard drive—from the previous day's patient studies, for example—they will be accessible quickly. The software should make it easy for you to distinguish between the patient images that have already been archived and those that have not. When you want to erase the now duplicate copies of the files that are on your acquisition system's hard drive, you need software that will tell you that you have already made copies of the files. Good software will not let you delete the only copy of your images. Your software should, when you ask for the images on any patient, tell you which disk it needs for access to the stored images.

ARCHIVING

The speed and frequency requirements of image access will determine the technology appropriate for archiving your images. Just as patient charts that have not been accessed for many years may be stored in the basement, images that are not likely to be needed soon may be put onto a less-expensive medium for archiving.

The creation of a CD-ROM is a little problematic. When a CD is being "burned," there can be no interruption of the data (image files) that are being sent to it. If there is an interruption, then the disk becomes defective and none of the information that had been recorded on it will be available. There are two factors in maintaining this flow of data from the hard drive to the CD-ROM recorder (CD-R).

The hard drive, as well as the overall computer system, must be fast enough to keep up with the CD-R. While the CD-Rs do have a file cache to hold a little information, the drive must basically be able to keep up with the writing process.

There will be data transfer delays whenever a file has been broken up and recorded onto different areas of the hard drive. This is called file fragmentation. Additionally, many small files need to be placed adjacent to each other on the hard drive from which the data are coming to keep the data flowing quickly.

Fortunately, there are solutions for these problems. One option is to create, on a separate and clean hard drive partition, a single large file that will then be transferred all at one time to create the CD-ROM. The CD-R software assists you in this process. Since the data are now one continuous file, there will be no delays in data transfer.

Another transfer method is to simply copy all of the desired files onto a clean hard drive partition. By moving the files and never erasing a file from this partition before making the burn, there will not be any file fragmentation. With this method, one hopes to avoid any delays in the data transfer.

It is also important to only use hard drives that use intelligent (and not thermal) recalibration. The intelligent recalibration feature ensures that the drive will not pause for self diagnosis and align itself while data are being transferred.

Screen savers should not be used since there may be an interruption in the transfer of data when they get turned on. Obviously, do not perform any other function on the computer while it is writing a CD-ROM. If the computer on which you are performing this CD-R function is on a network, don't forget to either take it off the network or make sure that any e-mail notices, for example, will not be posted to the machine and interrupt the flow of data.

As with any important file copying, make sure that you enable the software's *verify* function to ensure that the write was successful.

IMAGE COMPRESSION

There are both advantages and disadvantages to compressing (making smaller) your image files. Obviously they will take less space to store, and the ability to store more information in less space is important, since the expense of image storage is not insignificant. A compressed file also can be transferred more quickly over a computer network. Once the image has been transported, it can be uncompressed at the review station. Even considering the extra time needed to uncompress the image, it is still usually faster to ship compressed images and to uncompress them after the transfer. Recent images that may require image enhancements should be kept online in an uncompressed format.

It is important to understand that if the size of the image file is made smaller, there is the possibility that information may also be reduced. Best of all are the loss-less compression programs, which make the file smaller and then bring it back to its original size without the loss of any information. The original and reconstructed files will be identical. Other file compression methods actually remove information from the file. This is not a desirable situation, but it does permit the file to be made much smaller. These are "lossey-compression" schemes. The degree to which the file is made smaller and the method of file compression determine the amount of image degradation.

One disadvantage of lossey-compressed images is that they are not identical to the original images. This may have medicolegal implications as well as being a practical diagnostic problem. While they may be visually "close enough" for diagnostic work, there would be significant limitations to performing image enhancements and manipulations on a previously compressed image (Figure 7-28).

It is important medically, legally, diagnostically, and photographically to maintain high-quality, uncompressed original images. One way to manage the vast quantity of data that images comprise would be to have 3–6 months of patient data on the network at full resolution. Older records could be kept online in a compressed format to permit viewing (without manipulation) of the older images. If manipulation were to be required of an older image, then the original disk could be manually loaded onto the network to give access to the uncompressed file.

Image Access

After images have been acquired, the physician must review them for diagnostic information. Prints may be adequate for limited purposes, but image monitors are needed to show the images in their full brilliance. The image monitor literally has no substitute.

REVIEW STATIONS

The simplest solution is to use the acquisition system to review the images. While this is cost-effective in terms of initial equipment costs, if the practice is busy, it may hinder the utilization both of the staff and of the expensive image acquisition system.

If a physician is reviewing images on the fluorescein acquisition station, then the system may not be available for a study, and it cannot be put back into use until the review has been completed. While some systems let you "step out" of an ongoing study and review a case, it is advantageous to complete a fluorescein angiogram without interruption. If the practice is small and scheduling permits, a second image monitor may be installed in the laser suite if it is close to the angiography room. An A-B switch box could then send the signal to either monitor. Some monitors allow the signal to be "looped through" to another monitor. Obviously, this would tie up the acquisition system for the duration of the laser procedure, but it may be acceptable for small practices.

If the laser suite is too far away for the monitor signal to be sent, then another method of transferring the image(s) must be used. In concert with the decision of how the images will be transferred will be the decision of whether the review station will be a simple single-image station or a full-function review station (Table 7-9). If the photographer is going to enhance the images and get them ready for the physician in a manner similar to that in the darkroom, then the simple-image review com-

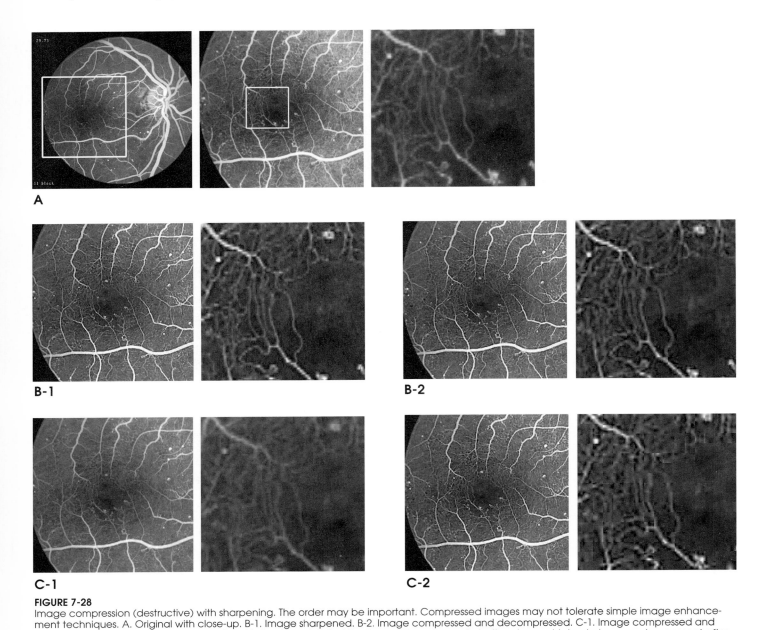

FIGURE 7-28
Image compression (destructive) with sharpening. The order may be important. Compressed images may not tolerate simple image enhancement techniques. A. Original with close-up. B-1. Image sharpened. B-2. Image compressed and decompressed. C-1. Image compressed and decompressed, and then sharpened (C-2). Notice how detail of the fine perifoveal vascularization does not tolerate image enhancement after an image has been compressed.

Table 7-9. Image Review Systems Based on Size of Retinal Practice

Size of Practice	Acquisition	Laser Room
Small	Acquire and review	Monitor only
Medium	Acquire and review	Simple computer review
Large	Acquire	Full review computer with network
Very large	Acquire	Network feed to laser and physicians' offices

puter may be sufficient. However, if the retinologist wants to enhance these images or to create his or her own image overlays, the review station should be a full-function system.

Images may be moved either by physically moving them with a floppy or an optical disk of images (the "sneaker-net"—running the disk down the hall) or with a cabled computer network. If the needs are simple, a sin-

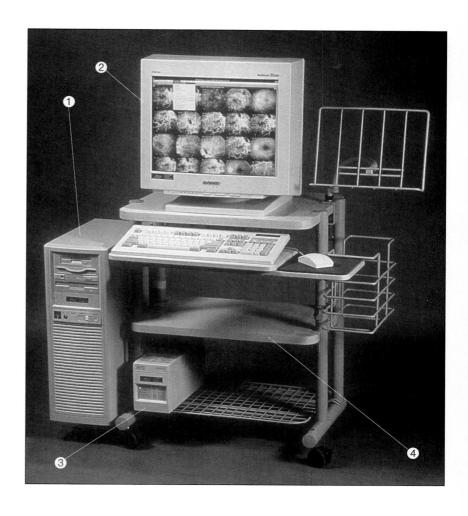

FIGURE 7-29
Floppy review station. (1) Computer with 3.5″-disk
drive. (2) High-resolution Multi-sync monitor.
(3) Isolation transformer with hospital-grade plug.
(4) Wheeled cart to hold components. (Courtesy of
Ophthalmic Imaging Systems, Inc.)

gle image that has been placed on a floppy disk can be loaded onto the
floppy review station. Since there is limited or no image manipulation at
this station, a low-end computer system with a single high-resolution monitor will provide an adequate system (Figure 7-29). Inexpensive software
will permit you to view most formats of image files. The network is faster
but requires some additional initial expense for setting it up. Which to
choose is purely an economic decision: time vs. money.

Networking Imaging Systems
There are many advantages to having diagnostic imaging systems connected to a computer network. The ability to have a centralized archiving system and to have the images from many sources available at
many workstations is obvious. The hardware to create the image
archives can be a single system that provides archival and retrieval
functions for imaging systems ranging from corneal topography to ICG
angiography. Access to such a system also means that more images can
be kept online for use at multiple desktops and examination rooms.
Having a single networked computer for archiving and printing
reduces the need for multiple printers. Integration of color fundus photographs and other images is possible with the addition of a slide scan-
ner or a color digital fundus camera. Images from corneal topography,
visual field machines, and magnetic resonance imaging and comput-
ed tomography scans are just some of the possibilities. All can also be

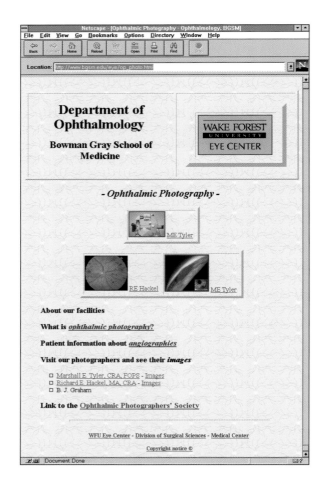

FIGURE 7-30
Ophthalmic Photography, Wake Forest University Eye Center, World Wide Web home page.

sent to printers and film recorders for slide making. The financial advantage in sharing expensive archiving and printing equipment is significant. With the introduction of online electronic medical records, the possibilities are literally infinite.

The ability to send images between offices in a timely manner may be useful. This is easier to accomplish when the images are already in electronic format. The Internet is a group of computer networks interconnected via high-speed data lines that forward information to a user's computer address. It permits transmission of text and/or images anywhere in the world where the network goes. Additional offices can be connected—admittedly at slower transfer speeds—with computer modems via telephone lines or radio links anywhere. Internet providers on a pay-for-service basis widen the outreach of those who wish to communicate via computers.

In 1994, ophthalmic photographers Joseph Warnicki and Paul Montague, respectively, set up the first ophthalmic photography list-server and file transfer protocol (FTP) sites on the Internet. These capabilities permitted interested ophthalmic photographers to send messages (typically news, questions, or answers) to other ophthalmic photographers around the world. The FTP site is a depository for images to be shared with other photographers. World Wide Web (www) home pages on the Internet provide additional image sharing capabilities (Figure 7-30). For home page addresses, contact the Ophthalmic Photographers' Society or use one of the web search engines.

Patient Flow

Patient flow through the photography area is different with electronic imaging. In a film-based fluorescein angiography clinic, as soon as the patient is finished, the film can be removed from the camera and another patient study can be initiated. In a digital angiography clinic, this may not be the case. One reason is that unless there is a full-featured review station available on a network, most of the printing process takes place at the acquisition camera workstation. This interferes with the ability to start another angiogram. In effect, the photographer is now doing darkroom work in the camera room. The implication of this change in timing one's work schedule is that, since the film does not get handed to the darkroom person, the camera is not available to photograph the next patient until the images are ready for the physician. There is time saved for the patient and the physician, but not necessarily for the photographer, who now must enhance, print, and archive the images.

If there is a full-featured review and printing station, then the camera can quickly be used for another angiogram. The images can be transported either on an optical drive disk or over a network. It takes less time (a few minutes) to write these images onto the disk or to put them onto the network than to review a case.

Equipment Selection

Digital ophthalmic imaging systems are expensive. Before you purchase one, we suggest you think about how your system is to be used in the clinic. Here are some things to think about.

Image quality is the prime concern of the retinologist as well as the photographer. Before choosing a digital ophthalmic imaging system, evaluate the image sharpness, both central and peripheral, as well as the tonal information, remembering that the manufacturers' promotional material will provide only the highest-grade images from the best patients. Ask other photographers about their experiences with the system you are considering, which fundus camera is used, and how it performs on patients with poor media.

The digital camera is the central control of the image quality that you will receive from your system. Review the technical section of this chapter to remind yourself of the imaging qualities that will be important to your clinical practice: exposure latitude, image saturation thresholds, tonal depth, and resolution. Obviously the optical components are also important. See Chapter 2 on fundus photography for guidelines on selecting a fundus camera. In analyzing the optical interface between the fundus camera and the digital camera, review the image quality for sharpness and evenness of illumination.

Evaluate the imaging software by attempting some of the tasks on the checklist in Table 7-10. Talk with other photographers who use digital systems. Be wary of photographers who have worked on, or even looked at, only one manufacturer's system. One very good photographer who had not previously worked on computers said about a particularly complicated software menu, "Well, it is better than the darkroom." Enough said? Remember this is a good tool—accurate, logical, convenient, and robust.

The user interface (fancy words for the software you must use to get the system to work) is the key to productivity. Your software should give you little interference in getting the images to assist the physician with high-quality diagnostic information. The interface should be logical and

Table 7-10. Imaging Software Task Check List

System startup
Startup and monitor calibration
Check date and time
Enter patient information. Check for information fields specific to your practice.

Image acquisition
What is the resolution of captured image?
Is resolution stored?

Image enhancement
Is there contrast stretching capability?
Is there sharpening capability?
Is there contrast enhancement (auto-burn and dodging)?
Can enhanced images be saved to the disk?
What imaging tools are available (overlay, zoom, MPS rings, etc.)?

Printing
What are the options for image layouts on a page?
Is adequate tonality recorded on the print?
Does tonality match the screen?
Is full-image resolution maintained to the printer?
Are the prints archival?
What is the cost of the printer and prints?

Storage and archiving
Does software ensure that images are not deleted without first archiving them?
Does software ensure that duplicate images are not created (unless you want them)?
What do the media cost?
What is the speed of the drives for writing and reading?
For image retrieval, which database fields can you look up?

Other considerations
Is there slide-making capability?
Can the image file be exported to other computer programs?
Can you export the patient database?
Is the UL-544 listed? Or is there a letter from the manufacturer stating that the system is built to meet or to exceed the UL-544 standard? In part, the standard requires that hospital-grade cord caps (plugs) be used and that the total ungrounded ground leakage be less than 100 µA (micro-amps).
Is the equipment layout clean and neat?
Will it fit into your room?
Are two phone lines available (one for the computer modem and one for the voice)?
Are the air conditioning and air flow adequate to condition the space into which this heat-producing equipment is going?
Are there two separate power circuits available for the imaging system (computer and the fundus camera flash power supply)?
Is the equipment energy efficient? Do the computer and the monitors go into a sleep mode to save electrical energy when they are not being used? Can you set the time of the sleep mode so that it will not interfere with angiography?

should make it convenient to complete frequently performed tasks. Menus should not require you to go through more than two levels to access these sections of the program. Drop-down menus make it easy to look at most of the choices. The program should respond to both mouse and keyboard for every command (see the sidebar "Of Mice and Photographers"). Entering data should make sense and should be easy. In some systems, there are two monitors. A separate image monitor allows software menu items to be viewed on a separate text monitor, which does not interfere with the images.

Good computer software should be intuitive and have clear menus. It is important to understand the strengths and weaknesses of the different systems you are considering. The menu is the road map to the imaging system's computer program. It will become either your friend and assistant or your antagonist and downfall. Pick your imaging system only after carefully analyzing its software.

Evaluate the software by considering the specific jobs that need to be accomplished. For example: Say that you need to go to your kitchen several times a day to get food and take it to your dining table in the next room. If the architect puts in a doorway, you could carry the food on a

Of Mice and Photographers

In working with images on computers, it is mandatory to use some type of pointing device. The most commonly used one is the computer mouse. This is a bar-of-soap-sized device that is held under the hand, palm down, and moved over a flat surface. There are one or more buttons on the top of the mouse so positioned that they can be pressed by the fingers. There is usually a wire connecting the computer and the mouse—hence the name, since the wire looks like a mouse's tail. Inside the mouse is a small ball, which is slightly exposed on the lower side of the mouse. This ball rolls on the desktop and sends rotation information to the computer. You see the results of this movement with the display of an arrow or cross-hairs on the computer monitor screen. With the mouse you can point at something on the screen and tell the computer that you wish to do something by pressing the appropriate mouse button. The computer can also understand the rapid pressing of a button twice as a request different from that made when the button is slowly pressed twice.

Another pointing device is a trackball. This is simply mouse technology that is turned upside down and lets you move the exposed ball with your thumb, while you use your fingers to press buttons.

Tablets use a mouse-like device that does not have a positioning ball but has a physical cross-hair on a plastic window. The tablet can sense where the cross-hair is. Tablets can also use a pencil-like pointer.

A light pen is a pencil-like light sensor that can recognize the spot on the monitor screen to which you are pointing. It has a switch built into the tip that, when pressed onto the screen, tells the computer that you wish to select the choice at which you pointed.

Touch screens are special monitors with built-in sensors that know where a finger is in contact with the screen. Touch screens do not have the precision of other pointing devices.

Table 7-11. Database Fields

Length	Field
11	Patient ID number
11	Social Security number (automatically placing dashes)
20	Last name
20	First name
15	Middle name
6	Date of birth (DOB)
1	Sex
1	Race
15	Diagnosis (primary); ICD-9
15	Diagnosis (secondary); ICD-9
15	Diagnosis (systemic disease)
10	Study (drug)
6	Date of procedure
5	Type of procedure: FA, ICG angiography, monochromatic, color, NFL
15	Physician (staff)
15	Physician (resident/fellow)
15	Physician (referring)
15	Referring source (group/practice name)
15	Photographer
1	Teaching quality T/F
72	Memo

tray and make a single trip into the dining room through the doorway. If the architect did not put in a doorway, but rather a 6-foot-high wall, you could learn to pole vault and carry one item at a time in a backpack to the table. This example might seem extreme, but that is how I felt using some of the early imaging software. I could accomplish a task but it required multiple steps and was not intuitive. I had to memorize arcane terms and remember the purpose of function keys without references even being included on the menu. Make sure that the system you choose does not have these kinds of problems.

Attention should be paid to reviewing sample ICG angiography late images to ensure that the system has adequate flash power, optics, and camera sensitivity images of these late phases. This also applies to SLO systems.

The date and time should be automatically entered from the computer's internal clock. It is good to have the date displayed so that you can check to ensure that the computer's internal clock and calendar are accurate.

The types of information that a photographer wants to enter into the database record may include the database fields (Table 7-11). Make sure that the diagnosis and the physicians can be changed to match a changing diagnosis on subsequent studies if that is important for your practice. Additional capabilities could include the automatic recording of eye, field of view, filters, flash output, digital camera gain, and so forth.

Each field should be long enough to ensure that the data your practice needs are sufficient to retrieve the patient's record. Keep in mind that this database may be the only computer database you have for retrieving patients and/or their images for teaching purposes, so discuss this with potential vendors before you purchase, buying only if the system will meet your needs.

Monochrome monitors are typically sharper than color monitors. Check the image for fine detail and don't forget that the timers on these small images can be difficult to read on a poor monitor. Typical presentation of contact sheets on a 20-inch monitor is five rows of images by

Table 7-12. Factors to Consider in Thinking About "Going Digital"

Economic factors
Time factors
Test availability—e.g., ICG angiography
New office, consider instead of a darkroom
You want the newest technology
Networking of images
Tele-medicine (remote clinics)
Patient convenience and education
Marketing

four rows of images. Some manufacturers use display boards that create a square display, which, of course, would not use the entire horizontal width of the monitor. Their boards typically display only 16 images.

An uninterruptable power supply (UPS) keeps the digital camera and the computer system powered in the event of an electrical power failure. The UPS has a battery strong enough to keep the computer running for 5–10 minutes if the main power goes off. Images in the RAM are volatile; thus, if the RAM loses power, the images will be lost. With an UPS, there is enough time for you to copy the images from the computer RAM onto the hard drive. Without a UPS, a power outage of less than a second could lose all of the recently acquired images and would also require the image acquisition program to be reloaded from the hard drive before additional images could be taken. The UPS is usually left plugged into the wall power outlet so that the internal battery remains charged and ready for use. If the power remains off, then the problems of taking additional frames are the same as those of conventional photography, since without power—lots of it—the camera flash cannot operate.

Cost Considerations

Technical equipment continues to be more sophisticated and powerful, although the prices have become more competitive. The original purchase price is only one of the factors in deciding if and when to "go digital" (Table 7-12). The job functions in the photography area are different. The photographer in the digital world typically edits, enhances, and prints his or her own images.

Cost considerations can be divided into categories: initial costs and training, yearly costs, and operating and updating expenses. The initial cost is the most obvious. Systems may include a fundus camera or may be adaptable to your existing fundus camera. Systems can come as a bundled package complete with a digital camera, the computer system (computer, imaging board, monitors, mass storage for images, and network connection), software, and specialized hardware (optical and computer interface), as well as a printer. There is usually an image review station in the laser suite.

Training by the vendor is important to quality and productivity, so do not ignore the need for (and the cost of) personnel training. Make sure that the training program will provide a specified amount of training at a time when the photographers are available. Installation time should not be included in the promised training time. One schedule might be to spend an evening learning about the system and its software before training with patients on another day.

Yearly costs include two major areas: the cost of the physical space for the equipment and depreciation of the software and hardware portions of the system. Your space costs may be less with an electronic system because you will not need to maintain the space for a darkroom. Equipment should be depreciated in 3–5 years. Software and hardware upgrades will help keep your system and photographers running at peak performance and capability. Hardware keeps getting better and will always need updating to provide the patients with access to the current imaging technology.

Analysis of your patient workload will assist you in selecting printers and storage/archiving methods for your imaging system.

Indocyanine Green Angiography

Patrick J. Saine

Ocular angiography with dyes other than fluorescein sodium has been explored.[17] The most clinically promising angiography technique for the posterior segment has been ICG angiography.

ICG has been used in medical imaging since 1956[18] and was first photographed in the eye by Kogure and Choromokos in 1969.[19] Flower and Hochheimer continued developing the procedure throughout the 1970s, with Destro and Puliofito updating it in the late 1980s.[20, 21] It was not until 1992, however, that Yannuzzi, et al. first described a practical method for achieving clinically significant ICG angiographic images.[22] Yannuzzi's work has led to ICG angiography becoming an important adjunctive technique to fluorescein angiography.[23]

This section describes the principles of of ICG angiography and provides a step-by-step procedure for performing it. It assumes that you are familiar with the physical and physiologic properties of ICG as discussed in Chapter 4, and with electronic fluorescein angiography.

Choroidal Angiography Versus Retinal Angiography

The principles of fluorescein angiography provide a framework for understanding ICG angiography. Both tests use a fundus camera to document ocular blood vessels after a colored dye has been injected intravenously. Fluorescein angiography documents the dynamic flow of fluorescein sodium primarily in the retinal vasculature (Figure 7-31); ICG angiography documents the staining characteristics of ICG in the choroid.

These complementary dyes have differing physical characteristics. Fluorescein sodium is a red, water-soluble dye that is excited by blue (465–490 nm) light and emits yellow (520–530 nm) light. ICG is a green, water-soluble, tricarbocyanine dye that becomes excited in the near infrared range: maximal excitation: 805 nm; maximal emission: 835 nm (Figure 7-32).

There are practical differences between these two dye tests. Fluorescein sodium is provided in solution while ICG must be dissolved shortly before use. Circulating fluorescein sodium can be recorded using either film or electronic media, whereas ICG angiography can only be recorded (practically) using electronic imaging. Different exciter and barrier filter pairs maximize the appropriate wavelengths for each test. As we shall see, the plane of best focus and timing is unique to each test. Dye changes during fluorescein angiography are visible in the optical viewfinder, while those during ICG angiography are not. Fewer complications and a less fatiguing flash intensity make patients more comfortable during ICG angiography.[18, 24]

However, the duration of ICG angiography (up to an hour versus 15–30 minutes for a complete fluorescein angiogram) balances the patient comfort scales. Procedures for obtaining optimal exposure vary between the two tests. Fluorescein angiography has a relatively constant dynamic range, which is captured within the recording range of either film or electronic imaging systems. ICG angiography has a much larger

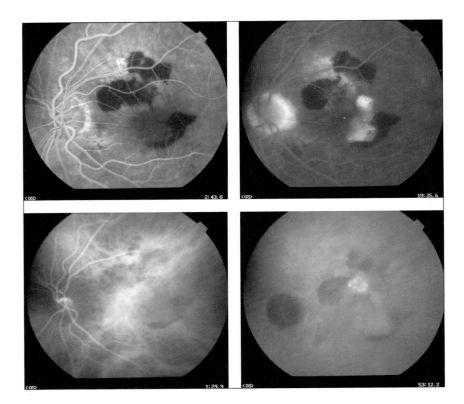

FIGURE 7-31
Four-up of fluorescein and ICG angiography of same patient.

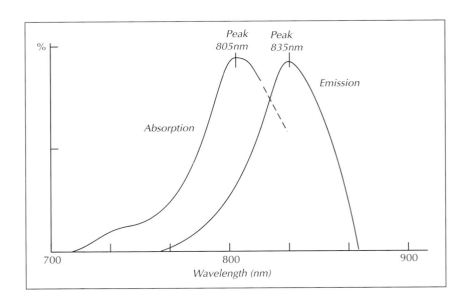

FIGURE 7-32
The excitation and emission spectra of indocyanine green dye.

luminescence range, which falls within the infrared portion of the spectrum. Both the flash and the electronic camera sensitivity must be manipulated throughout the procedure to obtain consistent tonal qualities throughout the study. One reason for the large range of fluorescence may be the difference in the percentage of each dye that is bound by proteins in the blood.[25, 26] Only half of the circulating fluorescein sodium is protein-bound; the rest remains independent to circulate freely through the blood. On the other hand, the over 90% of the ICG that will bind to protein begins by circulating freely, making the early post-injection photographs very bright. Within the first minute after the injection, however,

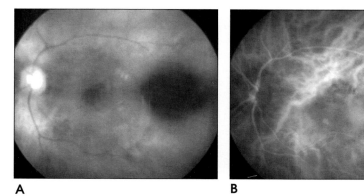

FIGURE 7-33
Red filter photograph (A) and ICG photograph (B) of same eye showing nevus and hypofluorescence.

A   B

Focusing with Infrared Radiation

The range of electromagnetic radiation extends from gamma rays and x-rays through ultraviolet, visible, and infrared radiation to radiowaves and microwaves. Our eyes, our optical instruments, and our recording media are all optimized for that small band of the electromagnetic radiation that we call visible light.

We record infrared radiation (IR) during ICG angiography. While its longer wavelength allows visualization through some pigments and thin hemorrhages, IR does not focus in the same plane as visible light. An additional 0.25% of the focal length added to the lens-film distance is a standard correction.[27] The red index mark on 35-mm interchangeable camera lenses simplifies this process. After the lens is focused, the indicated distance is shifted to the red index mark. Both the standard calculation and the index mark options for correction are impractical for fundus photography.

Two different strategies have been used to ensure the sharp focus of IR wavelengths in ICG angiography. Real-time IR-sensitive video viewing (with or without a barrier filter) is available on some systems. An IR-sensitive video camera replaces the viewfinder and displays real-time images on a video-resolution monitor. Advantages include feedback from real-time focusing. Capital expense and lower viewing resolution are obvious disadvantages.

A technologically simpler strategy is to bias the focusing system manually by adding two positive diopters to your reticule setting. In this instance, you will see a blurry reticule when looking through the viewfinder. Focus on the choroid while keeping the blurred reticule as blurry as it looked when you first viewed it. The instant feedback of electronic imaging makes this method practical. Inexperienced angiographers may have some initial problems, but the experienced ophthalmic photographer will readily adapt. Although this solution is admirably inexpensive, it introduces the potential for photographer error.

Whichever focusing system is used, target the focus to the choroid by visually dissecting the retina as described in Chapter 2. Focus past the retinal blood vessels and the pigment in the retinal pigment epithelium to the larger choroidal vessels. Remember that even with the best possible focus, the spongy choroid will always seem less sharp than the retinal blood vessels you are accustomed to imaging.

most of the ICG becomes protein-bound and thus unavailable for exposure. As the test continues, less and less ICG is available for fluorescence, creating a need for increased flash and camera sensitivity.

Performing Indocyanine Green Angiography

ICG angiography uses the same basic fundus camera techniques used in fluorescein angiography. This section delineates a step-by-step procedure for ICG angiography, based on the following "prepare, position, expose, and follow up" format (also discussed in Chapter 2). The experienced angiographer who is proficient in the electronic imaging of fluorescein angiography can quickly become successful in ICG angiography.

Conduct a step-by-step review before or during the procedure to help establish your routine. Post a copy of the steps near your fundus camera for easy reference.

Prepare and Position

1. *Perform color fundus photography.* Expose stereo photographs that document the status of the retina, including any hemorrhage and edema. After obtaining these photographs, switch from film to electronic image acquisition.
2. *Expose monochromatic images.* Capture green and red monochromatic images. The green images are establishing shots that provide landmarks for overlay and indicate the status of retinal blood vessels and hemorrhages. Use a low flash setting and normal camera sensitivity for the green photographs.

   The red monochromatic photographs provide a view of the choroid without ICG dye (Figure 7-33) and document potential hypofluorescent areas (e.g., nevus, dense hemorrhage, or dense pigmentation). Exposure with a red filter can be problematic: You may need to abandon the flash and carry out the exposure using only the viewing light and perhaps some gain in camera sensitivity. Empirical testing will lead to a correct exposure.
3. *Prepare the camera.* After these monochromatic photographs are obtained, prepare the fundus camera and electronic imaging unit for ICG angiography. Double-check the exposure (we suggest a high flash intensity: 300 w/s), camera sensitivity (high), infrared exciter and barrier filter position (in), aperture setting (fully open), and focus (see the sidebar on focusing with infrared light). Remember that the exposure values are suggestions only: Empirical experimentation will yield the proper starting point for your particular instrument.

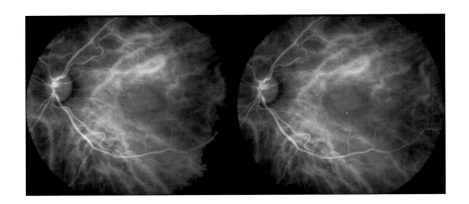

FIGURE 7-34
ICG angiography stereo pair clearly demonstrates the elevated, well-defined area of choroidal neo-vascularization beneath the retinal pigment epithe-lial detachment in a patient with choroidal neovascularization secondary to age-related macu-lar degeneration. (Courtesy of Dennis A. Orlock.)

Dual Injection

If fluorescein sodium and indocyanine green are both being documented in the ocular blood vessels, shouldn't you be able to make a single injection of both dyes for a combined angiography test? The answer is a resounding yes—and no. Interactions have not been doc-umented when these dyes have been mixed, but each test requires very different filters, focusing, and flash settings. Even so, dual ICG and fluorescein sodium angiography proce-dures can be practical. Multiple injection schemes include stopcock options, using a heparin lock or intravenous tubing, and even mixing the solutions in a single syringe (2 ml of 25% sodium fluorescein and 25 mg of ICG dilut-ed in 3 ml of solvent). The clinical needs of your specific practice will dictate the best method for dual angiograms. The single most important ingredient in these multiple angiography pro-cedures is timing. If compromises must be made, remember that the early fluorescein photographs are extremely important, as are the late ICG frames.

Practically speaking, if earlies of both pro-cedures are desired, then sequential injections are necessary.[28] The fluorescein angiogram may be embedded within the ICG angiogram either at the 2- to 5-minute or 10-minute level. Due to the large number of setting changes needed between the two procedures (exciter and barrier filter, exposure intensity, camera sensitivity, focusing, and viewing strategies), remember to doublecheck all controls before soliciting the fluorescein injection.

If only the fluorescein earlies and the ICG lates are requested, then the dyes may be mixed and injected simultaneously, with the fluo-rescein earlies and lates being captured immedi-ately and the ICG images beginning 10 minutes after the injection. While this is not ideal, it may be advantageous in some clinical settings.

Since it takes only 2–3 minutes more time, we recommend a dual-injection technique to permit the recording of the early phases of both the fluorescein and ICG angiograms.

Ascertain that the injection (25- or 50-mg ICG powder diluted in 3 ml of sterile aqueous solvent) and all necessary supplies are ready. Solicit an injection from the appropriate health care professional.

Expose

4. *Photograph the early phase.* As with your fluorescein technique, expose a control photograph and time the actual injection using pho-tographs. Stereo imaging during ICG angiography adds important visual information (Figure 7-34). Using established injection tech-niques, have the health care professional inject the patient with ICG (see the sidebar on dual injection). If you are viewing the retina through the ocular, there will be no visual indication of the dye. You will see instant feedback after the arterial phase on the computer image monitor. If your system is equipped with an infrared camera viewfinder with monitor, and you are viewing with a barrier in place, you may see the dye on the monitor. As with fluorescein angiogra-phy, begin capturing early images before you can see the dye.

   Constantly monitor the exposure during ICG angiography. ICG earlies will begin at about the same time as standard fluorescein earlies. Fluorescence will peak quickly (around 10–20 seconds) and then steadily decrease.

   Keep a hand on the exposure control. Your earliest choroidal images will be correctly exposed at 300 w/s. The ICG images will quickly become overexposed unless you rapidly decrease the flash setting. First reduce the camera gain (sensitivity) to zero. Then decrease the flash setting in full f-stop or greater increments. Continue to ride this wave of exposure, adjusting the flash setting all the way down to 18–25 w/s, if needed. The correct exposure will be a mov-ing target: With experience you will begin to anticipate the changes.

   There is some controversy over whether the earliest photographs are clinically significant, but because these pictures are the sharpest choroidal images and show the retinal blood vessels, we suggest that you include them (Figure 7-35). There will be few significant changes throughout the early images: edit this phase liberally, sav-ing only the sharpest and best exposures.

5. *Expose the late phase.* Continuously monitoring the instant feedback of electronic imaging, and increasing the flash setting and camera sensitivity as needed, continue to photograph the ICG at 2, 5, 10, 20, 40, and perhaps 60 minutes. The exact timing of the lates is open to interpretation. Some offices routinely expose 1-hour late images; some use a logarithmic timing series (2, 4, 8, 16, 30, and 60 minutes); others ignore the early photographs altogether.

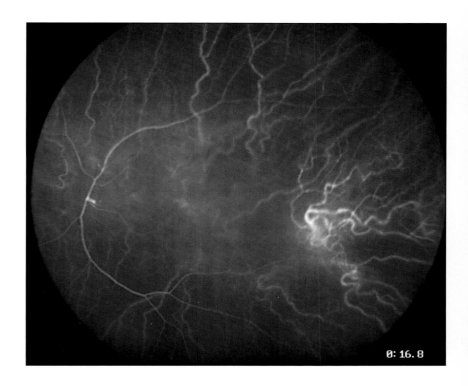

0: 16. 8

FIGURE 7-35
Early ICG angiogram showing choroidal and retinal blood vessels.

While the usefulness of early choroidal images is being debated, current clinical practice suggests recording the early choroidal and retinal phases until it is proved that they are not clinically useful. Thirty minutes may be the minimal time for the late phase images. The actual timing of your latest photograph is limited only by the tenacity of your imaging system.

The amount of illumination from ICG decreases dramatically as the time from injection increases. It is not unusual to have to maximize both the intensity of the flash and the sensitivity of the electronic imaging camera to provide adequate exposure for late photographs.

Late ICG photographs show a darkened disc where retinal blood vessels cannot be distinguished (Figure 7-36).

6. *Close the session.* Reassure patients that all went well. Release them with a smile, making sure that they feel fine and know where their next clinic stop is. Complete all paperwork, remembering to sign the chart.

7. *Complete the process.* Edit, save, and print a hard copy of the completed electronic angiogram. Take the time to evaluate your work for quality and to discuss the results with the physician. ICG angiography is still an emerging technology. Professional ophthalmic photographers keep informed of the cutting edge of ophthalmic imaging.

Additional Indocyanine Green Angiography Issues

ICG angiography has a very low rate of adverse reactions.[18] However, since ICG incorporates iodine in the dye preparation process, patients should be screened for iodine allergy. Because it contains iodine, ICG is contraindicated for use with the diabetic drug Glucophage (see Chapter 4). Although the dye does not pass through the placenta, fetal toxicity tests have not been performed, and thus this test should not be performed on a pregnant patient. The personnel, procedures, and supplies for systemic reactions to fluorescein angiography should be readily available.

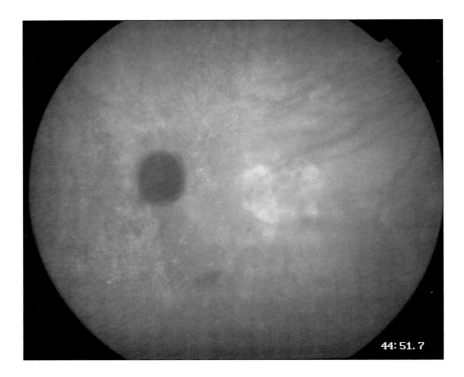

44:51. 7

FIGURE 7-36
Late image of ICG showing darkened disc; the retinal blood vessels cannot be visualized.

As with any exciter/barrier filter system, aging filters can result in pseudofluorescence. Autofluorescence has not been reported.

A technique for exposing late ICG photographs that includes retinal blood vessels as landmarks has been reported by Nyberg.[29] We suggest that the small amount of the ICG that remains in the original bottle is diluted and the patient is reinjected slowly. Photographs are exposed until the intensity of the retinal blood vessels matches the intensity of the choroidal blood vessels. Unwanted frames are deleted. The additional ICG in the various retinal blood vessels acts as anatomic landmarks.

Scanning Laser Ophthalmoscopes

The term *scanning laser ophthalmoscopes* (SLOs) refers to a group of ophthalmic instruments that have a number of elements in common. A number of different instruments use this technology, but first, some basics. There are two basic parts of the SLO that make it different from the conventional light sources (tungsten or flash). First, the light from the laser is scanned onto the subject in a manner similar to that in a television camera tube or television receiver (see Figure 7-3A). Second, the scanning laser does not simultaneously illuminate the entire subject, so the resultant total quantity of light is easily tolerated by the patient. Since there is only a small beam of light, it can be used through an undilated pupil (although a dilated pupil works better). Lasers typically have a monochromatic light source and therefore produce black and white images. The lasers scan 20–30 images per second, creating compatibility with video recorders. Unfortunately, the resolution of these systems is limited to video resolution.[31] As in conventional angiography, stereo images may be recorded using a lateral shift of the SLO and recording two images to produce a stereo pair.[32]

Laser beams can be modulated—that is, made brighter and dimmer—and since the laser beam is directed at only one portion of the retina at a time, a computer can be used to create a visual stimulus to the

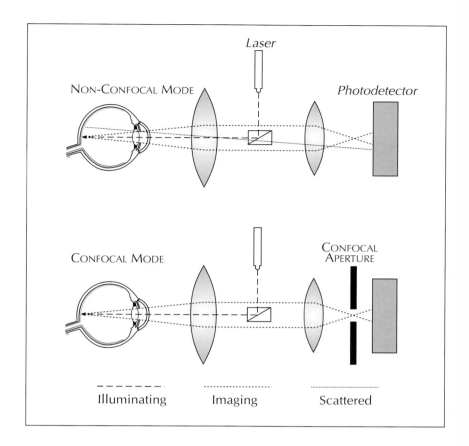

FIGURE 7-37
Scanning laser ophthalmoscope (SLO) schematic diagrams, including the aperture that is added to the confocal SLO.

patient—for example, the figure of a walking man, or words. At the same time the eye is receiving this image, the photoreceptor is measuring the reflective light from the retina and creating an image of the retinal vessels (minus the darker or lighter areas where the virtual image was presented to the patient). The resulting image permits you to examine the retina and the projected image simultaneously, which indicates the location of retinal functionality.[33]

Additional imaging capabilities are possible. In a confocal SLO (cSLO), an aperture is placed in front of the photo-detector to receive light only from the illuminated area of the subject. This increases contrast by reducing scattered light (Figure 7-37). cSLOs are used for fluorescein and ICG angiography (Figure 7-38). They can image these procedures with limited pupillary dilation. A disadvantage is the resolution limitation of these video-based systems.

The use of polarized light, with compensation for the polarizing properties of the cornea, has enhanced documentation of the nerve fiber layer (Figure 7-39).[34]

Retinal topography is achieved with yet another form of SLO. Since the depth of focus in the cSLO is small and precisely located, only the subject that is at the image plane of focus will be recorded. By acquiring a series of images that are sequentially "focused" from the anterior to the posterior levels in the retina (typically 32 images), a computer reconstruction of sharply demarcated retinal structures can be recreated in a three-dimensional computer map. Even though these systems use resolution images, it is the digital data that are being used for objective measurements. With this topographic information, different characteristics of the retina and optic nerve can be described (Figure 7-40). This is a quantitative process. Advantages to this technology are that a large pupil

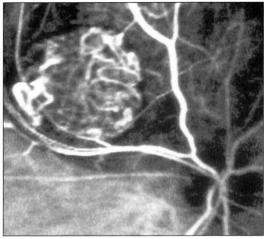

A

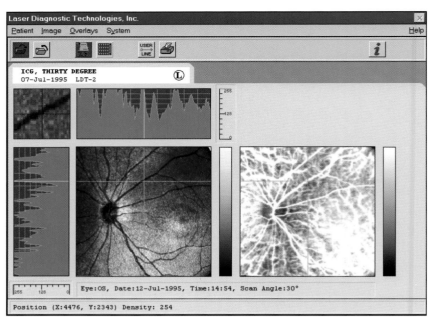

B

FIGURE 7-38
Fluorescein angiographic (A) and ICG angiographic images (B) from a scanning laser ophthalmoscope. (Courtesy of Laser Diagnostics, Inc.)

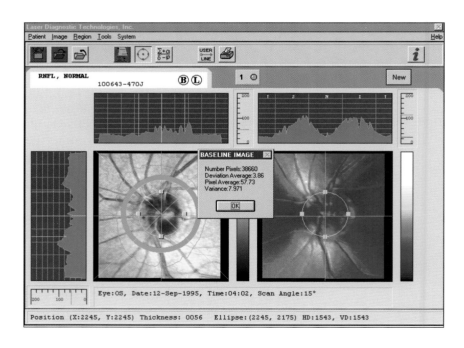

FIGURE 7-39
Nerve fiber layer (NFL) images using polarized light and a scanning laser ophthalmoscope. The computer analysis reveals areas of NFL dropout. (Courtesy of Laser Diagnostics, Inc.)

dilation is not required, as in stereo photographs, and the repeatability of the mapping process is good.[35]

Angiographies, both fluorescein and ICG, may be accomplished with SLO instrumentation. While often two SLO technologies and therefore two lasers are not incorporated into a single instrument, there is one instrument that simultaneously records both a monochromatic fundus and an ICG angiography image. Since they are in perfect registration, there is no need for the software to create image overlays. Some systems also use illumination information from the illumination detector to automatically adjust the illuminating laser during the ICG angiography procedure.

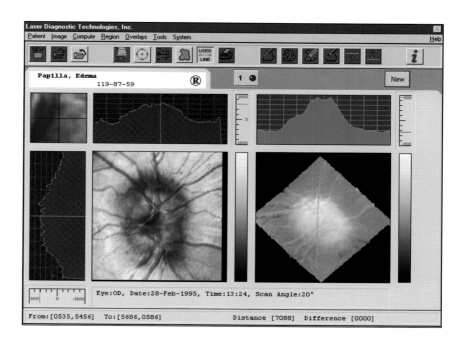

FIGURE 7-40
Retinal topography scanning laser ophthalmoscope
and a computer representation of the image.
(Courtesy of Laser Diagnostics, Inc.)

The technology of SLOs, with their properties of low light level and small pupil dilation requirements, will continue to evolve new imaging and measuring devices for the ophthalmic community.

Optic Nerve Analysis Systems

Quantitative measurement of the topography of the optic nerve can be achieved by passing multiple tangential slits of light across the nerve. A commercial product using this design, the Glaucoma-Scope (Ophthalmic Imaging Systems, Sacramento, CA) (Figure 7-41), was introduced in 1992. Twenty-five parallel planes of light are projected at an angle of 9 degrees onto the patient's optic nerve and imaged by a video camera. The video image is digitized with a computer, and the deviation of these straight lines, created by the variation in the depth of the optic nerve, is calculated. A computer program is then used to create a topographic map of the optic nerve and also can make a differential analysis of images taken on different dates.[30]

Fundus images taken with a digital camera or on slides that are scanned into a computer can also be analyzed by tracing the cup and disk and then making visit-to-visit comparisons. This also can be performed by alternately displaying two images that have been registered. This permits the clinician to track the optic nerve changes subjectively, a technique known as *flicker chromoscopy*.

Summary and Perspective

The advances in electronic imaging should not overpower the task that the ophthalmic photographer must accomplish. Deriving accurate and meaningful clinical and diagnostic information must be kept foremost in the mind of the photographer. Our ability to create images through a different modality should not lead to the instant demise of a current technology. If, however, the new technology provides more diagnostic information and

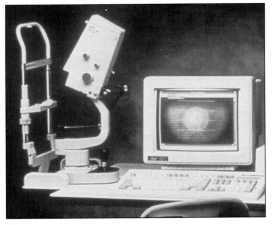

A

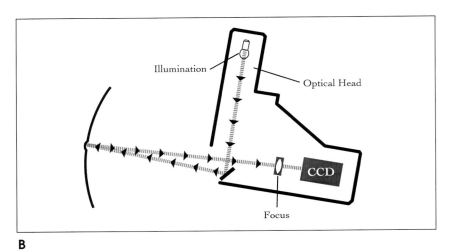

B

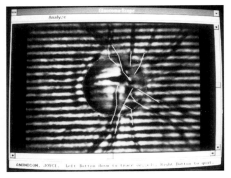
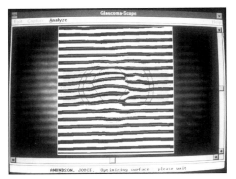
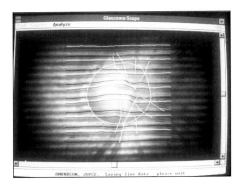

C

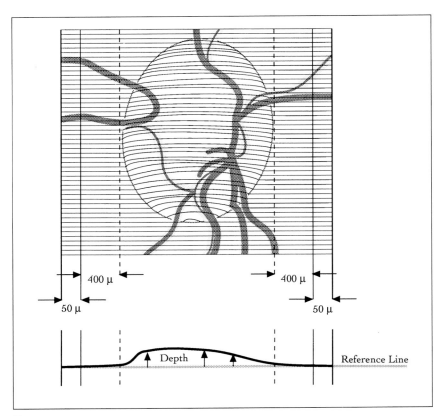

D

FIGURE 7-41
A. Glaucoma-Scope. B. Optical path. C. Image pro-
duced. D. Data acquisition. (Courtesy of Ophthalmic
Imaging Systems, Inc.)

at the same time improves timeliness, then so much the better. The ability to use computers to perform electronic imaging is a function of your aptitude for technical devices, your training with computers, the user interface of the imaging system you select, and, most important, your ability to integrate your knowledge of ophthalmic photography with new technology.

In the age of digital imaging, to be a proficient photographer, you should expand your knowledge to understand how to use computers. This does not mean that you will need to know how to program them, but the practical implication of using these tools is that you will need to be able to understand how work is accomplished when they are used. That basic understanding will put you in a better position to aid your practice in the efficient use of electronic images. Courses in computer theory and how to use applications will help. Remember that in today's ever changing world, employees "get a new job" every 10 years. This may not mean that you have a different title or that you will work somewhere else, but, particularly in this decade and the next, your responsibilities will change. If you learn and understand these and future new tools, you will be well served through the years to come.

Because the user interface is so important, it is paramount that the photographer be actively involved in selecting the system that will be used. It is well worth it to allow the major players who will be using the imaging system to actually see the functioning of the system and perhaps even to use it in a clinical setting before a selection is made.

With digital imaging systems, the flow of work through the photography unit will be different. How different will depend on how the system is configured. These are some of the factors: where and by whom are the images selected for printing? Where are the networked components? Is the review station full-featured? Are you moving images on floppy disks, prints, optical disks, or a network? An electronic angiography system may make dramatic changes in how the ophthalmologist and the office staff will function. Integration of computerized patient records and other diagnostic equipment is a serious consideration in how an office will handle image storage and retrieval systems.

One of the best positive outcomes that I have found is that patient communication and understanding of the situation is greatly increased. Instead of showing a patient a photograph of someone else's eye, the patient is able to see his or her own eye. The comprehension level that goes with the seeing of an image of one's own eye is monumental. Patients become participants in their health care and are able to better communicate with their physician. With an informed patient, there is better understanding and increased compliance, resulting in better patient outcomes and perhaps even lower health care costs.

References

1. Ridley H. Television in ophthalmology. Presented at the Sixteenth International Ophthalmological Congress (London). *Acta Ophthalmol* (Kobenhavn) 1951;2:1397.
2. Dallow RL. *Television Ophthalmoscopy: Instrumentation and Medical Applications*. Springfield: Charles C Thomas, 1970;1.
3. van Heuven WAJ, Schafer C, Mehu M. The use of low light level television in fundus imaging. *Mod Probl Ophthalmol* 1971;9:6.
4. van Heuven WAJ, Schafer C, Mehu M. The evolution of electronic recording systems for fluorescein angiography. Presented at the Twenty-Fifth Anniversary Congress, Retina Service, Boston, Massachusetts, 1972.
5. van Heuven WAJ, Schafer C. Televised Fluorescein Angiography. In K Shimizu (ed), *Fluorescein Angiography*. Tokyo: Igako Shoin, 1974;10.
6. van Heuven WAJ, Schafer C. Electronic imaging systems for fluorescein angiography. *Internat Ophthalmol Clin* 1974;14:31.

7. van Heuven WAJ, Mehu, M. The Clinical Applications of Televised Fluorescein Angiography. In JJ Justice (ed), *Ophthalmic Photography: International Ophthalmology Clinics*. Boston: Little, Brown, 16:2, 1976.

8. Yuhasz Z, Akashi RH, Urban JC, Mueller MMH. A new apparatus for videotape recording of fluorescein angiograms. *Arch Ophthalmol* 1973;90:481.

9. Kodak Megaplus Camera, Model 1.4 Users' Manual. Eastman Kodak Co, Inc., Digital Imaging, 151 State Street, Rochester, NY 14650

10. Beer PM. A laser printing option for digital angiography systems, 1994 [letter to the editor]. *Am J Ophthalmol* 1994;118:535.

11. Behrendt T, Wilson LA. Spectral reflectance photography of the retina. *Am J Ophthalmol* 1965;59:1079.

12. Behrendt T, Duane TD. Investigation of fundus oculi with spectral reflectance photography. *Arch Ophthalmol* 1966;75:375.

13. Russ JC. *The Image Processing Handbook*. Boca Raton, FL: CRC Press, 1992.

14. Todd H, Zakia RD. Photographic Sensitometry. In JM Sturge (ed), *Neblette's Handbook of Photography and Reprography; Materials, Processes, and Systems*. New York: VanNostrand Reinhold, 1977;165.

15. Macular Photocoagulation Study Group. Subfoveal neovascular lesions in age-related macular degeneration: Guidelines for evaluation and treatment in the macular photocoagulation study. *Arch Ophthalmol* 1991;109:1242.

16. Todd HN, Zakia RD. *Photographic Sensitometry. The Study of Tone Reproduction*. Hastings-on-Hudson, NY: Morgan & Morgan, 1969.

17. D'Anna SA, Hocheimer BF, Joondeph HC, Graebner KE. Fluorescein angiography of the heavily pigmented iris and new dyes for iris angiography. *Arch Ophthalmol* 1983;101:289.

18. Hope-Ross M, Yannuzzi LA, Gragoudas ES, et al. Adverse reactions due to indocyanine green. *Ophthalmology* 1994;101:529.

19. Kogure K, Choromokos EA. Infrared absorption angiography. *J Appl Physiol* 1969;27:154.

20. Bischoff PM, Flower RW. Ten years experience with choroidal angiography using indocyanine green dye: a new routine examination or an epilogue? *Doc Ophthalmol Proc Ser* 1976;138:3.

21. Destro M, Puliofito CA. Indocyanine green videoangiography of choroidal neovascularization. *Ophthalmology* 1989;96:846.

22. Yannuzzi LA, Slakter JS, Sorenson JA, et al. Digital indocyanine green videoangiography and choroidal neovascularization. *Retina* 1992;12:191.

23. Guyer DR, Yannuzzi LA, Slakter JS, et al. Digital indocyanine-green videoangiography of occult choroidal neovascularization. *Ophthalmology* 1994;101:1727.

24. Yannuzzi LA, Rohrer KT, Tindel LJ, et al. Fluorescein angiography complication survey. *Ophthalmology* 1986;93:611.

25. Wolfe DR. Fluorescein angiography basic science and engineering. *Ophthalmology* 1986;93:1617.

26. Baker KJ. Binding of sulfobromophthalein (BSP) sodium and indocyanine green (ICG) by plasma alpha-1 lipoproteins. *Proc Soc Exp Biol Med* 1966;122:957.

27. Sansone SJ. *Modern Photography for Police and Firemen*. Cincinnati: WH Anderson, 1971;312.

28. Miller K. Protocols for efficacious use of indocyanine green/sodium fluorescein angiography. *J Ophthal Photogr* 1993;15:63.

29. Nyberg WC. Re-injection technique for establishing landmarks in late phase ICG angiography. *J Ophthal Photogr* 1993;15:65.

30. Spaeth GL, Katz LJ, Baez KA, Nicholl JA. The Clinical Use of Image Analyses in the Diagnosis and Measurement of Patients with Glaucoma. In L Bonomi, N Orzalesi (eds), Glaucoma—Concepts in Evolution. Proceedings of an International Symposium held in Verona, Italy, June 16, 1991. Amsterdam, New York: Kugler Publications, 1991;71.

31. Woon WH, Fitzke FW, Chester GH, et al. The scanning laser ophthalmoscope: Basic principles and applications. *J Ophthal Photogr* 1990;12:17.

32. Frambach DA, Dacey MP, Sadun A. Stereoscopic photography with a scanning laser ophthalmoscope. *Am J Ophthalmol* 1993;116:484.

33. Timberlake GT, Van de Velde Druelde FJ, Julkh AE. Clinical use of scanning laser ophthalmoscope retinal function maps in retinal diseases. *Lasers Light Ophthalmol* 1989;2:211.

34. Retinal Nerve Fiber Thickness Measurements by Scanning Laser Polarmetry. AW Dreger, ED Bailey— Laser Diagnostics Technologies, Inc., 10467 Roselar Street, San Diego, CA 92121.

35. Allison AV, Giunta M, Chisholm L, et al. Reproducibility of topographic measurements of the macula with a scanning laser ophthalmoscope. *Ophthalmology* 1995;102:230.

Chapter 8

Fundus Photography and Fluorescein Angiography: Maximizing Diagnostic Information

Stephen J. Sramek

A. Introduction
B. Color Fundus Photography
C. Retinal and Choroidal Anatomy
D. Normal Fluorescein Angiogram
E. Abnormal Fluorescein Angiogram
F. Summary

Introduction

Fundus photography and fluorescein angiography provide information critical to the diagnosis and treatment of eye diseases. Although the concept is simple (take a picture of the retina), the process is complex. The different characteristics of equipment and patients will significantly affect your ability to provide the needed information to the clinician. To best accomplish this goal, the photographer needs technical training, knowledge of ocular anatomy, and an understanding of how fundus images are used by the clinician in the management of ocular disease. Earlier chapters in this book discuss technical aspects of retinal photography. The goals of this chapter are to review the pertinent ocular anatomy and to discuss the information required by the clinician from the point of view of the photographer. Photographers who understand the reason an image is required are able to assess the usefulness of their work, not just the technical quality. The more you understand about the process and the needs of the clinician, the better you will be able to contribute to and be part of the patient care team. This chapter does not attempt to provide a comprehensive discussion of the interpretation of fluorescein angiography, as there are other reviews that deal with this issue from the perspective of the clinician.[1,2]

What are the elements of the perfect fundus photograph or fluorescein? The correct eye, with focus at the correct level in the anteroposterior plane, at the correct location, with optimal field size and magnification, and, if a fluorescein angiogram, at the correct time. The correct eye and general location may or may not be apparent—and how does one determine what is "correct," "appropriate," or "optimal" for the other parameters? That is, how does one provide the maximum amount of information? Communication between the photographer and the clinician is key in this process. A large portion of the first 2 years of medical school are spent developing a vocabulary to allow further development of medical skills.

Although the photographer is not responsible for using clinical knowledge for diagnosis, treatment, or interpretation, at least a portion of this vocabulary is necessary to have a common ground for discussion. Information provided by the clinician is required by the photographer to best prepare to obtain the image. In this framework, basic clinical knowledge is as essential for the photographer as knowing the correct flash setting. Both are required for the most useful images.

There are several possible models of differing complexity within which the photographer may operate in the use of clinical data. One may use all of the following models at different times. The simplest framework, and the one inexperienced photographers use most, is to photograph the eye at the location that the clinician requests, always at the same magnification, focused on the retina, with fluorescein angiograms imaged in the same way—end of task. Following instructions from the person responsible for the medical care of the patient certainly cannot be faulted and should result in acceptable photographs most of the time. However, it makes the photographer a part of the camera, a button pushed by the clinician. Besides being less challenging and perhaps less satisfying for the photographer, it results in suboptimal images more often than one might think. For example, a colleague from another clinic complained to me after reviewing a set of photographs of a glaucoma patient that only included the macula. The physician marked "glaucoma" for the diagnosis, but during a busy clinic mistakenly circled the macula instead of the discs on the photo request form. The physician was quite upset that the photographer did not realize what was really needed, or did not at least question the request, even though the form was filled out incorrectly. Who hasn't heard, "Give me what I need, not what I ask for"? Further discussion revealed that the person was a part-time photographer at a satellite clinic with no experience and essentially no training. Education for both the physician and the photographer is an obvious solution to this kind of problem. This level of education and communication is the most basic, sort of the "Me Tarzan, you Jane" level—that is, glaucoma = nerve, diabetes = retina, etc.—and is the minimum that should be accepted by clinician or photographer.

Perhaps a more practical example is one in which a patient with proliferative diabetic retinopathy is sent to the photography department for photographs of the disc and macula, but neovascularization elsewhere (NVE) is present in field 3. Either the clinician missed the change or erroneously believed it to be within the field selected for photography. If the photographer can recognize the abnormality, he or she can choose whether to document the change. Recognition of what is abnormal is a model frequently used as a beginning strategy in medical education. It is based on the concept of a firm knowledge of what is normal to be able to recognize "anything else" as abnormal. Photographing whatever is identified as abnormal is a reasonably good strategy for a clinical photographer because it increases the chances that the image will provide the necessary information. An added advantage for the beginning photographer is that it does not require extensive clinical knowledge. Although one is working at a more sophisticated level within this framework, the technique has an inherent lack of sensitivity.

An unprepared mind (or one that is "unfocused") is limited in its ability to examine a problem or to find the appropriate steps needed for its solution. The concept is recognized in a number of areas. In psychology the principle surfaces in Stephen Covey's book *The Seven Habits of Highly Effective People* as habit number 2, "Begin with the end in mind." "To begin with the end in mind means to start with a clear understanding of your destination. It means to know where you're going so that you

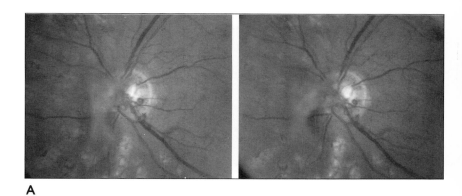

A

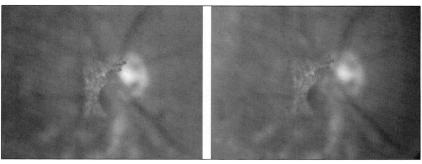

B

FIGURE 8-1
Information loss due to "improper" focus, not "poor" focus. The stereo pair in A is adequately focused at the level of the optic nerve. However, the clinician will not be able to adequately assess elevated neovascularization, which requires a different level of focus, shown in stereo pair B.

better understand where you are now and so that the steps you take are always in the right direction."[3] The principle is encountered by the medical student in the second year in Introduction to Physical Diagnosis or a similar course. A philosophy of examination from such a course that I have always remembered comes from a widely used textbook on internal medicine: "The detection of a few scattered petechiae, a faint diastolic murmur, or a small mass in the abdomen is not a question of keener eyes and ears or more sensitive fingers, but of a mind directed to be alert to these findings. Skill in physical diagnosis reflects a way of thinking more than a way of doing."[4] Detection of subtle changes—that is, maximizing information—increases with preparation of the mind before the task. The photographer needs to develop a "way of thinking" to complement the technical training to help prepare for the photograph.

The paradigm proposed in this chapter is based on the clinical use of the photograph. Remember the perfect photograph of the macula when the physician was interested in the optic nerve? Perhaps not as obvious, but just as important, is the technically perfect photograph focused at the level of the optic disc when the clinician is interested in documenting elevated neovascularization of the disc (NVD) in proliferative diabetic retinopathy. The blood vessels may be sufficiently elevated to be out of the plane of sharpest focus, and the photograph will not be very useful to the physician 4 weeks later when assessing the response of the NVD to panretinal photocoagulation (Figure 8-1). The photographer needs to have this information before taking the photograph. Therefore, a useful framework for preparing for a photograph is a categorization of its purpose— that is, *why* was the photograph ordered? Table 8-1 lists three common reasons clinicians order fundus photographs: documentation, diagnosis, and treatment. Briefly considering this table before actually taking a photograph is useful, especially for the inexperienced photographer. In the

Table 8-1. Purposes of Fundus Photography and Fluorescein Angiography

Documentation	Current status of a disease process
Diagnosis	Diagnostic pattern
	Rule out a diagnosis
Treatment	Localize the area to treat
	Assess the response to treatment

following examples I review these situations to demonstrate how the purpose of a photograph might affect the thinking of the photographer.

A common reason to order fundus photography is for documentation of the current status of a disease process. The images do not provide information in addition to the clinical examination but are to be used for later comparison to assess change. In many cases of retinal disease, treatment is guided by the results of national, multicenter randomized trials. In these trials, a certain level of change or "threshold" was necessary to allow the patient to enter the study. The common practice now is to wait until a patient has sufficient worsening of the ocular disease to the level of the initial study criteria. At that point the risks and benefits of treatment are clearly better than no treatment. The national studies pertinent to fundus photography and fluorescein angiography are the Diabetic Retinopathy Study (DRS),[5] the Early Treatment of Diabetic Retinopathy Study (ETDRS),[6] the Macular Photocoagulation Study (MPS),[7,8] and the Branch Vein Occlusion Study (BRVOS).[9,10] For example, the criteria of treatment for macular edema from the ETDRS describe retinal thickening (edema) threatening or involving the foveal avascular zone (FAZ), or hard exudate associated with retinal thickening threatening or involving the FAZ. Large areas of thickening or hard exudate that do not directly threaten the FAZ, often in field 3, also are an indication for treatment. What does this mean for the photographer? The most useful photographs within the context of the ETDRS are 30-degree stereo pairs that include the FAZ and any large areas of retinal thickening in field 3. The clinician reviewing the photographs will ask if retinal thickening or hard exudate with thickening that threatens the FAZ was underestimated or missed during clinical examination, or if, on comparison of photographs taken over a period of months, there has been progression in a borderline case. Clinically useful photographs hold the answers to these questions (Figure 8-2).

In addition to retinal and choroidal vascular diseases as examined in the national studies, another common situation requiring documentation involves a mass or pigmented lesion of the choroid. A choroidal nevus may be difficult to distinguish from a small choroidal melanoma. Documentation of growth on fundus photographs can be essential to management. In reviewing the photographs, one feature the clinician will examine is lateral extension of the lesion; therefore he or she will need to see all the margins of the lesion, and wide-field photographs may be useful (Figure 8-3). Failure to include the margins greatly decreases the usefulness of the image. Stereo will be helpful for an indication of thickening, although usually the clinician will rely on the ultrasound measurements to make this determination.

In some circumstances the diagnosis is apparent on clinical examination and the clinician uses fluorescein angiography in combination with fundus photography for the treatment of disease. For example, an elderly patient may present with vision loss, drusen, pigmentary changes, subretinal fluid, and hemorrhage on examination. The diagnosis is exudative age-related macular degeneration (ARMD), and the purpose

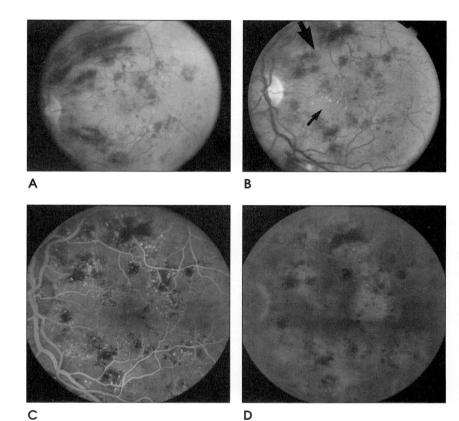

A   B

C   D

FIGURE 8-2
Documentation of disease progression and need for treatment. A. Fundus photograph of the left macula of a patient with diabetes at the initial consultation. Although numerous retinal hemorrhages are present, hard exudate is minimal and no thickening of the retina was apparent on contact lens exam. The patient was not a candidate for laser treatment based on ETDRS criteria. B. Two months later, although there has been some decrease in retinal hemorrhage (large arrow), there has been an increase in hard exudate (small arrow), and definite retinal thickening could be seen on clinical examination. C. Early-phase fluorescein angiogram used as a guide for focal laser treatment demonstrates numerous microaneurysms that leak in the late phase (D). Clinical photographs are essential to follow subtle but important changes, especially in patients with extensive disease.

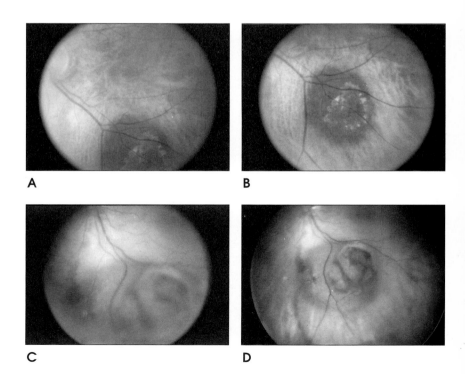

A   B

C   D

FIGURE 8-3
Document current status. Where's the edge? A, B. Thirty-degree fields showing a choroidal nevus/small melanoma. The image in A (field 5) is inadequate to follow this lesion for possible growth. Photographer needs to recognize importance of shifting fields to allow visualization of the entire margin (B). C, D. Large melanoma with subretinal hemorrhage. C. Entire lesion will not fit in a 30-degree field and is quite elevated, making focus difficult. D. A wide-angle photograph not only allows the entire lesion to be visualized, but the increase in depth of field provides more detail overall.

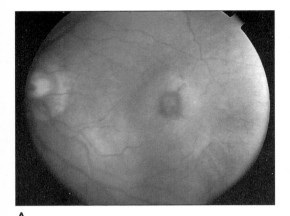

A

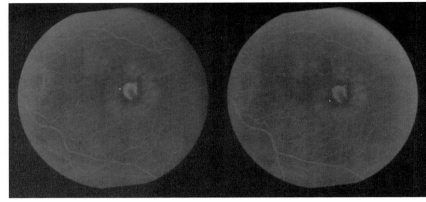

B

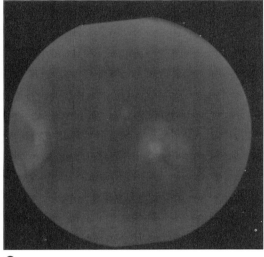

C

FIGURE 8-4
Localize area to treat. A. Fundus photograph of a 74-year-old patient who presented with metamorphopsia in her left eye shows a deep pigment ring and subretinal fluid. B. Stereo pair of early phase of fluorescein angiogram reveals a fan-shaped, deep hyperfluorescent lesion that leaks in the late phase. C. Early frame (B) was used to guide focal laser treatment.

of the angiogram is to locate the source of the leakage and to determine if the leakage is treatable based on the guidelines developed in the national studies. Three elements are essential for adequate assessment and treatment. They include the relationship of the leakage to the FAZ, the relationship of the leakage to the retina (intraretinal or deep to the retina), and the change with time in the intensity and pattern of leakage. Again, the purpose of the angiogram dictates the photographic technique. The standard angiographic technique described in earlier chapters fulfills these requirements nicely, providing stereo images in which the FAZ is visualized with high-quality early photographs (choroidal, early arterial). Imaging the early phase is crucial in this clinical setting because one of the frames in the early phase will guide laser treatment (Figure 8-4). Post-treatment photographs are used to assess the adequacy of coverage of the treated area. Finally, it is standard practice to repeat an angiogram after laser treatment to evaluate the response.

In other situations the diagnosis may not be apparent on clinical examination. For example, a patient presented with unexplained vision loss 3 months after uncomplicated cataract surgery. Visual acuity decreased from 20/20 to 20/80. Macular edema was present on clinical examination. Common diagnostic possibilities include the Irvine-Gass syndrome,[11] occult choroidal neovascularization, or a macular branch vein occlusion. The angiogram is essential to determine the diagnosis. Figure

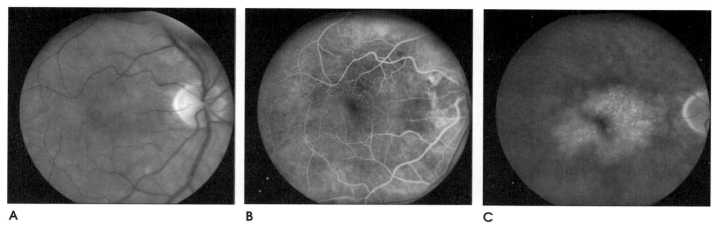

FIGURE 8-5
Diagnostic patterns in fluorescein angiography. Post–cataract surgery cystoid macular edema. A. "Red-free" photograph. B. Early venous phase of fluorescein angiogram demonstrates irregular hyperfluorescence at the level of the retinal vasculature. C. Late phase reveals typical pattern of cystoid edema and slight hyperfluorescence of disc.

8-5 shows a macular photograph of the patient. Although the clinical photograph is fairly unremarkable, the fluorescein angiogram demonstrates late intraretinal dye leakage and leakage from the disc (see Figure 8-5). These angiographic characteristics suggest post-cataract cystoid macular edema, or Irvine-Gass syndrome, which occurs in a small percentage of patients after uneventful cataract surgery. This situation is different from the previous example in that the late photographs are extremely important, as well as photographs of both optic discs for comparison and to assess leakage from the disc. An excellent arterial-phase photograph of a well-defined FAZ may be technically beautiful, but is not very helpful in the absence of 10-minute late photographs and late bilateral optic disc photographs when assessing this patient.

Color Fundus Photography

Understanding the purpose for which the image is to be used prepares the photographer to anticipate the outcome and allows the basic technique to be varied to obtain optimal results. In deciding where and how to obtain an image of the fundus, the photographer must, of course, begin with the request form sent by the clinician. At a minimum, the request should include a diagnosis and a location. If the request is unclear, the photographer should have the freedom to obtain additional information from the physician. By reviewing the purpose (see Table 8-1) and expected changes for the diagnosis, the photographer can then consider whether variations in the basic technique might be required. For example, are additional images required at different levels of focus, or perhaps different locations than on the request? Are 30- or 60-degree fields more appropriate? It may be helpful for the inexperienced photographer to develop a mental checklist to ensure that all technical aspects of the photograph are considered and logically chosen or excluded based on the clinical need as determined by the diagnosis. Table 8-2 is one possible guide. Review of the diagnosis, location, purpose, and technique should provide reasonable preparation to increase the probability of obtaining a photograph with maximum clinical value. A solid foundation in ocular anatomy and an understanding of the fundamentals

Table 8-2. Photographer Checklist

Angle of view	Normal, narrow, or wide-angle?
Field of view	Macula or disc? Mid- or far-periphery?
Level of focus	Vitreous, nerve fiber layer, retina, retinal pigment epithelium, or choroid?
Stereo	Is stereo technique helpful? Is it possible?
Filters	For angiography? For monochromatic photography?
Patient	Comfort? Lids? Cornea? Media?
Exposure	Standard? Or increase/decrease?
Advanced techniques	Slit fundus photographs with auxilliary lenses?
	Monochromatic fundus photography?

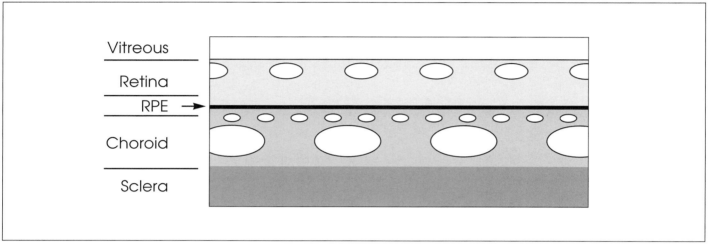

FIGURE 8-6
Simplified model of the posterior eye wall demonstrating the layering of retina, retinal pigment epithelium (RPE), and choroid.

of fluorescein angiography are needed for this process. The next section reviews aspects of ocular anatomy.

Retinal and Choroidal Anatomy

Fundus photographs and fluorescein angiography provide complementary information about ocular anatomy and ocular blood flow. Photographers need a working knowledge of ocular structures and blood circulation to assess the suitability of fundus photographs and fluorescein angiograms.

When interpreting fluorescein patterns, it is helpful to think of the posterior eye wall as a three-layered structure consisting of retina, retinal pigment epithelium (RPE), and choroid (Figure 8-6). Just behind these layers is the sclera, the opaque, tough, white, outer covering of the eye, while immediately in front of them is the optically clear vitreous. The blood supply to the eye can be divided into two distinct elements: the choroidal and retinal circulations. The retinal circulation is supplied by the central retinal artery, while the choroid is supplied from the ciliary arteries. It also is useful to consider that these two compartments are separated anatomically and functionally by the RPE, a barrier layer between the retina and choroid (Figure 8-7). As demonstrated below, the microanatomy of these compartments is different and determines the appearance of a fluorescein image. The layering of the eye and the

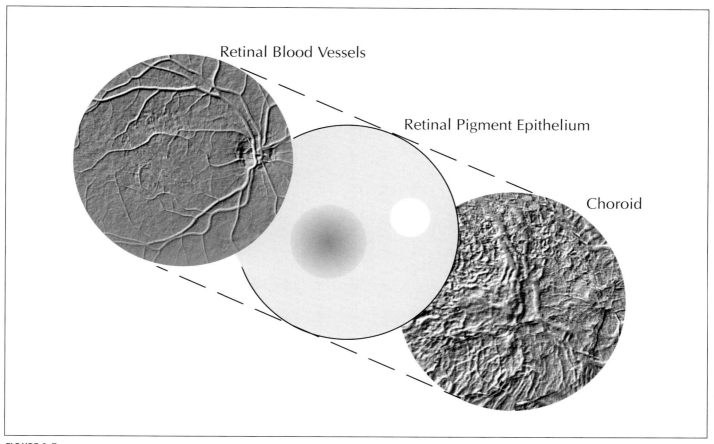

FIGURE 8-7
Retinal and choroidal circulation separated by the retinal pigment epithelium.

difference in blood vessel anatomy produces the different patterns as fluorescein passes through the eye.

The retinal layer consists of the light-sensitive photoreceptors, other nerve cells, support cells, and the *retinal circulation*. The source of the blood in the retina is the ophthalmic artery, a branch of the carotid. The blood vessels in the retina share a property with other blood vessels in the central nervous system—that is, there are specialized anatomic structures between cells called *tight junctions* (Figure 8-8A). Because of the tight junctions, there is only minimal leakage of blood components, fluid, drugs, and chemicals such as fluorescein through the blood vessel wall. Tight junctions are responsible for the *blood-brain barrier*, as well as a *blood-retinal barrier*. The retinal circulation behaves as a traditional vascular bed, with decreasing diameters of arterioles to the capillary level, and subsequent increasing diameters of the venous circulation.

Posterior to the retina is the RPE (see Figure 8-6), a single layer of pigment-containing specialized cells that perform a vital role in maintaining the health of the retina, particularly the adjacent photoreceptors. Bruch's membrane is a complex structure immediately posterior to the RPE that consists of the basement membranes of the RPE cells and cells from the choroid, as well as the layers between these cells. Damage to Bruch's membrane and the overlying RPE is important in the mechanism of vision loss in a number of diseases, including ARMD. The RPE, because it contains pigment, prevents visualization of the underlying choroid to varying degrees, depending on the pigment density. In the center of the normal macula there is an increased pigmen-

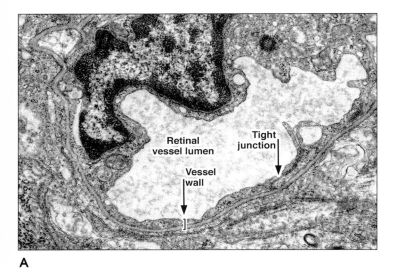

A

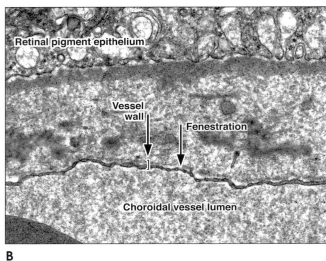

B

FIGURE 8-8
Electron micrographs of ocular blood vessels. A. Tight junction in a retinal capillary that forms part of a blood-retinal barrier. B. Fenestrations in a choroidal vessel that allow passage of small molecules into the extracellular space. (Courtesy of I. Wallow.)

tation in the RPE cells, recognized by the early pathologists and responsible for the name *macula lutea*.[12] This pigmentation typically masks the choroidal vessels. In contrast, in lightly pigmented individuals or individuals without pigment, such as in an albino, the choroid may be easily visualized.

The choroid is the layer of blood vessels between the RPE and the sclera. In addition to location, the anatomy of the *choroidal circulation* differs from that of the retinal circulation in several important ways. First, the choroidal vessels do not have tight junctions. In fact, the choriocapillaris or small choroidal vessels are fenestrated—they are built to leak (Figure 8-8B). As a result, small molecules such as fluorescein freely diffuse into the extravascular space. Substances that leak out of the choroid are prevented from entering the retina by the outer blood-retinal barrier, the RPE. Rather than a single arterial source as in the retina, the choroid is supplied by multiple long and short posterior ciliary arteries, which are branches of the ophthalmic artery. In an angiogram, the choroidal circulation fills earlier than the retinal circulation because of the supply from the posterior ciliary arteries. Finally, the choroid is not a simple progressive branching type of vascular bed as is the retina but consists of an interlocking network (anastomosis) of blood vessels that function as lobules (Figure 8-9).[13] The lobular arrangement of the choroid can sometimes be seen in the early phases of a fluorescein angiogram or in certain pathologic situations, but the pattern is rapidly lost because of dye diffusion through the fenestrated capillaries. Because of the multiple sources of arterial supply to the choroid, it is not as susceptible to occlusion by embolic disease as is the retinal circulation; however, the blood supply can be interrupted by a diffuse process. In fact, choroidal ischemia due to occlusion of posterior ciliary arteries can be an important angiographic finding in temporal arteritis, an inflammation that generally causes occlusion of a number of different arteries.

Except for the blood vessels, normal retina is optically clear. It has to be, since the photoreceptors are at the "bottom" of the retina, and light

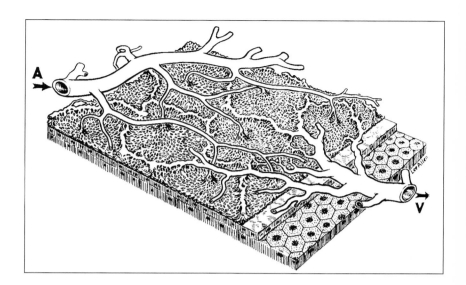

FIGURE 8-9
Classic drawing demonstrating the lobular structure
of the choroid. (Courtesy of Lee Allen.)

Table 8-3. Phases of the Normal Fluorescein Angiogram

Choroidal	Earliest recording of dye
	Retina relatively quiet except with cilioretinal artery
Arterial	Dye in arteries only
	Very short: less than 1–2 seconds
Arteriovenous	Arteries fill with fluorescein
	Laminar flow in veins
Venous	Veins generally brighter than arteries
	Veins are filled with fluorescein
Recirculation	Arteries and veins of equal brightness
	Fluorescence beginning to decrease
Late	Residual fluorescence (staining) of some normal structures
	Slow decrease in total fluorescence

must pass through the retina to these cells. The fundus appearance, then, is a combination of what is seen by looking through the retina and various amounts of pigment in the RPE, to the choroid. Differences in these layers is enhanced with fluorescein. In the next section knowledge of ocular anatomy is applied to understand the patterns seen in normal and abnormal fluorescein angiograms.

Normal Fluorescein Angiogram

A fluorescein angiogram documents a dynamic process in which fluorescein moves into the eye from the arterial circulation, interacts with anatomic structures both normal and abnormal, and leaves the eye via the venous circulation. It is important to recognize the patterns of fluorescence that emerge in a normal eye. The phases of the normal fluorescein angiogram are discussed in the following section and are briefly summarized for quick reference in Table 8-3.

Monochromatic green-filter photographs document in black and white the appearance of the retina just before injection of fluorescein (Figure 8-10A). After injection, fluorescence begins to appear in 10–20

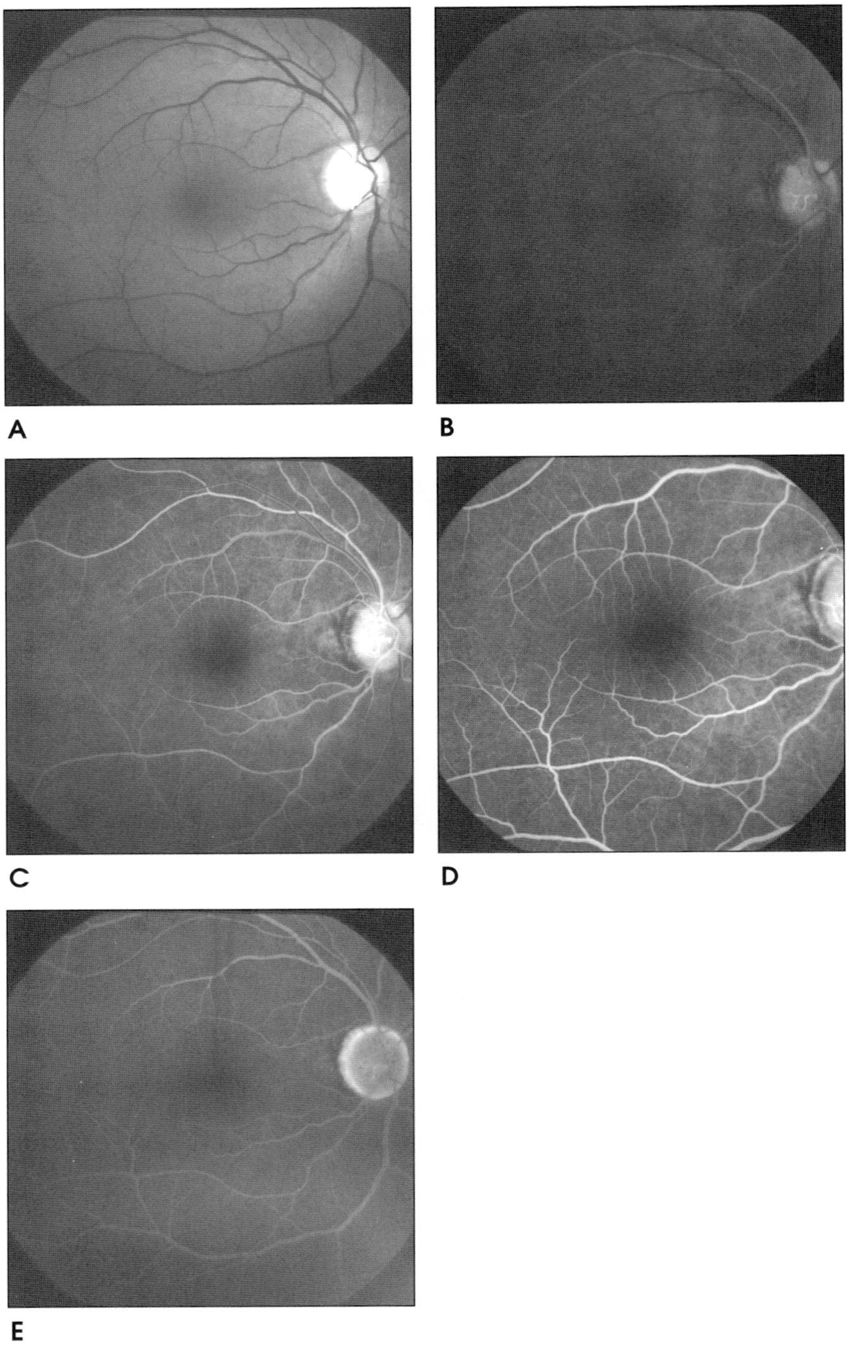

FIGURE 8-10
Normal fluorescein angiogram. A. "Red-free" photograph. B. Choroidal and early arterial phase. "Patchy," deep (on stereo) fluorescence characteristic of choroidal filling can be seen in the posterior pole. In the cup of the optic nerve an arteriole fills with the choroid and is a "cilioretinal" artery. Although the choroidal circulation is the first to fill, the delay in dye appearance in the retinal circulation is very small. Fluorescein is already present in other retinal arterioles but is not yet present in the venous system. C. Arteriovenous phase. Dye is now beginning to enter the veins and shows a laminar type of flow pattern. D. Venous phase. The intensity of the dye is greater in the veins than the arteries. E. Recirculation phase. Overall fluorescence decreases in intensity and tends to be equal in arteries and veins. (Normal fluorescein angiogram provided by Ophthalmic Imaging Systems, Inc.)

seconds, depending on the individual. The fluorescence that first appears in the eye is from the *choroidal* circulation. A diffuse or patchy choroidal filling can sometimes be seen immediately before the appearance of dye in the retinal circulation (Figure 8-10B). Any sense of structure in the choroid is quickly lost as dye rapidly diffuses from the fenestrated capillaries of the choriocapillaris into the surrounding tissue matrix. A retinal artery supplied from the choroid ("cilioretinal artery") provides blood to a portion of the macula as a normal bilateral anatomic variation in 15% of individuals, and up to 30% of eyes.[14] When present, cilioretinal vessels will fill with the choroidal circulation.

After the appearance of dye in the choroid, it next enters the retinal arteries (*arterial* phase), followed very rapidly by the veins over the next 1–2 seconds, the *arteriovenous* phase. Initially dye does not fill the veins but is visible along the edge of the vessel walls in a very characteristic pattern (Figure 8-10C). This pattern is a result of laminar flow of blood in the vessel. As anyone who fishes for trout knows, water (or blood) flows through a stream (or blood vessel) in one of two patterns—either laminar or turbulent. "In laminar flow, all the molecules of water move parallel to each other in a single direction. In turbulent flow, there are countless little eddies and whirlpools that move the water in all directions as the main current moves downstream."[15] When dye moves from the smaller venous branches into the peripheral "lamina" of fluid along the wall of the larger veins, it tends to move in a position that stays in constant relation to the vessel wall. After a short period of time, however, there is sufficient mixing of dye to cause the entire vessel to fluoresce.

In a normal eye, the central macula appears to be less fluorescent than surrounding tissue (Figure 8-11A). The decreased fluorescence is a consequence of two features of normal anatomy shown schematically in Figure 8-11B. First, retinal blood vessels are not found in a circular area approximately 500 microns (0.5 mm) in size in the center of the macula. This region is called the *foveal avascular zone* (FAZ) and includes the fovea, a specialized retinal section that contains a higher concentration of cones. The FAZ is responsible for the sharpest vision and is important to the clinician because it is a guide in laser treatment. In some individuals the perifoveal capillaries cannot be well visualized, but failure to do so does not necessarily indicate an abnormality. In addition to an absence of dye in retinal vessels in the FAZ, dye in the underlying choroid is not well visualized because the RPE contains a higher amount of pigment here compared to other regions.

As the angiogram progresses to the *venous* phase, fluorescence fills the veins and decreases in intensity in the arteries (Figure 8-10D). In the *recirculation* phase, dye that has already exited the eye through the venous system reenters, and the intensity of fluorescence in the arteries and veins is approximately equal (Figure 8-10E). Subsequently the overall intensity of fluorescence continues to decrease—the *late* phase—as dye is further diluted and excreted.

Abnormal Fluorescein Angiogram

Initially it is useful to characterize the findings in the abnormal fluorescein angiogram using the "second level" of clinical information discussed previously—concentrate on what differs from normal. With this starting point for analyzing a fluorescein angiogram, one must learn to recognize variations from the normal patterns as areas of either decreased fluorescence (*hypofluorescent*) or increased fluorescence (*hyperfluorescent*) (Table 8-4). A hypofluorescent area may be due either to an absence of dye or blockage of the dye by some other material such as blood (Figure 8-12A). A hyperfluorescent area compared to a normal eye can be due to an increase in the amount of dye, termed either *staining*, *pooling*, or *leakage*, or to better visualization of a "normal" amount of dye (window defects) (Figure 8-12B). Clinical examples can show how the purpose of the test emphasizes aspects of technique.

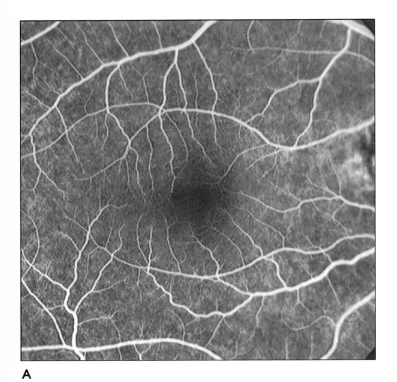

A

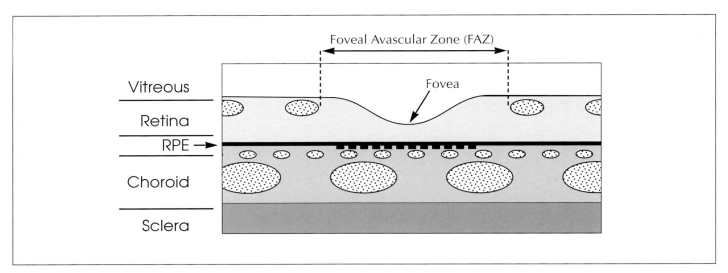

B

FIGURE 8-11
A. Early venous phase fluorescein photograph from a normal patient in which the perifoveal capillaries are well visualized. The dark central area is normal—the foveal avascular zone (FAZ). (Normal fluorescein angiogram provided by Ophthalmic Imaging Systems.) B. Line drawing illustrating the reason for the hypofluorescent central area in the normal macula. Retinal blood vessels are absent in this area, and there is an increase in pigment in the retinal pigment epithelium.

Table 8-4. Abnormal Fluorescein Angiogram Patterns

Hyperfluorescence	Window defect	Hyperfluorescence early, then slow decrease in intensity
		No change in shape or size over time
	Staining	Hyperfluorescence late
		No change in shape or size over time
	Leakage	Early hyperfluorescence with late increased intensity, diffusion, and enlargement of dye
	Pooling	Slowly developing hyperfluorescence with sharply demarcated borders
Hypofluorescence	Filling defects	Results from decreased vessel perfusion, red-free and color photographs may be normal
	Blockage	Material (usually blood) often visible on red-free or color photographs with shape or size corresponding to the area of decreased fluorescence

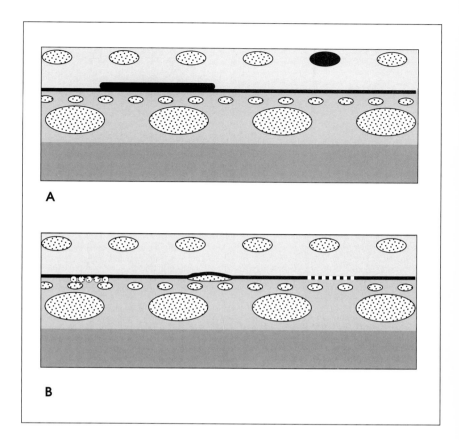

A

B

FIGURE 8-12
Line drawing illustrating hypofluorescent (A) and
hyperfluorescent (B) areas. A. Opaque material such
as blood prevents visualization of underlying fluorescein and is described as blocked fluorescence.
Absence of dye in normal structures can occur with
closure or obstruction of blood vessels. B. Three reasons for hyperfluorescence: absorption of dye by
drusen (staining), pooling of dye, and window defect.

A common cause of a window defect is loss of pigment in the RPE in
ARMD. The pigment loss allows visualization of the normal amount of dye
in the choroid as it moves beneath the RPE. A window defect is characterized by early hyperfluorescence during the choroidal phase, followed by a
progressive decrease in fluorescence through the later phases of the
angiogram as the choroid empties. An important characteristic is that the
shape of the defect is unchanged. Another cause of hyperfluorescence is
referred to as staining. Staining is the uptake of dye by a structure, usually
drusen that are abnormal deposits in Bruch's membrane common in ARMD.
Objects that stain behave the opposite of window defects—that is, drusen
are not particularly hyperfluorescent in early stages, but as the angiogram
progresses they become increasingly brighter. They are similar to a window
defect in that their size and shape generally do not change (Figure 8-13).

Remember that normal retinal blood vessels do not leak fluorescein
because of their tight junctions, and that although the choriocapillaris normally will leak, the RPE is a barrier that prevents dye from entering the retina. Retinal blood vessels or RPE that have been damaged by disease and
abnormal blood vessels that grow in response to certain disease processes
(neovascularization) leak fluorescein, which then accumulates in the tissue
space. Leakage and pooling are somewhat similar terms, as both refer to
hyperfluorescence caused by an increased amount of dye. Leakage is used
in any situation in which dye appears in an area where it is not normally
observed. Fluorescence increases in intensity and spreads diffusely during
the angiogram. The change in size and shape of the hyperfluorescence is
important in distinguishing this abnormal pattern from window defects or
staining where the pattern does not change, only the intensity. Leakage may

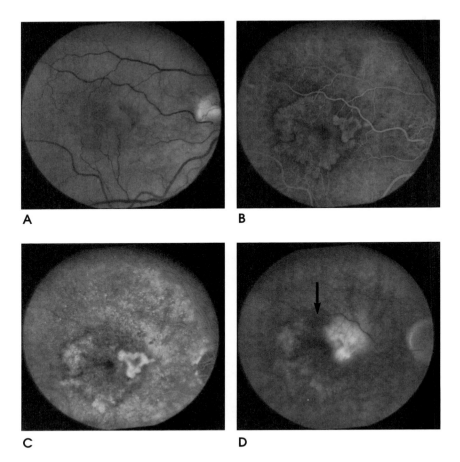

FIGURE 8-13
Clinical examples of hyperfluorescence. A. Fundus photograph of right macula of patient with macular degeneration. B. Early phase of angiogram shows a wide area of hyperfluoresence. C. In the midphase, hypofluorescence decreases in the center and increases on the edges. D. In the late phase the hyperfluorescence at the nasal edge diffuses and increases in intensity (leakage). Hyperfluorescence continues to decrease temporal to this, behaving as a window defect (arrow).

be from normal retinal blood vessels that have been damaged, abnormal blood vessels that have grown (retinal or subretinal neovascularization), or from damage to the RPE. Pooling is a type of leakage in which dye accumulates in a confined anatomic space—for example, intraretinal (cystoid macular edema), subretinal, or sub-RPE space. Because of the physical confinement of the dye, the edges of the hyperfluorescent area tend to be more sharply defined, and the fluorescence increases slowly because the dye is moving into a reservoir of fluid. The case presented in Figure 8-14 is interesting, because it demonstrates leakage from subretinal neovascularization, as well as pooling in an adjacent RPE detachment.

Hyperfluorescence due to dynamic stress on pre-existing normal pathways is often seen in vein occlusions. Figure 8-15 demonstrates dilated, normal vessels secondary to a central vein occlusion resulting in macular edema. The dilated vessels on the optic nerve are called shunt vessels and can be distinguished from neovascularization of the disc because shunt vessels will not leak in contrast to new vessels that leak profusely. In this particular case perfusion is fairly good—that is, we can see fluorescein in the perifoveal capillaries—and the patient is classified as having a nonischemic vein occlusion. In other cases the retina may be poorly perfused, resulting in hypofluorescent areas, indicating an ischemic vein occlusion.

Earlier in the chapter we examined two cases of hyperfluorescence due to the growth of abnormal vessels under the retina in ARMD—that is, choroidal neovascularization and subretinal neovascularization. The example also showed the progressive increase in fluorescein intensity and spread characteristic of leaky vessels. Another type of hyperfluorescence and leakage due to the growth of abnormal blood vessels occurs

FIGURE 8-14
Clinical example of leakage and pooling. A. Photograph of the right disc and macula of a patient with macular degeneration and decreased visual acuity. Hard exudate is apparent. Clinical examination revealed subretinal fluid and a solid elevation of the choroid consistent with a RPE detachment. B. In the early phase of the angiogram the RPE detachment is visualized as a round hypofluorescent area, the result of blockage of choroidal fluorescence by fluid within the detachment. Between the RPE detachment and the disc is an irregular area of early hyperfluorescence. C. A few seconds later the hyperfluorescence adjacent to the disc increases significantly, while only slightly in the RPE detachment. D. Late phase. The RPE detachment is a sharply demarcated, slowly filling area of hyperfluorescence due to pooling of dye within the confined space of the detachment. The adjacent choroidal neovascularization is visualized as an area of early hyperfluorescence and diffuse leakage in the subretinal and intraretinal space late in the angiogram.

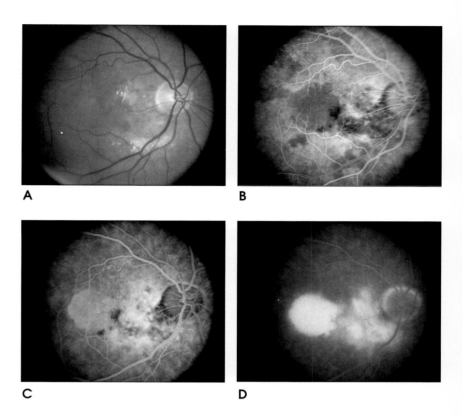

A

B

C

D

FIGURE 8-15
Clinical example of leakage from stressed "normal" retinal vessels. A. Clinical photograph of a central retinal vein occlusion, showing retinal hemorrhage, venous tortuosity, and dilated vessels on the optic nerve. B. At 20 seconds, laminar flow is still visible in the superotemporal vein. Capillary nonperfusion is mild. C. Late-stage fluorescein demonstrates diffuse leakage in the posterior pole and development of cystoid macular edema. Compare to a normal fellow eye in late phase (D). Also note "blocked" fluorescence by retinal hemorrhage in the fluorescein angiogram.

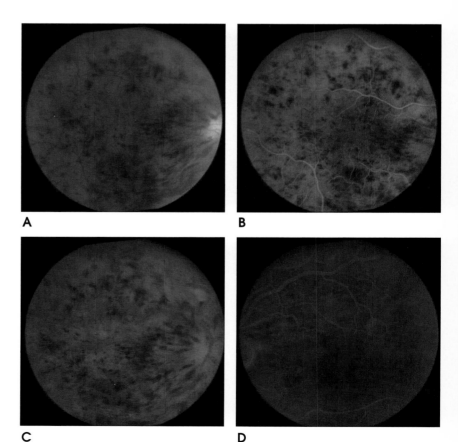

A

B

C

D

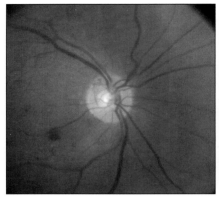
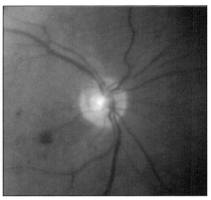

A

B

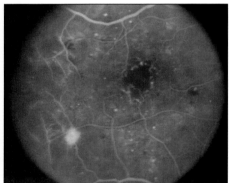
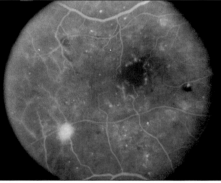
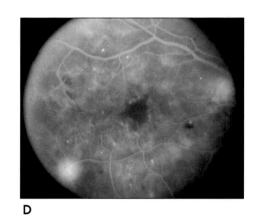

C

D

FIGURE 8-16
Clinical example of leakage from abnormal vessels, resulting in retinal neovascularization. A. Rubeosis iridis. The neovascular process is caused by ischemia that involves the retina. Color photograph provides baseline image for follow-up to help assess response of the eye to laser treatment. B. Stereo fundus photograph showing elevated NVD. C. Stereo pair from fluorescein demonstrates hypofluorescence due to severe loss of perifoveal capillaries—that is, ischemia. Elevated NVE are visible in the lower left and are beginning to leak into the vitreous. D. Single image showing late fluorescein leakage from NVE and NVD. Anterior segment photographs, fundus photographs, and the fluorescein angiogram all play an important role in assessing the amount of damage to the eye from the disease process and in following the response to treatment.

when the vessels grow from the retinal circulation as in proliferative diabetic retinopathy. Figure 8-16 is an example of diffusion of dye into the vitreous due to leakage from NVD and NVE.

Hypofluorescence, an absence of the normal amount of fluorescence, is due to either a decrease in the amount of dye or to an obstacle that prevents visualization of the dye underneath. An example of hypofluorescence due to absence of dye is seen in capillary dropout or ischemia secondary to diabetic retinopathy (Figure 8-17). In ischemia, the capillaries are closed and there simply is no dye to fluoresce. However, in blocked fluorescence, the dye is present but cannot be visualized because of the intervening material (see Figures 8-12A and 8-15B and C).

Summary

The purpose of this chapter has been to provide a framework within which photographers may apply their technical training to help the physician solve a clinical problem. The framework is based on the concept that photographs will be useful more often when the photographer is aware of the purpose of the photograph and is actively seeking specific changes, not

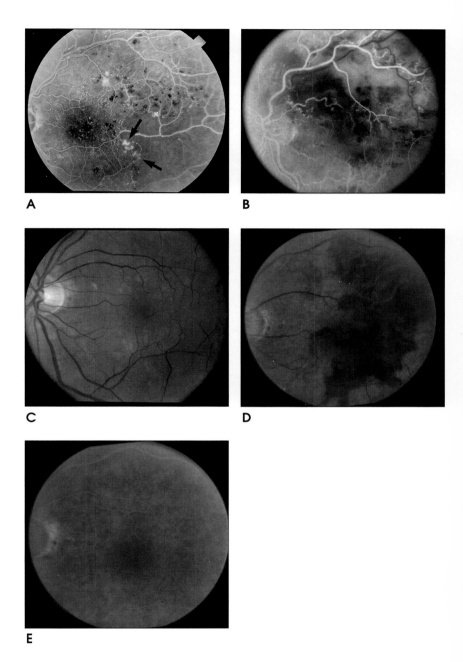

FIGURE 8-17
Clinical examples of hypofluorescence due to nonperfusion. A. Arteriovenous phase of fluorescein angiogram in a diabetic patient demonstrating capillary closure/nonperfusion in field 3 (temporal to FAZ). Arrows point to stumps of closed vessels on several dilated capillaries. B. Early frame from a patient with a superotemporal branch vein occlusion shows a large area of retinal nonperfusion distal to a section of blockage by retinal hemorrage. C, D, E. Because of the multiple ciliary arteries supplying the choroid and the interconnection of lobules, choroidal nonperfusion is uncommon. A diffuse process may, however, affect the choroidal circulation. The three frames here are from a patient who complained of "blotchy" vision and was referred with a diagnosis of impending macular hole. However, the fundus photograph shows several cotton wool spots indicating ischemia. The early phase of the fluorescein angiogram is remarkable for severe delay in filling of the choroid. On further questioning, the patient did admit to recent headaches, which lead to an evaluation for and confirmation of temporal arteritis. Temporal arteritis results in closure of vessels due to inflammation and is a diffuse process.

passively recording events. The ability to apply photographic technique in this manner requires an understanding of normal ocular anatomy, normal and abnormal fluorescein patterns, and clinical information and experience. Table 8-5 is included as a "jump start" for beginning and intermediate photographers who want to achieve this goal. It truly is a pleasure to have the photographer as an active participant on the medical care team.

Table 8-5. Disease-Specific Fundus Photography and Fluorescein Angiography

Age-related macular degeneration

Nonexudative	Colors	Drusen, pigment change. Severity of disease, absence of fluid or hemorrhage, change with time.
	Location	RPE disease; macula.
	FA	May be required to ensure absence of CNV.
	Other	
Exudative	Colors	Document subretinal fluid or hemorrhage in macula, response to treatment.
	Location	RPE disease; macula.
	FA	Demonstrate CNV; imaging of FAZ important for treatment. Used to decide if treatable and then to guide laser treatment. Occasionally diagnostic.
	Other	Stereo FA is very important—required for accurate diagnosis of CNV. The pattern alone is insufficient.

Artery occlusion

Colors	Retinal edema, possibly an embolus in an arteriole. May look normal weeks after the event.
Location	Retinovascular disease. Any field.
FA	To assess restoration of perfusion and ischemia, and determine prognosis. Include disc in field.
Other	

Acute multifocal posterior placoid pigment epitheliopathy (AMPPE)

Colors	Acute lesions are flat and white; resolve without pigment changes. (see Serpiginous Choroiditis)
Location	RPE/choroid; Posterior pole.
FA	Acute lesions block early in the study with late staining.
Other	

Birdshot

Colors	Retinal edema, papilledema, depigmented areas, progressing to numerous deeply depigmented patches showing choroidal vessels.
Location	RPE/choroid. Depigmentation scattered in posterior pole, often sparing macula.
FA	Macular edema may be present. Early choroidal lesions not visible.
Other	

Central serous retinopathy

Colors	Fluid under RPE and/or neurosensory retina.
Location	RPE; Macula.
FA	Occasionally to rule out choroidal neovascularization. Occasionally to guide treatment in recurrent, persistent, or bilateral cases.
Other	Stereo is important since leak is deep. Also can show elevation of neurosensory retina. Document with green filter.

Choroidal nevus/tumor

Colors	Document extent of lesion. Assessment of growth. Assist diagnosis in some cases. Red filter may help define borders and assist in focusing.
Location	Choroid; any field. A choroidal lesion but may be highly elevated; focus on base of lesion for extent, apex of lesion to indicate depth. Wide-angle view may be useful.
FA	May be used to image tumor vascularization.
Other	Stereo helpful to give some indication of elevation; differential focusing for stereo.

Coats disease

Colors	Serous retinal detachment; often massive amounts of hard exudate.
Location	Retinovascular disease; macula or periphery.
FA	Diagnostic. Demonstrates areas of involvement with irregular vessel dilation, leakage, and nonperfusion.
Other	Wide angle may be useful. May require FA during EUA for young children.

Cytomegalovirus retinitis

Colors	Retinal hemorrhage, multiple gray and white retinal lesions in active disease. Progresses to area of atrophic retina with underlying RPE disturbance. Wide angle useful.
Location	Retinitis; any field.
FA	
Other	

Diabetic retinopathy

Nonproliferative	Colors	Microaneurysms, retinal hemorrhage, hard exudate, cotton wool spots, edema. Assists in determining progression of change, decision to proceed with focal laser treatment of macula, assessing response to treatment.
	Location	Retinovascular disease. FAZ most important since indication for treatment is HE or thickening that involves or threatens it. May use other fields to document severe NPDR or IRMA, which indicate a higher progression to PDR.
	FA	Important in distinguishing edema from other causes or vision loss due to ischemia. Imaging of FAZ important to guide treatment.
	Other	Stereo very important in colors and FL to help assessment of thickening.
Proliferative	Colors	Status of NV, progression, response to retinal photocoagulation. Condition of macula can be crucial, since traction by fibrous tissue important in proceeding to surgery.
	Location	Retinovascular disease. Can be any field, at the edge of a field or elevated or obscured by hemorrhage.
	FA	May demonstrate unsuspected NV. Occasionally used to assess amount of ischemia.
	Other	Stereo can be important for evaluation of NV or macula.

Glaucoma

	Colors	Cupping, disc notches, splinter hemorrhages.
	Location	Stereo pairs of optic discs.
	FA	Not applicable.
	Other	Clinician following cup-to-disc ratio.

Juvenile macular degeneration

Flecked retina	Colors	Deep RPE changes or deposits.
	Location	Macula, mid-periphery.
	FA	Silent choroid in Stargardt's disease and fundus flavimaculatus; diagnostic.
	Other	

Macroaneurysm

	Colors	Serous retinal detachment, retinal edema, hard exudate; retinal, subretinal, or vitreous hemorrhage.
	Location	Retinovascular disease; posterior pole.
	FA	May leak, be occluded, or obscured by hemorrhage.
	Other	May or may not be treated with laser depending on evidence of bleeding or progressive hard exudate in macula.

Macular holes

	Colors	Status, response to treatment.
	Location	Vitreoretinal interface, but generally with RPE changes. Macula.
	FA	Pattern characteristically a deep window defect. Occasionally mild, late leakage in retina surrounding the hole.
	Other	Stereo, higher magnification; slit-beam photography often useful to demonstrate a full-thickness hole. Occasionally an operculum.

Multiple evanescent white dot syndrome

	Colors	Multiple small, gray-white patches composed of tiny white dots.
	Location	RPE. Posterior pole.
	FA	Late staining, possible disc leakage.
	Other	Dots resolve without residual RPE changes.

Myopic macular degeneration

	Colors	Pigment disturbance, lacquer cracks, possible hemorrhage; document severity of changes.
	Location	Macula.
	FA	Rule out choroidal neovascularization in a patient with hemorrhage.
	Other	Important for level of leakage. May need plus diopter focusing range.

Ocular histoplasmosis syndrome
(and simulating disorders: multifocal choroiditis and panuveitis, punctate inner choroidopathy)

	Colors	Document deep RPE changes, chorioretinal scar.
	Location	Choroid. Macula, mid-periphery.
	FA	Imaging of FAZ with suspected choroidal neovascularization. Guide treatment of choroidal neovascularization if present.
	Other	

Post-cataract cystoid macular edema

	Colors	Mild macular edema may be difficult to show.
	Location	Retinovascular disease; macula.
	FA	Diagnostic. Rule out choroidal neovascularization, other patterns of leakage in FAZ. Bilateral late disc photos helpful.
	Other	Stereo important to demonstrate leakage from the retina.

Table 8-5. (continued)

Preretinal membranes

	Colors	Demonstrate amount of retinovascular distortion. Used to study anatomy in presurgical evaluation.
	Location	Vitreoretinal interface; macula. Blue or green filters may highlight NFL changes.
	FA	Helpful to assess amount of retinovascular distortion and presence of edema. Rarely will demonstrate another diagnosis such as occult choroidal neovascularization or branch vein occlusion.
	Other	Stereo extremely helpful. High magnification may be useful.

Pseudoxanthoma elasticum

	Colors	Angioid streaks.
	Location	Choroid; posterior pole.
	FA	May be needed for CNV.
	Other	

Serpiginous choroiditis

	Colors	Acute lesions are flat and white; resolve with extensive RPE changes (see AMPPE)
	Location	RPE/choroid; peripapillary.
	FA	CNV not infrequent.
	Other	

Temporal arteritis

	Colors	Show swollen or pale disc in optic neuropathy.
	Location	Disc, posterior pole.
	FA	Delayed filling of choroid helpful in diagnosis in absence of prior ischemic optic neuritis.
	Other	

Trauma/retinal detachment/choroidal detachment

	Colors	May be photographed for documentation.
	Location	May require external or slit-lamp photography.
	FA	Chorioretinal shunts may develop.
	Other	

Vein occlusion

	Colors	Document quadrants involved with hemorrhage, evidence of ischemia (e.g. cotton wool spots), macular edema, presence of NV or vitreous hemorrhage. Treatment decision for macular edema based on FA and visual acuity (VA). Patients with VA 20/40 or worse due to macular edema with good perfusion are candidates for focal laser in BRVO.
	Location	Retinovascular disease; any field. NV may be elevated.
	FA	Imaging of FAZ for treatment. In BRVO wide angle or "survey FA" to assess ischemia in CRVO.
	Other	

RPE = retinal pigment epithelium; FA = fluorescein angiography; CNV = choroidal neovascularization; FAZ = foveal avascular zone; EUA = exam under anesthesia; HE = hard exudate; NPDR = nonproliferative diabetic retinopathy; IRMA = intraretinal microvascular anomalies; PDR = proliferative diabetic retinopathy; NV = neovascularization; NFL = nerve fiber layer; BRVO = branch vein occlusion; CRVO = central retinal vein occlusion.

References

1. Gass J, Donald M. *Stereoscopic Atlas of Macular Diseases Diagnosis and Treatment* (3rd ed). St. Louis: Mosby, 1987;1.
2. Schatz H. Fluorescein Angiography: Basic Principles and Interpretation. In AP Schachat, RP Murphy, A Patz (eds), *Medical Retina*. St. Louis: Mosby, 1989;3.
3. Covey SR. *The 7 Habits of Highly Effective People*. New York: Simon & Schuster, 1989;98.
4. Isselbacher KJ, Braunwald E, Wilson JD, et al. (eds). *Harrison's Principles of Internal Medicine* (13th ed). New York: McGraw-Hill, 1994;2.
5. Diabetic Retinopathy Study Research Group. Indications for photocoagulation treatment of diabetic retinopathy, DRS Report No. 14. *Int Ophthalmol Clin* 1987;27:239.
6. Early Treatment of Diabetic Retinopathy Study Research Group. Photocoagulation for diabetic macular edema, ETDRS Report No. 1. *Arch Ophthalmol* 1985;103:1796.
7. Macular Photocoagulation Study Group. Krypton laser photocoagulation for idiopathic neovascular lesions: results of a randomized clinical trial. *Arch Ophthalmol* 1990;108:832.
8. Macular Photocoagulation Study Group. Persistent and recurrent neovascularization after laser photocoagulation for subfoveal choroidal neovascularization of age-related macular degeneration. *Arch Ophthalmol* 1994;112:489.
9. Branch Vein Occlusion Study Group. Argon laser scatter photocoagulation for prevention of neovascularization and vitreous hemorrhage in branch vein occlusion: a randomized clinical trial. *Arch Ophthalmol* 1986;104:34.

10. Branch Vein Occlusion Study Group. Argon laser photocoagulation for macular edema in branch vein occlusion. *Am J Ophthalmol* 1984;98:271.

11. The Miami Study Group. Cystoid macular edema in aphakic and pseudophakic eyes. *Am J Ophthalmol* 1979;88:45.

12. Nussbaum JJ, Pruett RC, Delori FC. Historic perspectives—macular yellow pigment: the first 200 years. *Retina* 1982;1:296.

13. Hayreh S. The choriocapillaris. *Albrecht v Graefes Arch klin exp Ophthal* 1974;192:165.

14. Justice J Jr, Lehmann RP. Cilioretinal arteries: a study based on review of stereo fundus photographs and fluorescein angiographic findings. *Arch Ophthalmol* 1976;94:1355.

15. Rosenbauer T. *Reading Trout Streams. An Orvis Guide.* New York: Lyons & Burford, 1988, 10.

Chapter 9

Fundus Photography: Descriptive Interpretation

Patrick J. Saine and Timothy J. Martin

Introduction

Examining your initial fundus photographs is a bit like reviewing travel snapshots taken in a foreign land. You'll remember having taken the trip (the photographs in front of you are proof that you were there), and yet the images seem strangely different. Upon reviewing them, you will discover new shapes, colors, and details that you may have failed to notice at the moment of exposure. And the more you study the images—the more you'll see!

This chapter uses fundus images of common retinal characteristics to orient you to the new landscape you will be photographing. Our intention is a short introduction to the visual characteristics of the normal and diseased fundus; this chapter is not meant to be a comprehensive guide to retinal abnormalities. You can learn more about the retina by reviewing your clinical photographs with your referring physician, by studying a comprehensive fundus atlas, and by attending continuing education seminars in ophthalmic photography. A greater understanding of the eye in normal and diseased states will enhance your fundus photography results.

Landmarks in the normal fundus and its variations begin the chapter. Abnormal maculae and optic discs are described, as are vascular abnormalities and various types of hemorrhages. We conclude with a potpourri of retinal abnormalities and a look at fundus photographs after retinal surgery.

The Normal Fundus

The easiest fundus landmark for orientation is the optic disc (Figure 9-1). This somewhat oval, pink structure is located nasally to the central visual axis. The optic disc is made up of a number of elements entering or leaving the eye:

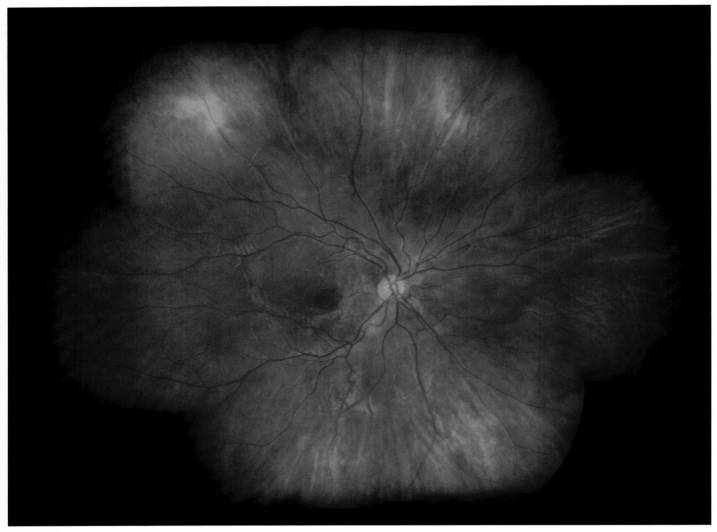

FIGURE 9-1
Normal fundus (a FundusMap, a multi-image computer composite photo-illustration by Richard E. Hackel).

1. *Blood vessels*: The central retinal artery emerges from the center of the disc and immediately divides to deliver blood to the four quadrants of the retina. The superior and inferior temporal branches (arcades) sweep around the fovea and roughly define the macula. The retinal veins form a similar pattern as they exit the eye at the optic disc. The optic disc can therefore always be found by tracing these vessels to their point of convergence.
2. *Axons (nerves):* The optic disc contains more than a million axons; these "wires" are cell processes that begin throughout the inner retina and sweep toward the optic disc, making a right-angle turn to exit the eye on their way to the brain. The fine capillaries that support these axons give the disc its pink color. These axons—"end on"—make up the neural rim of the optic disc, which in most individuals surrounds a central, whitish depression of variable size (the optic cup).

The optical center of the retina is the fovea. Photoreceptors are highly concentrated here to deliver the sharpest, clearest vision. The fovea is centered between the temporal vascular arcades and can be identified as a circular pigmented area slightly larger than the disc. The large number

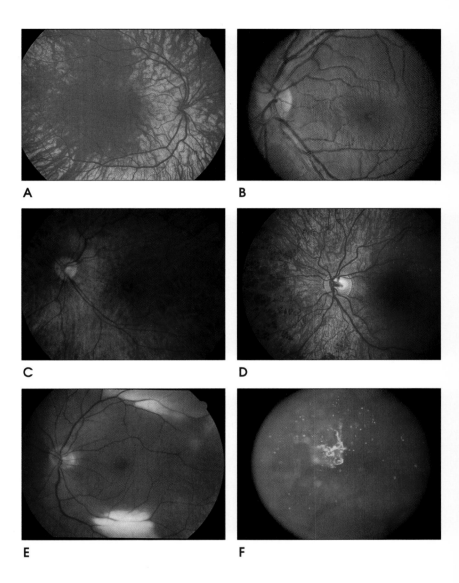

FIGURE 9-2
Normal variations. A. Blonde fundus. B. Highly pigmented retinal pigment epithelium (RPE). C. Tigroid fundus shows variations in RPE. D. Congenital hypertrophy of the RPE. E. Myelinated nerve fiber layer. F. Asteroid hyalosis.

of axons extending radially from the center of the fovea cause a mound of increased retinal thickness, often identified by circular light reflexes on the smooth, innermost transparent retinal layer (the internal limiting membrane). To provide the clearest optical performance, axons from the temporal retina are carefully routed around the fovea. This strategy is the basis of the arc-shaped pattern of the nerve fiber layer. The axons can often be seen as fine striations sweeping toward the disc, especially above and below the disc, where the nerve fiber layer is thickest.

In lightly pigmented patients, the deeper choroidal circulation is evident. These vessels have a more random pattern and do not normally communicate with retinal vessels.

The Fundus: Normal Variations

The pigmentation (and thus transparency) of the retinal pigment epithelium (RPE) may vary considerably among normal individuals, generally correlating with the degree of pigmentation elsewhere (skin, hair). Thus, in the blonde fundus, the choroidal vessels are easily seen (Figure 9-2A). In darkly pigmented individuals, all choroidal details are hidden by the relatively opaque RPE (Figure 9-2B) In some subjects, there may be marked variations of pigmentation within the same fundus (Figure 9-2C).

Congenital hypertrophy of the RPE (Figure 9-2D) appears as characteristic areas of darkly pigmented "spots." This finding does not cause visual symptoms but is important because it must be distinguished from melanoma or other pigmented fundus lesions.

As the axons exit the eye, they acquire an insulating coating (myelin), which increases the speed and efficiency of data transfer. Occasionally, otherwise normal individuals will show aberrant myelinization of axons in the nerve fiber layer, producing the feathery, superficial, white areas, extending along the path of the nerve fiber layer (Figure 9-2E).

In asteroid hyalosis, opaque white concretions are scattered throughout the vitreous. Despite their impressive appearance, they generally do not cause visual symptoms, although they can interfere with visualization of the retina (Figure 9-2F).

The Posterior Pole

As opposed to the water-tight retinal vessels, the vessels in the choriocapillaris are inherently "leaky," though the RPE prevents this fluid from entering the subretinal space by providing the outer blood-retinal barrier. Bruch's membrane is a complex layer between the RPE and the choroid and is composed of elements from the base of the RPE and the choriocapillaris. A number of diseases damage Bruch's membrane and the RPE. In age-related macular degeneration (ARMD), fluid may collect under the RPE, appearing as "soft drusen" (Figure 9-3A). Fluid also collects under the RPE in central serous retinopathy, a disease of young patients, and breaks through the RPE to collect under the neurosensory retina (Figure 9-3B). Discontinuities in Bruch's membrane occur in many clinical entities, allowing choroidal vessels to grow into the sub-RPE and subretinal space (subretinal neovascular membrane). ARMD is a common cause of subretinal neovascularization and hemorrhage (Figure 9-3C).

Myopic individuals of any age may also develop choroidal neovascular membranes. It is thought that in such large, myopic eyes, Bruch's membrane is stretched tenously thin (as suggested by the failure of the RPE to reach completely to the disc margin, resulting in a "myopic halo" around the disc), and is prone to breakage (Figure 9-3D).

Many different diseases may cause the retinal vessels to become leaky, allowing blood components to seep into the deep retinal tissues. As the fluid portion resorbs, chalky-white hard exudates or "edema residues" are left behind. In the fovea, the dense radiating axons (Henle's nerve fiber layer) enclose the edema and create radial or wedge-shaped patterns. In other areas, rings of edema residue encircle the leaky spots (Figure 9-3E). Diabetic retinopathy is a very common cause of hard exudates.

Many ocular disorders may be associated with the growth of membranes at the innermost level of the retina. Contraction of these membranes results in macular pucker, or wrinkling, distorting vision (Figure 9-3F).

The Optic Disc

In glaucoma, visual field defects result from axonal death. Axonal loss can be identified in the fundus as loss of the nerve fiber layer striations and enlargement of the central cup in the optic disc (Figure 9-4A). In other forms of optic atrophy, the optic cup may remain unchanged, but

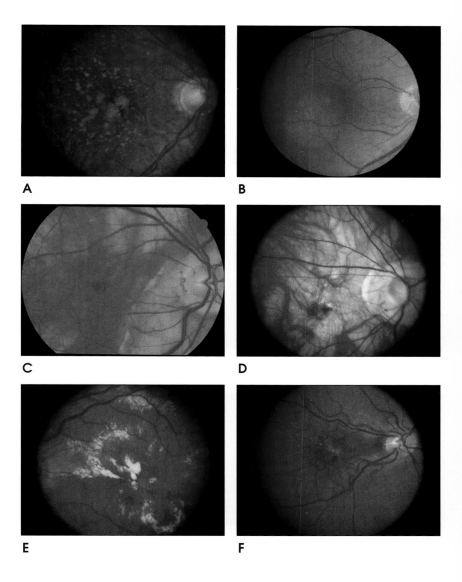

FIGURE 9-3
The posterior pole. A. Age-related macular degeneration with soft drusen. B. Central serous chorioretinopathy. C. Subretinal neovascularization. D. Myopic halo or scleral crescent. E. Circinate retinopathy. F. Epiretinal membrane.

other forms of optic atrophy, the optic cup may remain unchanged, but the normally pink neural rim becomes pale (Figure 9-4B).

Acute disorders of the optic disc often result in swelling of the axons or supporting tissue, causing elevation of the disc and blurring of the disc margins (Figure 9-4C). The cerebrospinal fluid that bathes the brain and spinal column also surrounds the optic nerve right up to the globe. Intracranial diseases can raise the pressure of this fluid and can cause bilateral disc swelling. Other common causes of disc swelling include anterior ischemic optic neuropathy and optic neuritis.

The optic disc may also be elevated by rock candy–like hyaline material buried in the axons of the optic disc. Visual field loss can occasionally result, but the finding is usually benign. In older individuals, this refractive material can often be seen poking through the surface of the disc (Figure 9-4D). In young patients, the material may be completely buried, and the disc elevation may be difficult to distinguish from true disc swelling (Figure 9-4E).

Congenital malformations of the optic disc (such as this optic nerve coloboma) can result in bizarre appearances with variable visual disfunction (Figure 9-4F).

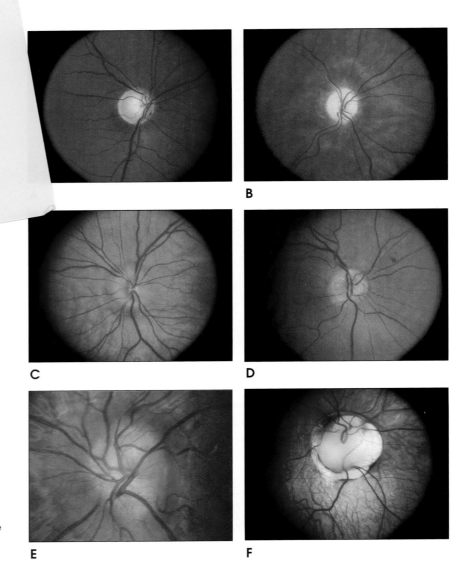

FIGURE 9-4
The optic disc. A. Glaucomatous optic nerve.
B. Optic atrophy. C. Optic disc edema. D. Drusen of
the optic nerve. E. Buried drusen. F. Coloboma of the
optic nerve.

Vascular Abnormalities

Infarction of the retina can occur if intravascular material lodges in the central retinal artery or its branches. Hollenhorst plaques are cholesterol crystals that commonly originate in the large carotid arteries in the neck and can be seen as glistening white, refractile material, often at arterial bifurcations (Figure 9-5A). More proximal blockage of the central retinal artery can be identified acutely as an opaque, pale, macular swelling accentuating the choroidal red of the foveola, known as the "cherry red spot." Following infarction, the normally transparent arterial wall becomes opaque, appearing as a ghost vessel (Figure 9-5B).

Retinal ischemia from vascular disorders such as diabetes may incite neovascularization. These new blood vessels grow into the vitreous from the disc (NVD) (Figure 9-5C) or elsewhere (NVE) (Figure 9-5D), resulting in vitreous hemorrhages and traction retinal detachments. A common early sign of ischemic diabetic retinopathy is segmental narrowing of retinal veins, creating venous beading. Figure 9-5E shows venous beading in a patient with radiation retinopathy.

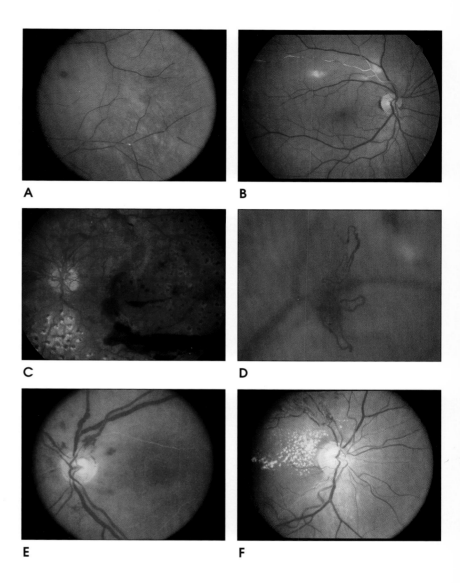

FIGURE 9-5
Vascular abnormalities. A. Hollenhorst plaque.
B. Retinal ghost vessel. C. Neovascularization of the
optic nerve. D. Neovascularization elsewhere (NVE).
E. Venous beading secondary to radiation. F. Arterial-
venous crossing change. (E and F courtesy of Tim
Bennett.)

Systemic hypertension causes stiffening and thickening of the retinal arterial walls, resulting in segmental narrowing, as well as the appearance of venous discontinuity at artery-vein crossings (A-V nicking) (Figure 9-5F).

Retinal Hemorrhages

Hemorrhages may occur at any retinal level. The shape of the hemorrhages is determined by the orientation and shape of the surrounding tissue structures at that level. Blood beneath the sensory retina (subretinal) can separate layers and spread out (Figure 9-6A). Dot and blot hemorrhages are rounded by the deep structures in the retina (Figure 9-6B). The orientation of the nerve fiber layer creates elongated flame-shaped hemorrhages (Figure 9-6C). Blood on the surface of the retina (preretinal) obscures retinal details (Figure 9-6D), with its shape determined by the apposition of the vitreous hyaloid face and the forces of gravity (Figure 9-6E).

Figure 9-6F is a fundus photograph depicting the characteristic trauma-induced hemorrhages that occur in the "shaken baby syndrome."

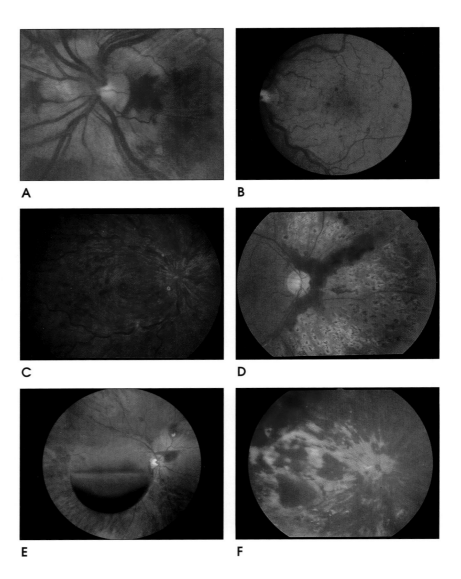

FIGURE 9-6
Retinal hemorrhages. A. Subretinal blood. B. Dot-and-blot hemorrhages. C. Nerve fiber layer hemorrhages. D. Preretinal hemorrhage. E. Boat-shaped hemorrhage. (FundusMap by Richard E. Hackel.) F. Shaken baby syndrome. (F is courtesy of Tim Bennett.)

Retinal Potpourri

Presumed ocular histoplasmosis syndrome (POHS) presents with punched-out chorioretinal scars and peripapillary atrophy (Figure 9-7A). Patients are generally asymptomatic unless they develop a third common finding: macular choroidal neovascualar membranes.

Fluffy, superficial, white "cotton-wool" spots represent swelling and opacification of the nerve fiber layer and may obscure the retinal details. These are likely areas of focal nerve fiber layer ischemia and are common in diabetic, hypertensive, and human immunodeficiency virus (HIV) retinopathy (Figure 9-7B).

A common cause of blindness in HIV-infected patients is cytomegalovirus (CMV) retinitis (Figure 9-7C). Prompt treatment may prevent its progression to multiple retinal holes and retinal detachment.

Choroidal nevi (Figure 9-7D) are similar to moles on the skin. They are common and generally benign but must be distinguished from choroidal melanomas.

Angioid streaks are radial cracks in Bruch's membrane (Figure 9-7E). Because they are red and radiate from the disk, they may be mistaken

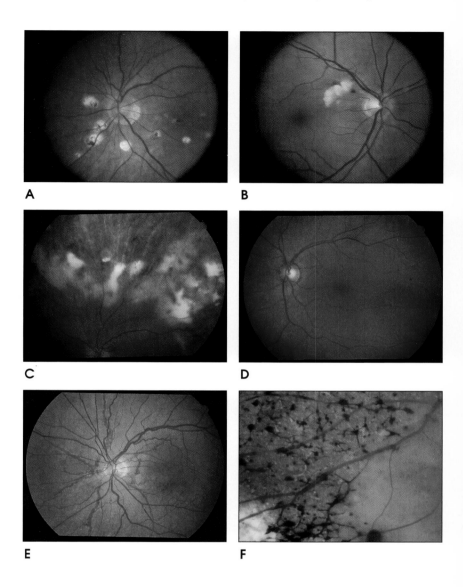

FIGURE 9-7
Other retinal appearances. A. Presumed ocular histo-
plasmosis syndrome (POHS). B. Cotton-wool spots.
C. Cytomegalovirus (CMV) retinitis. D. Choroidal nevi.
E. Angioid streaks. F. Retinitis pigmentosa.

for blood vessels (thus, "angioid"). Choroidal neovascular membranes
may develop.

Retinitis pigmentosa represents a spectrum of retinal degenerative disorders, often characterized by a peculiar "bony spicule" pigmentation of
the peripheral retina (Figure 9-7F).

The Surgical Fundus

Neovascularization in ischemic vascular disorders (especially diabetes)
can frequently be prevented by selective destruction of the ischemic retina with laser photocoagulation. Fresh laser spots appear as pale, "soft"
white spots (Figure 9-8A), with time developing into well-defined white
areas with variable pigmentation (Figure 9-8B).

Macular holes may develop if abnormal vitreous attachment and traction creates a "divot" in the foveola. A cuff of retinal detachment is frequently seen (Figure 9-8C).

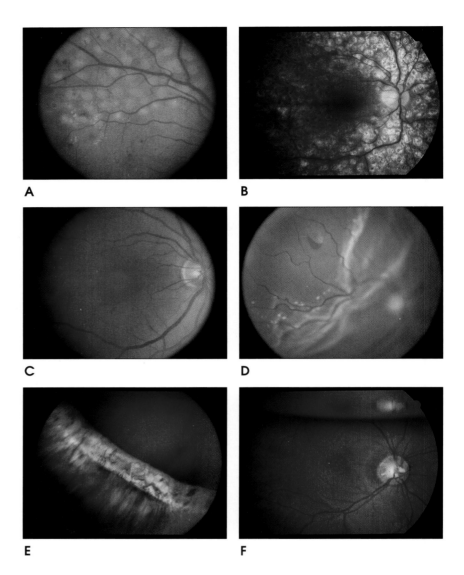

FIGURE 9-8
The surgical fundus. A. Laser treatment. B. Laser treatment with time. C. Macular hole with operculum. D. Retinal detachment. E. Retinal appearance of a scleral buckle. F. Silicone oil vitreous replacement.

Any break in the sensory retina may allow vitreous fluid to seep underneath, causing a retinal detachment (Figure 9-8D). Surgery is required to close the break, often by using an external element to indent the globe beneath the break (Figure 9-8E). In complicated cases, viscous silicone oil may be required to mechanically "steam roller" the retina back into position (Figure 9-8F).

Ophthalmic photography integrates specialized photographic procedures with the clinical needs of the ophthalmologist. As important as fine tuning your technical skills, successful ophthalmic photographers understand how and why their photographs are used.

Appendix A

Abbreviations for the Ophthalmic Photographer

AAO	American Academy of Ophthalmology
AC	anterior chamber
ACL	anterior chamber lens
AIDS	acquired immune deficiency syndrome
AION	anterior ischemic optic neuropathy
ALK	automated lamellar keratoplasty
ALP	argon laser photocoagulation
AMPPE	acute multifocal placoid pigment epitheliopathy
ANV	angle new vessels
APD	afferent pupillary defect
ARMD	age-related macular degeneration
ARN	acute retinal necrosis
ASAP	as soon as possible
ASCC	anterior subcapsular cataract
ASORN	American Society of Ophthalmic Registered Nurses
ATPO	Association of Technical Personnel in Ophthalmology
AVM	anterior venous malformation
BAO	branch artery occlusion
BDR	background diabetic retinopathy
BID	twice a day
BLL	both lower lids
BOPA	British Ophthalmic Photographic Society
BP	blood pressure
BRAO	branch retinal artery occlusion
BRVO	branch retinal vein occlusion
BUL	both upper lids
BVO	branch vein occlusion
C/D	cup to disk ratio
CAO	central artery occlusion
Cat.	cataract
CC	color correction (filter)
CC	cubic centimeters
$\overline{C}C$	with correction
CD-ROM	compact disk-read only memory
CF	count fingers
CME	cystoid macular edema
CMV	cytomegalovirus
CNVM	choroidal neovascular membrane
COA	certified ophthalmic assistant
COAG	chronic open-angle glaucoma
COMS	Collaborative Ocular Melanoma Study
COMT	certified ophthalmic master technician
COPRA	certified ophthalmic photographer and retinal angiographer
COT	certified ophthalmic technician
CPR	cardiopulmonary resuscitation
CR	chorioretinal

CRA	central retinal artery
CRA	certified retinal angiographer
CRAO	central retinal artery occlusion
CRVO	central retinal vein occlusion
cSLO	confocal scanning laser ophthalmoscope
CSME	clinically significant macular edema
CSR	central serous retinopathy (choroidopathy)
CVO	central vein occlusion
CVOS	central vein occlusion study
DM	diabetes mellitus
DOB	date of birth
DR	diabetic retinopathy
DRS	Diabetic Retinopathy Study
Dx	diagnosis
ECCE	extracapsular cataract extraction
EI	exposure index
EM	electron microscopy
EOM	extraocular movement
ER	emergency room
ERM	epiretinal membrane
ETDRS	Early Treatment of Diabetic Retinopathy Study
EUA	examination under anesthesia
f/u	follow up
FA	fluorescein angiography
FAZ	foveal avascular zone
FOPS	fellow of the Ophthalmic Photographers' Society
FP	fundus photographs
gtt	drop
H&D	Hurter & Driffield (characteristic curve, film)
HCL	hard contact lens
HIV	human immunodeficiency virus
HM	hand motion
Hx	history
ICCE	intracapsular cataract extraction
ICG	indocyanine green
IDDM	insipidus diabetes mellitus
IN	inferior nasal
INV	iris new vessels
IOFB	intraocular foreign body
IOL	intraocular lens
ION	ischemic optic neuropathy
IOP	intraocular pressure
IR	infrared
IRMA	intraretinal microaneurysm
ISO	International Standards Organization (film speed)
IT	inferior temporal
IV	intravenous
IVFA	intravenous fluorecein angiography
JCAHPO	Joint Commission on Allied Health Personnel in Ophthalmology
JOPS	Japanese Ophthalmic Photographers' Society
JPCNV	juxtapapillary choroidal neovascularization
K	Kelvin (color temperature)
LASIK	laser-assisted in situ keratomileusis
KLPC	krypton laser photocoagulation
LLL	left lower lid
LP	light perception

LUL	left upper lid
MA	microaneurysm
ME	macular edema
ML	milliliters
MM	malignant melanoma
MPS	Macular Photocoagulation Study
N/I	no improvement
N/V	nausea and vomiting
NAG	narrow-angle glaucoma
ND	neutral density
NFL	nerve fiber layer
NL	normal
NLP	no light perception
nm	nanometer
NPDR	nonproliferative diabetic retinopathy
NV	near vision
NV	veovascularization
NVD	neovascularization at the disc
NVE	neovascularization elsewhere
OD	ocular dexter (right eye)
ONH	optic nerve head
OPS	Ophthalmic Photographers' Society
OS	ocular sinister (left eye)
OU	ocular uterque (both eyes)
P/O	postoperative
PA	physician assistant
PC	posterior chamber
PCL	posterior chamber lens
PDR	proliferative diabetic retinopathy
PED	pigment epithelial detachment
PH	pinhole (visual acuity)
PK	penetrating keratoplasty
PO	by mouth
POAG	primary open-angle glaucoma
POHS	presumed ocular histoplasmosis syndrome
PPDR	preproliferative diabetic retinopathy
Pre-op	preoperative
PRK	photoreactive keratectomy
PRM	preretinal membrane
PRMF	preretinal macular fibrosis
prn	as needed
PRP	panretinal photocoagulation
PSC	posterior subcapsular cataract
PTK	photo-therapeutic keratectomy
PVD	posterior vitreous detachment
PXE	pseudo-xanthoma elasticum
QD	every day
QH	every hour
QID	four times a day
R/O	rule out
RAM	random access memory
RD	retinal detachment
RK	radial keratotomy
RLF	retrolental fibroplasia
RLL	right lower lid
ROM	read only memory
ROP	retinopathy of prematurity

RP	retinitis pigmentosa
RPE	retinal pigment epithelium
RPED	retinal pigment epithelium detachment
RUL	right upper lid
Rx	prescription
S/P	status post
SB	scleral buckle
S̄C	without correction
SCL	soft contact lens
SLO	scanning laser ophthalmoscope
SLR	single lens reflex
SN	superior nasal
SRNV	subretinal neovascularization
SRNVM	subretinal neovasular membrane
ST	superior temporal
STAT	immediately
Sx	symptoms
TAPP	applanation pressure by tonometry
TID	three times a day
TTL	through the lens
Tx	treatment
UV	ultraviolet
Va	visual acuity
WA	wide angle
WNL	within normal limits
Ws	watt seconds
WYSIWYG	"what you see is what you get"

Appendix B

Professional Societies of Interest to the Ophthalmic Photographer

Association Espanola de Technicos Especialistas en Fotografia Cientifica (AETEFC)
Senor Manuel Soler Martinez, President
5 Congreso International de la Imagen Cientifica
Plaza Luc de Tena, No. 13
28045 - Madrid
Spain
Tel: +34 1 539 7768

Biological Photographic Association (BPA)
1819 Peachtree St. NE, Suite 620
Atlanta, GA 30309
Tel: 404-350-7900

British Institute of Professional Photography (BIPP)
Ralph Marshall, Secretary of Medical Group
Fox Talbot House
Amwell End
Mare Herts SG 12 9HN
United Kingdom
Tel: 0920 464011, FAX 0920 487056

British Ophthalmic Photographic Association (BOPA)
c/o Richard Hildred
Medical Imaging
The Priory Hospital
Priory Road
Birmingham B5 7UG
United Kingdom

Deutsche Gesellschaft fur Photographie (DGPh)
Horst Wesche
Unfallchirurgische Klinik
Fotodocumentation
Medizinische Hochschule Hannover
Konstanty-Gutschow-Strasse 8
D-3000 Hannover 61
Germany
Tel: 0511-532-3842

European Federation of the Scientific Image (EFSI)
Jean Pierre Stepanow
12, Rue Forest 13007
Marseille
France
Tel: 91 38 2030

Foreninge fur Medicinsk och Tecknisk Fotografi (FMTF)
Ole Roos
Department of Biomedical Communications
Sahlgren Hospital
413 45 Goteborg
Sweden
Tel: 031 60 2326

Institute of Medical Illustrators (IMI)
Gillian Lee
15 Little Plucketts Way
Buckhurst Hill
Essex Ig9 5QU
United Kingdom
Tel: 081 504 0076

Japanese Ophthalmic Photographers' Society (JOPS)
C/O Chika Kanagami
Department of Ophthalmology
School of Medicine
Kyorin University
6-20-2 Shinkawa Mitaka City
Tpkyo 181
Tel: +81-422-47-5511

Nederlandse Vereniging voor Medische Audiovisuele Communicatie (NV-MAC)
Secretariaat
Schaepmanlaan 17, 5344 BA Oss
Tel: 04120-23357

Ophthalmic Phototographers' Society (OPS)
OPS Membership Office
Barbara J. McCalley
213 Lorene
Nixa, MO 65714
Email: OPSMember@aol.com
Tel: 417-725-0181; 800-403-1677

Royal Photographic Society (RPS)
Andrew Rolland
Department of Medical Photograph
St. George's Hospital
Blackshaw Road
London SW17 0QT
United Kingdom
Tel: 081 672 1255 ext. 51462/56101

Selskabet for Medicinsk of Biologisk (SMBI)
Preben Holst
The John F. Kennedy Institute
Department of Medical Genetics
G1 Landevej 7
Dk-2600 Glostrup
Denmark
Tel: 4245 2228 ex. 224

Societe Francaise d'Iconographie Medicale et Scientifique (SFIMS)
Jean Pierre Delmas
Service Audio-Visual
Faculte de Medecine Lyon Sud
69921 Oullins Cedex
France
Tel: 78 51 0826

Appendix C

Companies of Interest to the Ophthalmic Photographer

General

Agfa, Division of Miles
100 Challenger Road
Ridgefield Park, NJ 07660
201-440-2500

Akorn, Inc.
100 Akorn Drive
Abita Springs, LA 70420
504-893-9300
800-535-7155

Alcon Laboratories, Inc.
6201 South Freeway
Ft. Worth, TX 76134
817-293-0450

Angioloth Premium Films
80 Oak Street
Newton, MA 02164
617-964-6341

Omega/Arkay
191 Shaffer Ave.
Westminster, MD 21157
800-777-6634

Becton Dickinson & Co.
One Becton Drive
Franklin Lakes, NJ 07417-1881
201-847-6800

Byers Industries Inc.
6955 Southwest Sandburg Street
Portland, OR 97223
503-639-0620

Canon USA Inc
1 Canon Plaza
Lake Success, NY 11042-1119
516-328-5000
http://www.usa.canon.com/medical

Ciba Vision Ophthalmics
11460 Johns Creek Pkwy.
Duluth, GA 30136
404-418-4101

Carl Zeiss Canada Ltd.
45 Valleybrook Dr.
Don Mills, ON M3B 2S6
800-387-8037

DA-LITE Screen Co., Inc.
PO Box 137
Warsas, IN 46581-0137
800 622-3737
219-267-8101

Eastman Kodak Co., Inc.
343 State Street
Rochester, NY 14650
800-235-6325
716-724-4349

FUJI Photo Film, USA, Inc.
555 Faxter Road
Elmsford, NY 10523
800-755-3854
914-789-8145

Heidelberg Engineering
5661 Palmer Way, Suite G
Carlsbad, CA 92008
800-931-2230
619-930-3570

Humphrey Instruments, Inc.
(A company of the Carl Zeiss Group)
PO Box 5400
2992 Alvarado Street
San Leandro, CA 94577
800-227-1508
800-341-6968 Customer Service

Ilford Photo Corp.
70 W. Century Road
Paramus, NJ 07653-1490
201-265-6000

Insight Instruments Inc
175 E. Crystal Lake Ave.
Lake Mary, FL 32746
800-255-8354

Interzeag, Inc.
100 Otis St.
Northboro, MA 01532-2438
508-393-5726
800-627-6286

Justice Ophthalmics
825 Ridge Lake Blvd.
Suite 300
Memphis, TN 38120
800-842-1574
901-683-9896

Konica USA, Inc.
440 Sylvan Avenue
Englewood Cliffs, NJ 07602
201-568-3100
800-285-6422

Kowa Optimed, Inc.
20001 South Vermont Avenue
Torrance, CA 90502
800-966-5692
310-327-1913

Laser Diagnostic Technologies, Inc.
9550 Waples St., Suite 105
San Diego, CA 92121
800-722-6393
619-558-9144

New Vision Technology
653 Hutchison Street
Vista, CA 92084
619-941-5500

Nikon Inc. Instrument Group
1300 Walt Whitman Rd.
Melville, NY 11747-3012
516-547-8500

Ophthalmic Imaging Systems, Inc.
221 Lathrop Way, Suite I
Sacramento, CA 95815
800-338-8436
916-646-2020

PAR Technology Corp.
220 Seneca Turnpike
New Hartford, NY 13413
800-448-6505

Polaroid Corp.
575 Technology Square
Cambridge, MA 02139-3587
617-386-2000

Acklands Safety Supply
90 W. Beaver Creek Rd.
Richmond Hill, ON L4B 1E7
905-731-5516

Taylor-Merchant Corp.
212 West 35th Street
New York, NY 10001
800-223-6694
212-757-7700

Technical Enterprises
1401 Bonnie Doone
Corona Del Mar, CA 92625-1717
800-903-8326
714-644-9500

Tomey Technology, Inc.
325 Vassar Street
Cambridge, MA 02139
800-358-6639

TTI Medical
7026 Koll Center Pkwy, Suite 207
Pleasanton, CA 94566-3105
800-322-7373
415-484-0700

Topcon America Corporation
65 West Century Road
Paramus, NJ 07652
800-223-1130
201-261-9450

3M Photo Color Sys. Div.
3M Center
Building 223-4N-11
St. Paul, MN 55144
800-695-3456
612-733-7742

Stereo Supplies and Equipment Manufacturers

3-D Concept
Jon Golden
Roundwood Road Productions
16 Roundwood Road
Newton, MA 02164
617 332-5460
email: JGoldenRRP@aol.com
Products: RBT stereo mounts (4, 5, 7, 8 perf. and full-frame mounts), RBT stereo cameras and projectors

3D-Magazin (German)
Oerter Puett 28
D-45621 Haltern, Germany
+49 (2364) 16107, FAX +49 (2364) 169273
email: 3D-Magazin@stereo.s.bawue.de
Website: http://www.tisco.com/3d-web/3dmag/3dmag.htm
Products: Magazine about stereoscopic imaging. Includes test of stereo equipment (cameras, viewers), book reviews, etc.

Adobe Photoshop
1585 Charleston Road
PO Box 7900
Mountain View, CO 94039-7900
American Paper Optics
2005 Nonconnah Blvd., Suite 27
Memphis TN 38132
910-398-6111, 800-767-8427, FAX 910-398-6119
Products: 3D glasses

American Paper Optics
2005 Nonconnah Blvd., Suite 27

Memphis TN 38132
800 767-8427
Products: stereo glasses: Polaroid, red-blue

Argraph Midwest
PO Box 1556
Elk Grove Village, IL 60007
Products: Samigon Professional Filter Holder

DA-LITE Screen Co. Inc.
PO Box 137
Warsaw, IN 46581-0137
800-622-3737, 219-267-8101; FAX: 219-267-7804
Products: Projection screens

Double Vision 1995
Visual Software, the 3D Software Co.
Woodland Hills, CA
Eastman Kodak Co.
Kodak Park, Rochester, NY 14650
800-242-2424
Products: Projectors (2 × 2)

Heureka! (3D mail order catalog)
Feiedrich-Kahl-Strasse 8
D 60489 Frankfurt am Main, Deutschland (Germany)
069/78 88 88, FAX 069/78 77 77
Products: Books, projectors

Larson Viewer
P. O. Box 0192
Sheboygan, WI 53082
Products: 2 × 2 slide viewer

LenTec Corp.
4850 River Green Parkway
Duluth, GA 30106
404/497-0727
Products: Lenticular prints

New Vision Technology
653 Hutchison Street
Vista, CA 92084
619-941-5500, FAX 619-941-3934; email: ThreeD@ats.com
Products: Viewmaster reel production, Viewmaster viewers, 3-D Calc, PC software for calculating stereo base

Nidek Incorporated
2460 Embarcadero Way
PO Box 50488
Palo Alto, CA 94303
800-223-9044
Products: stereo fundus camera

Polaroid Corporation
Polarizer Division
1 Upland Road
Norwood, MA 02062
800-225-2770
Products: Polarizing filters

Reel 3-D Enterprises, Inc.
PO Box 2368
Culver City, CA 90231
310-837-2368, FAX 310-558-1653
Products: 2- ×2-inch transparency viewers, 3-D slide viewers, side-by-side print viewers, precision 2- × 2-inch slide mounts, projector polarizers, polarized 3-D glasses, books

Rocky Mountain Memories 3D
2200 Creststone Court
Fort Collins, CO 80525
http://www.frii.com/rkymtmem/
joel.alpers@symbios.com

Stereo World
National Stereoscopic Association, Inc.
Box 14801
Columbus, Ohio 43214
Products: magazine and books

StereoGraphics, Inc.
PO Box 2309
2171 East Francisco Blvd.
San Rafael, CA 94901-5536
415-459-4500; FAX: 415-459-3020
www.stereographics.com
Product: LCD glasses

Synthonics, Inc.
818-707-6000
800-497-0787
www://www2.synthonics.com/synthonics
synthonics@synthonics.com
Product: 3D Maker (anaglyph software)

Taylor-Merchant Corporation
212 West 35th Street
New York, NY 10001
212-757-7700, 800-223-6694, FAX 212-695-1265
Products: Folding stereo viewers (two 2 ¥ 2 slides or Realist duplicates), Stereopticon print viewer

Technical Enterprises
1401 Bonnie Doone
Corona Del Mar, CA 92625-1717
714-644-9500, 800-903-TECO
Products: TECO-Nimslo split-frame 35-mm camera, split-frame viewers

Digital Imaging Equipment

Alcon Ophthalmic
Fort Worth, TX 76134
Canon USA, Inc.
Rodenstock SLO
One Canon Plaza
Lake Success, NY 11040
516-488-6700

Eastman Kodak Co., Inc.
Digital Imaging
151 State Street
Rochester, NY 14650
800-235-6325

Fargo Electronics, Inc.
7901 Flying Cloud Drive
Eden Prairie, MN 55344
800-258-2974

FUJI Photo Film, USA, Inc.
555 Faxter Road
Elmsford, NY 10523
800-378-3854

Humphrey Instruments, Inc.
(A company of the Carl Zeiss Group)
PO Box 5400
San Leandro, CA 94577
800-341-6968

Laser Diagnostic Technologies, Inc.
9550 Waples Street, Suite 105
San Diego, CA 92121
800-722-6393, 619-558-9144; FAX: 619-558-9145

Texas Optical, Inc.
22007 Chesterwick
Houston, TX 77450
info@txoptical.com

Index